Reflex Zone Therapy for Health Professionals

For Churchill Livingstone:

Publishing Manager: Inta Ozols
Project Manager: Gail Murray
Project Development Manager: Valerie Dearing
Designer: George Ajayi
Illustrator: Ethan Danielson

Reflex Zone Therapy for Health Professionals

Ann Lett RM (South Africa) RNT
Principal, British School — Reflex Zone Therapy of the Feet,
Wembley Park, UK

Foreword by

Hanne Marquardt SRN

Principal, International School for Reflex Zone Therapy of the Feet,
Königsfeld-Burgberg, Germany

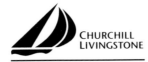

CHURCHILL
LIVINGSTONE

EDINBURGH LONDON NEW YORK PHILADELPHIA ST LOUIS SYDNEY TORONTO 2000

CHURCHILL LIVINGSTONE
An imprint of Harcourt Publishers Limited

First published 2000

ISBN 0 443 06015 0

British Library Cataloguing in Publication Data
A catalogue record for this book is available from the British Library

Library of Congress Cataloging in Publication Data
A catalog record for this book is available from the Library of Congress

Note
Medical knowledge is constantly changing. As new information becomes available, changes in treatment, procedures, equipment and the use of drugs become necessary. The author and the publishers have, as far as it is possible, taken care to ensure that the information given in this text is accurate and up to date. However, readers are strongly advised to confirm that the information, especially with regard to drug usage, complies with the latest legislation and standards of practice.

The publisher's policy is to use paper manufactured from sustainable forests

Printed in China

Contents

Foreword

It is with pleasure that I write the foreword to Ann Lett's book *Reflex Zone Therapy for Health Professionals*. Since she first attended my school in 1980 to participate in a course, I have appreciated both her and her work. By that time the predominance of reflexology as a widely practised form of elementary, either pleasant or painful, self-help had given way to an organised and structured therapy which had been developed during my many years of practice. Reflex zone therapy matured further in the school which evolved as a response to a growing demand by physiotherapists, hospitals and rehabilitation centres for practitioners who had attained a recognised therapeutic competence. Mrs Lett returned to many courses thereafter as an interested, critical and thoughtful therapist. She incorporated all that she learned in the school into her practice as nurse, tutor and midwife.

I passed over to her the administration of a new training school in the UK, for her to manage independently. Thanks to her personal, teaching and professional ability, the UK school soon acquired its good reputation. From its inception, she concentrated on teaching this method to her colleagues and those who had already completed their professional medical or paramedical training. Recognising the complexity and many layers of disorder inherent in all illness and incorporating this knowledge in treatment distinguishes reflex zone therapy from reflexology. For this reason, reflex zone therapy has always been taught to people working in the medical field.

At about the same time, between 1982 and 1986, we founded a school in Israel together. With equal engagement she devoted herself to establishing a school in Spain. Ann Lett has enhanced the reputation of reflex zone therapy, and helped it to gain greater acceptance by orthodox medicine in the UK. She has been involved in a number of associations whose concern has been to raise the standard of complementary therapies in Europe.

In this book she has condensed her many years of experience in a practical and well-structured manner, and has documented the professional, legal and ethical requirements very well.

The term 'reflexotherapy' is applied to many different groups and models of care in the English-speaking countries. I hope that for them and all students of reflex zone therapy this book will set a standard for their work and treatment. Several decades have been spent working on the feet in all my teaching schools. Much of the potential that lies in this treatment method has been reached and developed in the UK, thanks to Ann Lett's endeavours. Her experience is made available to those who are seriously interested in advancing their patients' treatment in the manner which is personally and therapeutically called for.

Ann Lett's book deserves a wide audience, and I wish it every success.

Hanne Marquardt

Preface

In the West, a rising tide of chronic illness and a growing awareness of the complexity of many drug interactions has turned the attention of the general public towards different patterns of care. Reflex zone therapy (RZT) affords a way of treating the whole person through the small surface of the feet. Its effects upon the ground regulating system are to support all physiological and psychological mechanisms and, where specific function is defective, to stimulate innate healing abilities when these have deteriorated.

The ability of the human body to repair itself is one of our greatest assets in the constant human struggle for biological survival. This recuperative process is aided by rest, circumscribed exercise, careful nutrition, abstinence from certain foods, and medicines from plants and herbs, all under the watchful eye of the physician. Then there is the surgeon's knife or needle, and the therapeutic effect of touch.

Because of its supportive effect, the pressure technique of RZT can be given to people of all ages whatever their state of health or illness. While it may be used as first aid to relieve pain and muscle spasm, or during a series of treatments to relieve specific physical complaints, its primary purpose is to strengthen and support all function. The experience of stress relief which it gives is a reflection of its deep and pervasive effect—lightening the load on debilitated systems and, over time, improving their capacity. It may by itself be sufficient to restore well-being, but is most effective when seen as but one of the factors by which health is sustained. RZT may be used both in partnership with other therapies, and as a complementary adjunct to orthodox medicine. It

may also need to be supported by relevant and well-chosen advice on breathing, nutrition, rest and exercise.

RZT should not be invasive, does not perforate the skin, does not complicate the disease picture of the recipient by introducing any other preparations, and is simple, portable and effective. Only the simplest of equipment is needed, and it is comparatively straightforward to learn and to practise.

The organisation of this book is as follows. The first section describes the basis and theory of RZT, its historical development, its contemporary spread and its uses. It then examines the scientific basis of its action.

Section two looks at the basics of RZT practice. First the practical issues involved in preparing for practice are detailed—the room, the equipment needed, the keeping of records and the legal position of the therapist. Then the course of treatment is considered. A course of treatment consists of assessment, treatment and follow-up. The initial assessment includes the taking of a history, informing the patient about what the treatment involves and what results can be expected, visual examination and palpation of the reflex zones of the feet to discover tissue changes. After the assessment, the findings must be interpreted and a decision about the best course of treatment reached. This process necessitates an awareness of both the uses and the limitations of RZT, the contraindications and the conditions in which caution must be applied, whether of a systemic nature or of localised abnormalities in the foot. It is also necessary to decide upon the order of treatment where there is more than one complaint, and its extent. The treatment method itself comprises a variety of different strokes, holds and pressure techniques that either tonify and stimulate or sedate and disperse the tissues. A general order and procedure for treatment is suggested, and modifications to this general pattern necessary in particular conditions are suggested. The variety and extent of reactions to the treatment are then discussed, and advice is given on a follow-up procedure. Finally, this basic treatment can be supplemented with other techniques — using reciprocal (or cross) reflexes where the primary zone cannot be treated directly, the treatment of interference fields and scars, and the technique of manual neurotherapy.

Section three details the reflex zones of the body. The major reflex area is on the feet, and each of the organ systems, and their assessment and treatment, using one or both hands, is described and illustrated extensively. The reflex areas of the hands, the back and the oronasopharynx and teeth are then described in turn.

The final section looks at the use of RZT in different groups of people. These include pregnant women, children, elderly people and those with life-threatening illnesses such as cancer.

Although there are many ways in which the feet can be treated, RZT offers a framework in which treatment can be safely and effectively offered, interpreted and given. Its growing use amongst those whose training has been in the care of the sick is testimony to its capacity, and it is in the hope of providing for the beginner some simple guidelines, derived from experience, that this book is written.

The distinguishing marks of a good therapist are knowledge, skill, experience and discretion. A good training lays the foundations for safe practice, after which the therapist learns in, and from, practice how to hone her skills in observation, listening for the hidden cues, and giving the appropriate therapy. When giver and receiver collaborate in giving each other a clear explanation of procedure and progress, the improvements which follow are consolidated and there is less likely to be a recurrence of the debility. Good practice is safe and supportive for the patient, and does not make undue physical demands on the posture, spine, hands or joints of the therapist. Good practice in any discipline acknowledges the totality of the person, recognising that thoughts, feelings, physical strengths and weaknesses form an indivisible whole, in which there are a myriad distinctive constitutional and reactive capacities for each individual.

■ *"The universe, the earth we live on, and the bodies we inhabit alike beat to the eternal rhythm of some cosmic pulse. Philosophers and poets have known intuitively what science has observed, measured and recorded; almost everything in the world we know moves in tides and cycles."*

BENJAMIN F. MILLER AND RUTH GOODE 1961

Wembley Park 2000   Ann Lett

Acknowledgements

I would like to acknowledge my grateful thanks to Hanne Marquardt for the good foundation given me and many others in reflex zone therapy; also the contribution of colleagues within her school: Trudi Kaiser, Uta Greiner, Dr Montserrat Noguera, Elizabeth Feuz, Gila Livne, and all other teachers. Catherine Rachem has been an invaluable teacher and friend, full of insight and wisdom, and made many helpful suggestions whilst I was writing.

I am indebted also to Yana Stajno, Ursula Wright, Dr Koni Witzig and Dr Gordon Latto, who have generously shared so much of their experience and given me much help in the past.

Sister Elizabeth Feuz, Sister in Charge of the Labour ward at the Frauenspital in Berne, Switzerland, for 20 years, pioneered there the practice of RZT in midwifery as it is now used in the maternity unit. She has generously shared her knowledge and experience, and her observations provide the foundations for Chapter 12. Today there are many midwives who have incorporated RZT into their maternity care in appropriate circumstances; I am grateful for their continuing contribution.

Anni Hogg, Sally Martin, Mary Price, Rixa von dem Bussche, Cherry Bond (who coined the term still-holding) and Lucy Bell all gave valuable help with this book.

My thanks are also due to Adrian for introducing me to reflex zone therapy, to Francis for his help with interference fields, and to Eric Danger for much helpful advice. I would like to thank Christine Wyard for her advice and careful revision of the text, and Valerie Dearing for her patience and support throughout the writing process. Thanks also to Beni Barda and Kevin Brown for taking the photographs, and Ethan Danielson for doing the illustrations. Hanne Marquardt, N. Gosch and A. Froneberg kindly allowed me to use their helpful diagrams.

What is reflex zone therapy?

1

The development and theory of RZT

Introduction — what is reflex zone therapy?

Reflex zone therapy (RZT) is the simple application of touch by one person to the feet, hands, back or head of another. Yet for all its simplicity of approach it has the capacity to illuminate much about the health of the receiver, to relieve pain and discomfort and, when appropriately given, may be a means of restoring health.

Our appearance, demeanour and temper are in a measure interwoven with the manner in which we have been fashioned and how we feel. When our eyes lose their lustre, skin becomes dry or scaly, hair loses its shine and becomes brittle, or there are changes in skin colour, we and others can see that we are not well. We suspect also that all is not well if we lose our appetite, feel excessively tired, lose interest in our surroundings, can't concentrate or feel unusually irritable. Illness is characterised by both signs and symptoms. Signs of illness are objective pieces of evidence which show a departure from normal, for example blueness of the lips or a discoloured or frothy sputum. Symptoms, such as shortness of breath, malaise or pain, give us the subjective experience of illness, and are less easily quantified.

RZT depends on the premise that body changes which occur when there is less than perfect function in any part are reflected on the mirror of the surfaces of the feet, hands, back and face. In other words, our skin covering, as well as nails, eyes and hair, is an important indicator of how well we are faring within ourselves, and can provide early clues to the nature of our ailments when we fall below par.

The first signs of illness are often unnoticed or disregarded until discomfort, limitation of movement or pain begin to interfere with the routine of normal daily activity. Yet these signs are detectable from the earliest stage of illness in the reflex zones of the body surface. They are visible to the discerning eye and can be discovered by a discriminating touch, the basis of the palpation technique.

Further to this, those zones indicating internal imbalance or overt illness are treated with a variety of gentle strokes and dynamic movements, using thumbs or fingers, to stimulate the body's own healing and self-balancing mechanisms.

As with any other method, RZT has advantages and limitations. A capable therapist is able to extend it to its full potential, recognises its limitations and, knowing these, is aware of the responsibility for referring onwards when necessary.

The aims of RZT are:

- to discover from a careful examination of the reflex zones whether there is any evidence of latent disease
- to prevent such illness from developing where possible
- to relieve symptoms without masking any serious underlying illness
- to support the body's natural healing mechanisms
- to promote relaxation, and
- to enhance, in combination with other therapies where indicated, all treatment.

History

Our human physiology has not changed over the past few thousand years. Those factors which promote health and those which erode well-being can and do change in detail over the centuries, but not in principle. The effects of touch as a means of communication, support and healing have been attested to by all cultures since prehistory.

Touch is an instinctive response to pain, and has been adapted to promote healing through many and varied forms, including massage and pressure (both Western and Oriental systems), osteopathy, physiotherapy and reflex zone therapy amongst many others. Usually practical and empirical experience has come first, to be explained in due course by the expanding body of knowledge in anatomy and physiology. In consequence, some of the above therapeutic modes are upheld by a more complete system of knowledge, while for others it is less comprehensive. All have a place amongst the healing arts, innovative healers having from earliest times evolved effective and culturally adapted ways in which to relieve the sick.

Although the feet have been used for massage and treatment by many cultures and peoples, the written and oral records of this practice which survive to date are sketchy and incomplete, and we can only guess at those methods which were used centuries ago. Yet, despite the obscurity in which past practice is shrouded, the observable and often lasting benefits of RZT have over the course of this century given relief and comfort to many, and growing confidence to its practitioners.

The many forms of practice and schools of thought from various individuals have given rise to the different terms zone therapy, reflex zone therapy, reflexotherapy, reflex therapy and reflex zone massage, all of which are included in the collective term 'reflexology'.

Early history and antecedents

Whether reflex zone therapy was first used in the Orient or in Egypt and Assyria we do not know. Ancient pictographs from these civilisations suggest that the feet were a source of information and possibly treatment.

The West

Massage is known to have been practised in the Orient before the birth of Christ, and was prescribed in the West by physicians in Greece and Rome, as was mentioned by Plato (375BC). The opinions of early writers on Greek medicine (Alcmaeon of Croton, Sicily 470BC, Heraclitus 540BC, Parmenides of Elea 515BC, Pythagoras, Sicily 530BC) are difficult to interpret. Their views on health and sickness are similar to those found in the Hippocratic corpus 440–340BC (Baas 1889, Lloyd 1978, Porter 1997, Singer 1962). It is the opinions and comments of Plato (427–347BC) about Hippocrates that are best known to us, as dialogue and debate were a vital part of Greek intellectual life. Philosophical speculation about nature included debate about sickness and health.

Hippocratic medicine was cautious, had a good knowledge of and observed closely both surface anatomy and its changes, and depended on detailed observation and reason. Plato refers to these Hippocratic virtues of reason over magic, a theme that is fully developed in the Timaeus (375BC). The human frame was constructed with a purpose — the soma affected the psyche. Behaviour can be determined by organic weakness or deficiencies; madness could have a physiological cause. Health depended on self-control in diet, exercise and massage as practised by trainers of gymnasts. (Sophrosyne — soundness of mind in a healthy body — was the ideal. But it was more the Greek admiration for athleticism that produced instructors in exercise, diet and massage.)

Celsus (AD30) wrote in Latin eight books of medicine and, like Hippocrates, stated that medicine required not just experience but also reason. He wrote about medicine, drugs and surgery for all parts of the body, and very importantly detailed the four cardinal signs of inflammation doctors must be alert to after surgery: pain, redness, heat and swelling (rubor, calor, tumor and dolor), to which has been added the fifth — loss of function (Singer 1962, p. 54). Celsus was the first major Latin author, and he was followed by Galen, AD129–216. Both authors incorporated ideas of diet, exercise, rest and body massage within regimes of care (Baas 1889, Porter 1997, Singer 1962).

The Orient

More than 4000 years ago in the Orient, traditional Chinese medicine (TCM) codified a system of treatment in which was acknowledged an intimate relationship between the internal systems of the body and its outer surfaces, and which embraced a different model of the person's relationship to the world or universe.

Oriental philosophy and cosmology was shaped by Taoism and Confucianism, which held that the cosmos is a whole — eternal, uncreated yet constantly recreating itself, in which everything is related to everything else under the interaction of the two fundamental polar yet complementary principles called Yin (female, dark, etc.) and Yang (male, light, etc.). All natural phenomena were also classified according to their physical composition, being either liquid, mineral, earth, heat or plant. A further classification into the natural 'elements' or 'phases', of Wood, Metal, Water, Fire and Earth, was then made.

Human beings are a microcosm of this macrocosm, therefore in their physiological and psychological make-up one can observe all the elements, movements, patterns, changes, relationships and forces of the universe. Like the larger universe, human beings are suffused with Qi (Chi) (sometimes translated as 'essential or vital energy', though there is no precise conceptual translation), Blood (which is not the Western understanding of a physical fluid, but rather its qualities such as transport and nourishment), Essence, Spirit and Body Fluids. The archetypal principles of Yin and Yang are always present too, in constant interplay, and all change is effected by shifts in their balance within any given situation.

When an indescribably harmonious coexistence, movement and functioning of any one of the above is disrupted, the disruption spreads to affect all the other components which make up the whole. The result is called a 'pattern of disharmony' in the East, and sickness in the West. According to this view, no sign, symptom or event can be isolated and viewed on its own, but only interpreted and subsequently treated in the context of its relationship to the whole.

An example of this is acupuncture which, although only one of the pillars of TCM, is the one which is best known in the West. In its diagnostic methods, changes which are taking place internally must be discerned by observing outward changes — by looking, listening, smelling, asking and touching. Much emphasis is given to visual examination of the tongue and its surface, and to the complex art of pulse taking, both of which help to reveal the prevailing pattern of disharmony.

Access to internal functions, organs and structures is gained through meridians. Meridians are invisible channels or pathways which connect the interior of the body to its exterior. Qi (Chi) and blood course through meridians, whose pathways link all capacities, organs and structures, and it is along or through these channels that 'information' about their dynamic relationship flows.

Of these channels, the most important (in acupuncture) are the 12 organ meridians and 8 extraordinary vessels, of which both the Governor (major Yang) and Conception (major Yin) Vessels are considered to be major meridians. (As the function of each organ, as well as its relation to the vital substances and all other organs and structures in the body, is considered more important than its anatomical structure, named meridians do not always correlate to a Western construct of the body's anatomy.)

In this way each meridian serves many more functions and parts of the body than the organ whose name it bears. Acupuncture points (*tsubos*), or pressure points, occur at intervals along each meridian. These structures allow access to the meridian, the functions and organs it serves, and the vital substances.

Treatment aims to restore imbalance in function of internal organs, as well as that of the emotions and the mind. A TCM practitioner may choose between needling, pressure, or local heat — either as moxibustion, in which a substance (primarily mugwort, *Artemesia vulgaris*) is burnt just above the skin, or as cupping to apply suction to one or more specific points on the chosen meridians. The intention is to effect a change in the pathway, thereby influencing the vital substances and subsequently influencing energy patterns and relationships of all functions, organs and structures maintained by that meridian. In this fashion, intervention on the surface of the body is used to bring about deep internal changes.

The TCM conception did not depend on the extending knowledge of anatomy, physiology, biochemistry and pathology, which are the hallmarks of Western scientific discipline. Also, in the latter the physical, psychological and spiritual factors often appear to be separated in considering both the causation and treatment of illness. This perceived emphasis on technical brilliance to the exclusion of other factors may account in part for the modern cry for 'wholism', although good doctors everywhere have always (and still do) give full consideration to every aspect of the effect of illness on the life of their patients. Traditional Oriental medical systems do not recognise this separation of the emotional disposition and activity from the body's physical function.

Modern developments in scientific understanding

The tradition of therapies involving touch remained obscure in the West until about two centuries ago when, in Sweden, Professor Per Henrik Ling (1859) devised a system of remedial massage and gymnastics, based on his clinical observations of the relationship between internal organs and specific areas of the skin. His prescriptions were so effective that for a century and a half they enjoyed a reputation for excellence throughout Europe and Professor Ling's work was being acknowledged in English textbooks until the middle of the 20th century (Johnson 1897).

Reflexes

In Edinburgh, Professor Robert Whytt (1714–66) confirmed 17th century observations that the spinal cord was integral to *reflex action* such as blinking and coughing, and that such action is carried out without conscious control or awareness (Whytt 1765, Whytt 1768). In London, the eminent neurophysiologist Marshall Hall (1790–1857) deduced that the nervous system was composed of many *segmental reflex arcs* (Figs 1.1 and 1.2), and showed that the spinal reflex arc could function even if the spine was injured or severed (Hall 1833, 1836, 1838, 1839, 1842, 1850).

Referred pain

On the other side of the Atlantic Ocean, in 1834, two brothers, W. and D. Griffin, observed that clinical disease states changed the structure and function of one or more vertebrae (1834, 1845). In the last half of

Anterior aspect

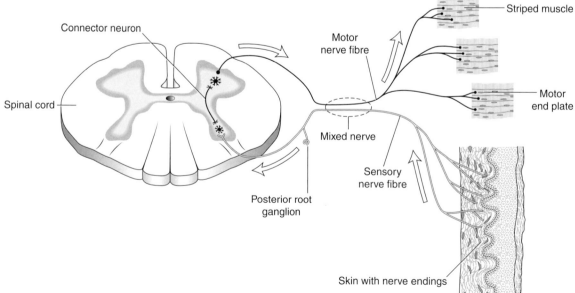

Fig. 1.1 *The basic three-neuron ipsilateral arc (After Anthony & Thibodeau 1983, with kind permission of C V Mosby)*

the 19th century, Dr Andrew Still further shaped these ideas in his American practice to develop the discipline of osteopathy (Still 1902, Northrup 1979).

The term 'transferred pain' (which we now call referred pain) was first coined by three Americans; J. Ross (1881), Dana (1899) and Abrams (1904).

Together they distinguished between the differential diagnoses of visceral disease (which could be made on the spinal column), when pain and sensitivity of the vertebrae is bilateral; and intercostal neuralgia, when it is unilateral. The first European reference to referred pain was made by Sir Henry Head in 1893.

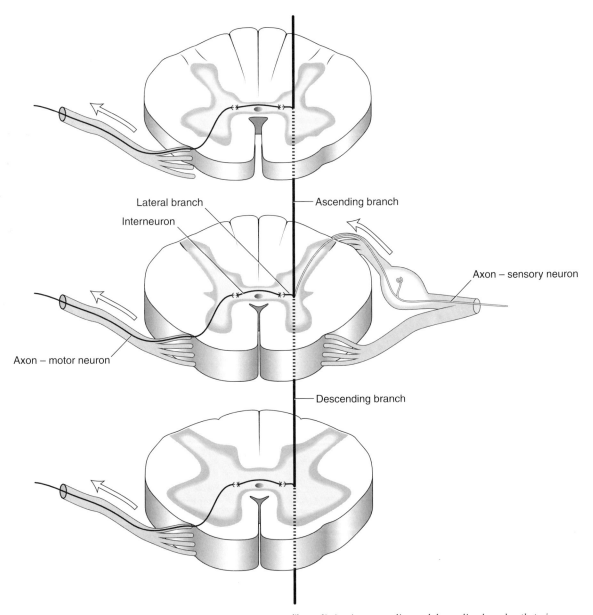

Fig. 1.2 *Intersegmental contralateral reflex arc, showing a sensory fibre splitting into ascending and descending branches that give rise to lateral branches which synapse with their respective interneurons (After Anthony & Thibodeau 1983, with kind permission of C V Mosby)*

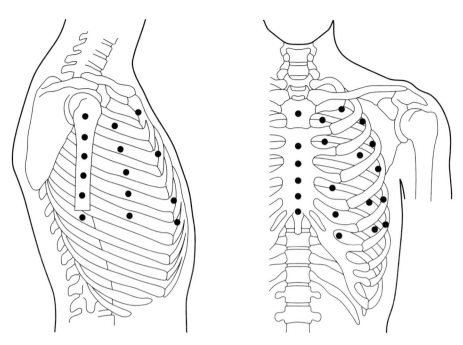

Fig. 1.3 *'Trigger points' described by Dr Weihe in 1886 (From Gleditsch 1983, with kind permission of MBH & Co.)*

Trigger points and kinetic chains

'Trigger points' were first described by Dr A. Weihe in 1886 (Fig. 1.3). These are specific points on the skin which become sensitive to pressure when an organ becomes diseased. There is a different pattern of trigger points on the skin for each organ, and diagnosis can be facilitated by palpating the trigger points to discover which are painful.

Although the concept had not then been developed, we now know that trigger points become painful along 'kinetic chains'. Kinetic chains are groups of muscles which are mobilised in the performance of any complex movement such as walking or talking, and form a pattern of use which is individual to each person. Although we all use the same groups of muscles for similar activities, each of us walks and talks distinctively. One of the best-known trigger points lies at the tip of the right scapula, and is frequently the presenting symptom when stones are forming within the gall bladder or when it becomes inflamed. In the early stages of this condition mobilising the muscles of the right shoulder gives rise to pain, whilst in acute conditions the pain arises suddenly and spontaneously, and can be severe and debilitating.

Today painful trigger points and the areas to which their pain is usually referred are increasingly well defined (Fig. 1.4). Travell & Simons (1983, 1992) demonstrated that there is a specific pattern of trigger point pain referral for each muscle in the body. The relationship of trigger points to internal organs and functions is emphasised today in treatment using applied kinesiology.

The routes by which pain is referred may provide interesting clues as to why some pinpoint size reflex zones in the feet may be painful in specific conditions. When pain is referred from a myofascial trigger point to a muscle, it causes painful spasm in that muscle. This can lead to the formation of painful secondary myofascial trigger points, called 'satellites', which in turn radiate their effect to still further distant myofascial trigger points. It is just possible that the reflex zone at the junction of the scaphoid, talus and cuneiform bones becomes painful when there is sacroiliac joint strain or pain because satellite myofascial trigger points have become enmeshed in the network of referred pain. The pain in the reflex zone recedes as the spasm or strain on the muscle is relieved.

The existence of 'latent myofascial trigger points', which are not painful except on firm palpation, was

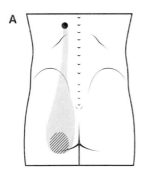

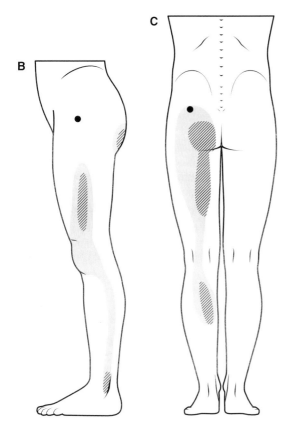

Fig. 1.4 *The pattern of pain referral from a trigger point (●) in: A the longissimus thoracic muscle; B either the gluteus medius or minimus near to the attachment of these muscles to the great trochanter; C the posterior part of either the gluteus medius or minimus muscles (From Baldry in Filshie & White 1998, with kind permission of Churchill Livingstone)*

found by Sola & Kuitert (1955) when they were conducting a routine examination of muscle in fit, young and symptomless adults. The input of very little further trauma was needed to convert these latent myofascial trigger points into painful trigger points.

The capacity of the body to give early warning signs of any impairment of function in palpable, external locations, and for these to become more urgent in accordance with any deterioration, cannot be underestimated.

Pain transmission and inhibition

Suggestions about how pressure or needling deactivate trigger points are based on the 'gate control' theory of pain perception, first proposed by Melzack & Wall (1965). According to recent research (Baldry 1998) pain messages arise from the activation of nociceptors (peripheral nerve receptors which receive and transmit noxious stimuli) in skin and muscle, and travel via 'C' nerve fibres through the dorsal horn up the spine to the brain (reticular formation, thalamus, then cortex). These impulses can in certain conditions be abolished by stimulating cutaneous and subcutaneous Aδ nerve fibres (mechanothermal nociceptors in the skin), for instance with dry needling (acupuncture). This procedure blocks pain input to the spine by activating enkephalinergic inhibitory interneurons in the dorsal horn. The mechanism underlying this 'gate control' theory of pain inhibition is detailed in Figure 1.5. Since free β-endorphins and also seemingly met-enkephalin (endogenous opioids) are released when an acupuncture needle is inserted or when pressure is applied to an appropriate *tsubo*, it may yet be shown that pressure on painful reflex zones or myofascial trigger points has the same effect. (Current research in this area is discussed further in Chapter 2.)

Reflex signs of disease

Over the centuries ever more information was garnered by physicians who noted which external signs and symptoms were caused by which disturbances of internal function. These conclusions led to a description of the 'reflex signs of disease' towards the end of the 19th century. These were not outward signs such as lacklustre eyes or pallid

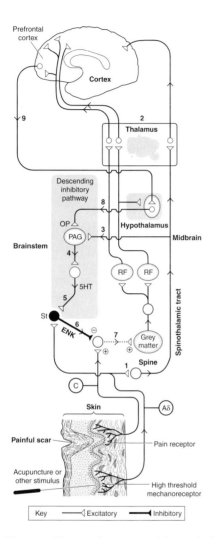

Fig. 1.5 *Diagram to illustrate the gate control theory of pain control and the serotonergic mechanism of acupuncture and manual therapies. Thumb pressure or needling causes information to be transmitted along Aδ nerve fibres and then up the spine to the thalamus (**1**), from where it is further projected up to the cortex (**2**) and becomes conscious. In the midbrain (hypothalamus) these axons give off a collateral branch (**3**) to the periaqueductal grey matter (PAG). The PAG projects down to the brainstem (**4**) and this in turn sends serotonergic (5HT) fibres to special cells called stalked cells (St) (**5**); these last cells trigger an enkephalinergic (ENK) mechanism (**6**) to prevent noxious (pain) information arriving along C fibres from skin nociceptors from being transmitted to cells deep in the spinal grey matter and thence up to the brain reticular formation (RF) (**7**). The PAG is also influenced by opioid endorphinergic fibres descending from the hypothalamus (**8**) (OP = opioids), which in turn receives projections from the prefrontal cortex (**9**) (After Thompson & Filshie 1993, derived from Bowsher 1992 (see Fig. 11.3, p. 118), with kind permission of Oxford University Press)*

complexion as described earlier, but discrete physiological changes (see p. 12) occurring in the temperature, sweat secretion and behaviour of hairs on the skin resulting from projection within a given spinal segment via the sensory motor system.

A reflex picture of disease noticed by Dr Voltolini in 1883 involved a change in the consistency of nasal mucous membranes in pregnant women. He subsequently discovered other small but significant changes in these membranes for other diseases. Yet the first known European description of a small area of the body providing a mirror image of all its organs and structures was given by Dr W. Fliess in 1893. In this depiction specific areas of the roof, floor, lower and middle musculature of the nose corresponded to particular visceral organs (Fliess 1893, 1926).

In 1893, Sir Henry Head, a neurologist working in London (and who is remembered in 'Head's zones'), was the first person to describe the reflex signs of disease, showing how any disturbance of internal function is quickly reflected to an external body surface, thereby giving notice of disorder. According to Head, internal organs are not well supplied with pain receptors and when their function becomes impaired they cannot transmit pain impulses to conscious areas in the brain. Instead, they send urgent messages of discomfort to the related skin (dermatome) (see Fig. 1.6), subcutaneous tissues (sclerotomes) and muscles (myotomes) of the segment to which they belong, and it is in these areas that pain is first perceived.

For this reason the pain of pleurisy or of biliary colic is first felt at the uppermost tip of the right shoulder blade, and the warning signs of angina are perceived in the neck, left shoulder girdle or arm, and sometimes the stomach.

Head's zones are areas of:

- reflex (distant)
- cutaneous (of the skin)
- hyperaesthesia (increased sensitivity) and
- hyperalgesia (diminished sensitivity to pain)

which result from visceral disease. He had already in 1893 described the sensory nerve roots involved in each segment of the body, and since then a defined area of skin supplied by a spinal nerve has been called a dermatome (Fig. 1.6).

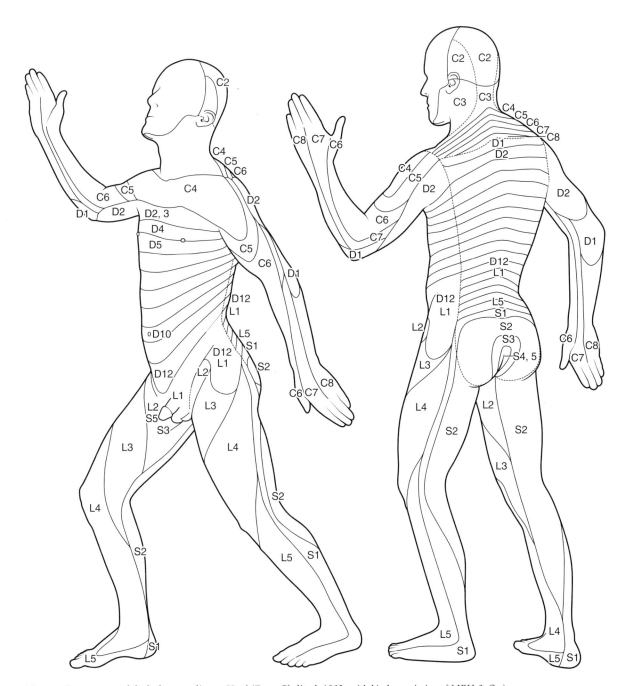

Fig. 1.6 *Dermatomes of the body, according to Head (From Gleditsch 1983, with kind permission of MBH & Co.)*

The researches in 1892 and 1893 of Dr (later Sir) J. Mackenzie, a colleague of Sir Henry Head, greatly refined the understanding of the segmental organisation of the body. A segment is that area of skin, subcutaneous tissue and muscle which receives its nerve supply from a particular level of the spinal cord (see Fig. 1.6). He described subcutaneous tissue and muscle which receives its nerve supply from a particular level of the spinal cord. He also described which areas of muscle were innervated at any given level within the spinal cord, since when they have been called myotomes. By testing for different sensations on the skin, any delay or abnormality in perception enables the physician to decide which nerve root is damaged, and at which level.

Between 1896 and 1921 Head and Mackenzie described the two directions in which impulses travelled:

- viscerocutaneous impulses carry information from viscera to skin
- cutaneovisceral impulses carry information from the skin to the viscera
- viscerovisceral pathways carry information from one organ to another.

When the functions of an organ are impaired, an alteration to the autonomically controlled functions in the related segment follows. Sir James Mackenzie is also remembered in Mackenzie's point, which is a point of tenderness in the upper segment of the right rectus abdominis muscle which becomes present in disease of the gall bladder.

In the same way, but the reverse direction, afferent nerves carry impulses mediated by touch, heat, cold, massage, water, poultices and the like to the internal organs. To obtain the desired effect, the right stimulus has to be applied precisely to the right place, with due regard to its intention, strength and duration. These pathways are not under conscious or voluntary control and, unless they are severed or diseased, they appear as functioning pathways for a lifetime.

The reflex signs of disease, mediated through the autonomic nervous system, can appear in any segment, depending on the stage the illness has reached, and are now recognised as follows:

- in the skin, which becomes pale, cold and clammy, with the appearance of gooseflesh and a raised dermatographia due to vasoconstriction and flushing due to vasodilatation
- in subcutaneous tissue, which becomes shiny, oedematous and dense; as the tension within the tissues increases they become less pliable and more difficult to 'roll' because persistent vasoconstriction has adversely affected tissue

perfusion, leading to poor oxygen and nutrient supply (trophic changes)
- in the muscles, which become less contractile; their trigger points become sensitised owing to trophic changes
- in the joints, with degenerative changes appearing in ligaments, capsule and cartilage, and reduction of synovial fluid leading to painful and restricted movement
- in the organs, whose function becomes impaired as a result of reduced circulating blood and tissue fluids.

Such changes in the colour and texture of the skin, or sweating, are present from the earliest stages of disease, albeit that they are little noticed on cursory examination. These tissue changes may become irreversible if the disease process is not halted and reversed.

It is not understood why the workings of the body should be reflected as a mirror image in the feet, nor why there should be either changes in the skin or autonomic nervous system reactions when reflex zones in the feet are palpated if the organs to which they correspond are underfunctioning. (These are not those zones described by Sir Henry Head, but they are reflex signs of disease.)

Development of tissue layers

To understand why treatment should have such an organised effect, we need to look at the development of the fetus. Before the somites develop, the embryo is formed of ectoderm and the disc-like endoderm (Fig. 1.7). Within the ectoderm a groove (called the primitive streak) appears at what will be the tail end, and 'funnels' towards the future head (Fig. 1.7a). The embryo is now made up of two equal halves, each of which will, from this point, be a mirror image of the other. At the same time a cellular rod-shaped structure, called the notochord, is formed at the cranial end of the primitive streak, and grows between the ectoderm and endoderm towards what will be the head (Fig. 1.7b). Mesoderm (from which all future tissues are developed) then grows out from the sides of the primitive streak into regularly arranged blocks called somites (or segments) (Fig. 1.7c), leaving the ectoderm and endoderm in contact with each other at just two places: the

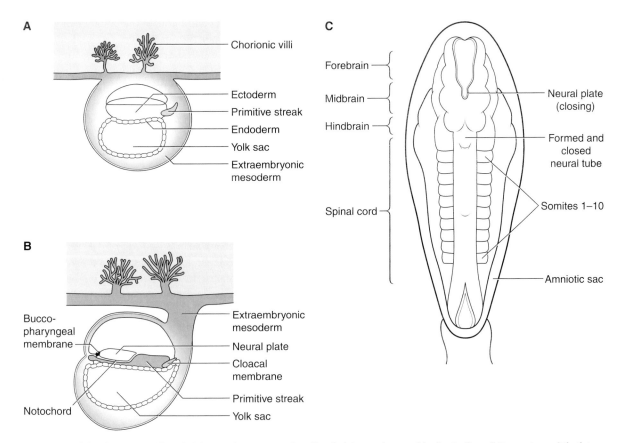

Fig. 1.7 *Fetal development:* **A** *The primitive streak appears at the tail end of the ectoderm and begins to 'funnel' its way toward the future head.* **B** *The notochord forms at the cranial end of the primitive streak and grows between the ectoderm and endoderm toward the future head.* **C** *Mesoderm grows out from either side of the primitive streak to form somites — the future segments. The ectoderm and endoderm remain connected at the buccopharyngeal and cloacal membranes.*

buccopharyngeal membrane and the cloacal membrane. It is possible that the reason why the central and autonomic nervous systems can be so readily influenced on this superficial surface of the body is the result in part of embryonic development in the first weeks of life.

The ground regulating system

Most recently Professor Pischinger has put forward a theory of how the physiological functions and biological tasks of connective tissue are organised, bringing about neurohumoral regulation via a system entitled the ground regulating system (GRS)

(see Ch. 2). Therapies such as acupuncture, shiatsu, massage, osteopathy and RZT, when applied to parts of skin and subcutaneous tissues whose structure and function show any departure from normal, are shown to strengthen the regulating capacity of this system.

The development of modern reflex zone therapy

William Fitzgerald

Towards the end of the last century Dr William Fitzgerald, an ear, nose and throat (ENT) specialist from Connecticut, America, began to experiment with the practice of zone therapy. He reported successful treatment in a wide variety of complaints, and in 1917, in collaboration with Dr Edwin Bowers, he wrote Zone therapy. This was the first published Western book describing a particular kind of pressure applied to skin or mucous membranes with the intention of relieving pain or symptoms at some distance away from the point of pressure. (Prof. Henry Head (1893, 1920) and Dr Mackenzie (1893, 1921) had both described successful treatment of gastric and eye disturbances by the application of mustard seeds and other poultices to the related segmental 'trigger points' as part of their great output of medical writing.)

Dr Fitzgerald concentrated his treatment on parts of the head, ears, nose, tongue and throat, as well as the abdomen, hands and feet. His division of the body into 10 equal zones — five on each side of a median line running from the feet up to the head and across the chest and back down to the hands, or vice versa from hands to feet, on both anterior and posterior aspects of the body (Fig. 1.8) — provided the original, simple framework by means of which reflex zones to organs and structures could be related to one another and described within their longitudinal zones. His early diagrams drew a line through the centre of each respective zone, with zone 1 being closest to the midline, and zone 5 being the most lateral. The diagrams were later simplified, dividing the body into two equal halves at the midline, with 4 imaginary lines on either side, thus dividing each half of the body into 5 equal zones. The connections so postulated were empirical, having at that time no known anatomical or physiological basis.

Joseph Riley, Eunice Ingham and Doreen Bayly

Dr Joseph S. Riley continued with and promoted the work of Dr Fitzgerald, refining specific points for treatment in his book Zone therapy simplified, published in 1919. One of his pupils was the American masseuse, Eunice Ingham. She applied those methods described by Drs Fitzgerald and Riley which did not demand their medical training, and found that discomfort frequently accompanied pressure to some areas of the feet. This discomfort was not uniform, but varied according to the

constitution and complaints of the person being treated. In her book Stories the feet can tell (1938) were published the first descriptions of treatment confined to the feet. This was followed by a second volume: Stories the feet have told (1951). A pupil of Eunice Ingham, Doreen Bayly, popularised the treatment in the UK in the 1960s.

Hanne Marquardt

In Germany, Hanne Marquardt, after training as a nurse, developed in 1958 a keen interest in the results claimed for 'compression massage' touch/treatment to the feet which had been made by Eunice Ingham, and she undertook a serious study of the subject. By imposing Dr Fitzgerald's 10 longitudinal zones on to the anatomical structure of the feet she enabled reflex zones to be located with greater precision. She also described and imposed three transverse zones: one at the level of the shoulder girdle, one over the waist line and one at the level of the pelvic floor, and related them to anatomical landmarks on the feet (Fig. 1.9) (see also p. 16). (The longitudinal and transverse zones were later combined into a 'zone grid' — Fig. 1.10.) The early charts were amplified, with many new reflex zones on both dorsum and sole being added (Marquardt 1984, 1993).

Hanne Marquardt developed a remarkable competence in what she now termed 'reflex zone therapy'. Her more complete and organised depiction of the 'zone map' on the feet has since been widely acknowledged and used. She realised how closely the small 'seated human form' in the feet reflected the complex, global totality of a person (Fig. 1.11). Her professional colleagues quickly acknowledged her ability and skill, and at their request she began to give training courses in 1967. By 1985 there were affiliated schools in Denmark, Holland, Switzerland, the UK, Israel, Spain, Italy and eastern, northern and western Germany. Physiotherapists, midwives, and naturopathic, osteopathic and acupuncture practitioners started to learn and practice RZT as an adjunct to their professional training.

Walter Froneberg

Walter Froneberg, who had been a pupil of Mrs Marquardt, had a particular interest in the nervous

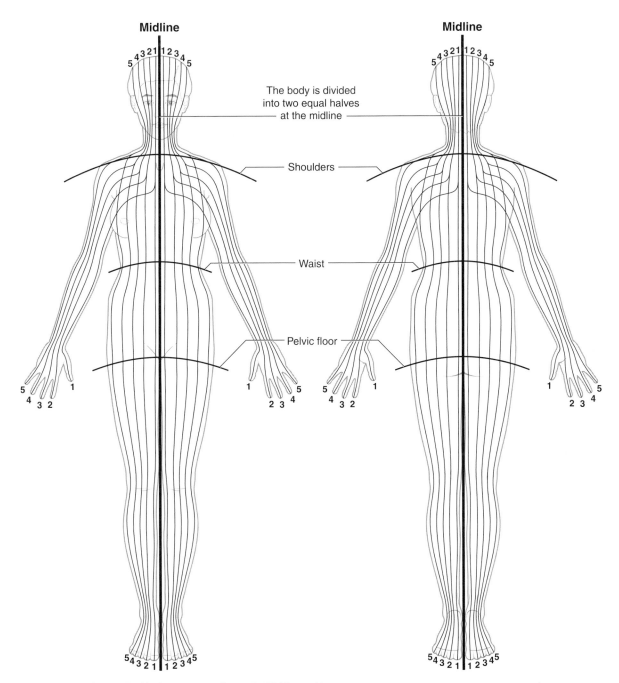

Fig. 1.8 *The 10 longitudinal body zones according to Dr W. Fitzgerald*

system. His work on people in whom there had been damage to nerve pathways led him to the discovery of several reflex zones to motor nerves and major muscle groups. In his continuing practice over the

next decade he identified reflex zones to the autonomic nervous system, uterine supports, and muscles of the eyes and teeth. His work gave rise by 1980 to a form of treatment, 'manuelle neurotherapie'

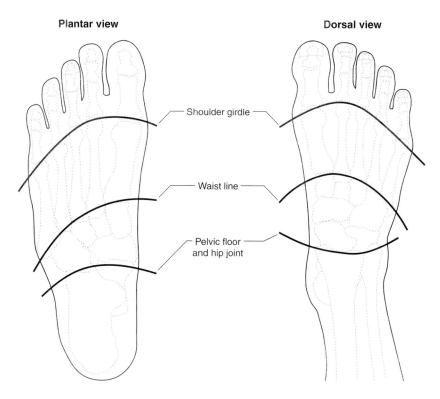

Fig. 1.9 *The three transverse zones in the feet (After Marquardt 1984, reproduced with kind permission)*

(manual neurotherapy), which could be used when nerve pathways were maimed or functionally impaired.

Present state — 1980 onwards

Reflexology in any of its variant forms has always been widely used in the Far East. It is increasingly used in the Americas, in India and in Europe, where it has become considerably better known over the past 30 years. In Western Europe, RZT has over the past 40 years been taught to people who already have a professional training in the care of the sick, and continues to be valued by givers and receivers. Properly used, it enhances other treatments, and may diminish the need for medicines. Over the past three decades there has been a gradual incorporation of complementary therapies into nursing, physiotherapy, midwifery and occupational therapy practice. The bodies which regulate these professions allow the use of complementary therapies, but demand that practitioners:

- are well taught
- are personally accountable in all circumstances
- are able to justify their choice of therapy, whether orthodox or complementary, and
- avoid any abuse of their privileged relationship with patients.

To date, however, the practice of RZT and reflexology is unregulated. An individual is generally protected under the common law of England (it was King Alfred (c AD893) who first decreed in his Book of laws, or dooms, 'What ye will that other men should not do to you, that do ye not to other men') against ignorance and malpractice from anyone professing to give care. There is not, as yet, any legislation by a national or international body to:

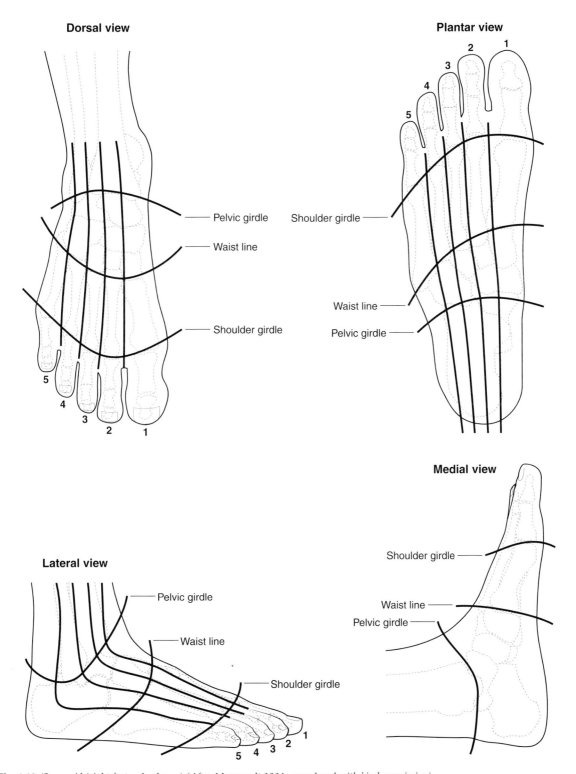

Fig. 1.10 *Zone grid (right foot only shown) (After Marquardt 1984, reproduced with kind permission)*

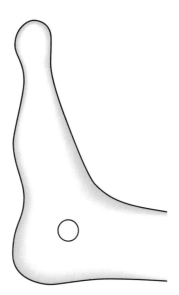

Fig. 1.11 *Diagram showing the miniaturised sitting human form reflected in the reflex zones in the feet (Reproduced with kind permission of Hanne Marquardt)*

- lay down commonly recognised standards of practice
- organise a syllabus
- oversee its teaching
- arrange for the examination and licensing of successful candidates
- allow them to practise as long as agreed standards are maintained
- make provision for complaints from the public and
- discipline any person found to be negligent in their duty towards those for whom it professes to care.

Tentative steps are being taken towards setting up such a body. A national consensus on the content of the syllabus, length of training and form of apprenticeship or experience learning under supervision has still to be reached.

Of the Western European countries reflexology appears to be most widely used in Denmark, where 40% of the population are known to have had experience of the therapy. Since 1977 a number of short studies to examine and document the effects of

reflexology have been made by the Danish Reflexologists Association (Eriksen 1993, Feder et al 1988, Johannessen 1993, 1994, Launso 1993).

In the UK the oncology department at Hammersmith Hospital in London was one of the first to practice, in an orthodox setting, complementary therapies which had been pioneered at the Bristol Cancer Centre. A recent survey shows that the services most in demand are for reflexology and massage (Bell 1996, Burke et al 1994).

In London, The Royal London Homeopathic Hospital, Mount Vernon and the Royal Marsden Hospitals were in the vanguard, being soon followed by other hospitals and hospices nationwide. Many support groups and day care centres have found that a balance of allopathic and complementary care is helpful, whether by lessening the need for drugs such as inhalers, laxatives, muscle relaxants and sedatives, or by more effective pain and symptom relief.

However, RZT is not only for those suffering from catastrophic illness and trauma. It is increasingly used in individual physiotherapy, maternity, intensive care, specialist units and general wards, where nurses, physiotherapists and midwives have been working to discover where, when and how it should most usefully be given.

Conclusion

Neither RZT nor any of the complementary therapies are at the 'cutting edge' of modern Western medicine. Their place is not in accident and emergency units, operating theatres or research laboratories. Their place is rather in the community, to build up a person's resilience, to detect early any changes in well-being, to foster recovery in illness, alleviate discomfort, pain and infirmity, and to complement all other care.

If the claims made for RZT are not too extravagant, if it is appropriately used and if its practitioners do not pretend to a knowledge which they do not have then it will have more to offer in the future.

References

Abrams A 1904 The concussional vertebral reflexes. American Medicine Publishers, Philadelphia, pp 115–118

Alfred the Great *c* AD893 Dômbôc (doom or judgement book). Quoted in Hodgkin R H A history of the Anglo Saxons, 3rd edn, vol 1. Oxford University Press, Oxford, pp 59, 67

Anthony C P, Thibodeau G A 1983 Textbook of anatomy and physiology, 11th edn. C V Mosby, St Louis, pp 238–239

Baas J H 1889 History of medicine. J H Vail, New York, p 138

Baldry P E 1998 Trigger point acupuncture. In: Filshie J White A (eds) Medical acupuncture: a Western scientific approach. Churchill Livingstone, New York, p 38

Burke C, Macnish S, Saunders J, Gallini A, Warne I, Downing J 1994 Clinical oncology, the development of a massage service for cancer patients. The Royal College of Radiologists 6:381–385

Bell L 1996 Complementary therapies and cancer care. Complementary therapies in nursing and midwifery 2:57–58

Dana C L C 1899 In: Baker W M, Harris V D Handbook of physiology, 15th edn, revised by Coleman W, Dana C L. William Wood, New York, pp 559–566

Eriksen L 1993 Reflexology and research. Danish Reflexologists Research Association Research Committee, Vallensbaek

Feder E, Liisberg G, Lenstrup C, Roseno H, Taxbol D 1988 Reflexology in relation to birth. Danish Reflexologists Association Research Committee, Vallensbaek

Fitzgerald W H, Bowers E F 1917 Zone therapy. I W Long, Columbus

Fliess W 1926 Nasale Fernleiden. Deutsche Verlag, Leipzig

Fliess W 1893 Die nasale Reflexneurose. Bergman, Wiesbaden

Froneberg W 1980 Reflexzonentherapie: Nerven, Muskeln, Statik, Bewegung. Eigenverlag W Froneberg, Mönchen-Gladbach

Gleditsch J M 1983 Reflexzonen und Somatotopien als Schlüssel zu einer Gesamtschau des Menschen. W B V Biologisch-Medizinische Verlagsgesellschaft, MBH & Co KG, Schorndorf

Griffin W, Griffin D 1834 Observations on functional affections of the spinal cord and ganglionic systems of nerves, in which their identity with sympathetic, nervous and imitative diseases is illustrated. Burgess and Hill, London, pp 147–168, 201–202, 212–215

Griffin W, Griffin D 1845 Medical and physiological problems being chiefly researches for correct principles of treatment in disputed points of medical practice, 8 vols. Sherwood, Gilbert & Piper, London, pp 60–73

Hall M 1833 On the reflex function of the medulla oblongata and spinalis, on the principle of tone in the muscular system. Abstracts of the papers printed in the Philosophical Transactions 1880–1884 (1830–1837): 210

Hall M 1836 Lectures on the nervous system and its diseases. Sherwood & Piper, London

Hall M 1838 Lectures on the nervous system and its diseases. W. Taylor, London

Hall M 1839 Extract from a lecture on the nervous system. J Mallett, London

Hall M 1842 On the mutual relation between anatomy and physiological pathways in therapeutics and in the practice of medicine. Baillière, London

Hall M 1850 A synopsis of the spinal system. Lancet 1:469–472, 495–496, 521–522, 554–557

Head H 1893 On disturbance of sensation with especial reference to the pain of visceral disease, part 1. Brain 16:1–133, 127

Head H 1894 On disturbance of sensation with especial reference to the pain of visceral disease, part 2. Brain 17:339–480

Head H 1920 Disorders of sensation in the skin arising from visceral disease. Studies in Neurology. Oxford University Press, London, p 328

Head H, Rivers W, Sherren J 1905 The afferent nervous system from a new perspective. Brain 28:99–115

Hodgkin R H 1952 A history of the Anglo Saxons, 3rd edn, vol. 2. Oxford University Press, Oxford, p 602

Ingham E 1938 Stories the feet can tell. Ingham Publishing, New York

Ingham E 1951 Stories the feet have told. Ingham Publishing New York

Johannessen H 1993 Reflexology in Denmark — an overview. Danish Reflexologists Association Research Committee, Vallensbaek

Johannessen H 1994 The hologram approach to reflexology. Danish Reflexologists Association Research Committee, Vallensbaek

Johnson T 1897 The Swedish system of physical education in medical and general aspects. Wright, Bristol

Launso L 1993 A description of reflexology practice and clientele in Denmark. Danish Reflexologists Association Research Committee, Vallensbaek

Ling P H 1859 Ling's educational and curative exercises, 3rd edn. Baillière, London

Lloyd G E R (ed) 1978 Hippocratic writings. Penguin, Harmondsworth. First published 1950 by Blackwell, Oxford

Mackenzie J 1892 Cutaneous tenderness in visceral disease. Medical Chronicle. John Heywood, London, XV: 302

Mackenzie J 1893 Some points bearing on the association of sensory disorders and visceral disease. Brain 16:321–354

Mackenzie J 1909 Symptoms and their interpretations. Shaw and Son, London, pp 37, 68

Mackenzie J 1920 Symptoms and their interpretations, 4th edn. Shaw and Son, London, pp 48–56, 74–83

Mackenzie J 1921 The theory of disturbed reflexes in the production of symptoms of disease. British Medical Journal Jan 29:143–147

Marquardt H 1984 Reflex zone therapy of the feet, 1st English edn. Thorsons, Northampton

Marquardt H 1993 Praktisches Lehrbuch der Reflexzonentherapie am Fuss. Hippokrates Verlag GmbH, Stuttgart

Melzack R, Wall P D 1965 Pain mechanisms: a new theory. Science 150:971–979

Northrup G W 1979 Osteopathic medicine an American reformation. American Osteopathic Association, Chicago, p 45

Plato *c* 375BC Timaeus, with an English translation by Rev. G Bury, 2nd edn, 1942. William Heinemann, London, pp 241–243

Porter R 1997 The greatest benefit to mankind. Fontana Press, London, pp 51, 55–64

Rasmussen et al. 1988 Danish Reflexologists Association Research Committee, Vallensbaek

Riley J S 1919 Zone therapy simplified. Health Research, Mokelumne Hill, CA

Ross J 1881 A treatise on diseases of the nervous system. Churchill Livingstone, New York pp 29–61

Singer C, Underwood E 1962 A short history of medicine, 2nd edn. Clarendon Press, Oxford, pp 27–41

Sola A E, Kuitert J H 1955 Myofascial trigger point pain in the neck and shoulder girdle. North West Medicine 54:980–984

Still A 1902 The philosophy and mechanical principles of osteopathy. Hudson Kimberly, Kansas City, p 121

Thompson J W, Filshie J 1993 Tens and acupuncture. In: Doyle D, Hanks G, MacDonald N (eds) Oxford textbook of palliative medicine. Oxford University Press, Oxford, ch 4–2–8

Travell J G, Simons D G 1983 Myofascial pain and dysfunction. The trigger point manual, vol 1. Williams & Wilkins, Baltimore

Travell J G, Simons D G 1992 Myofascial pain and dysfunction. The trigger point manual, vol 2. Williams & Wilkins, Baltimore

Voltolini R 1883 Der Krankheiten der Nase und des Nasenrachenraumes: nebst einer Abhandlung über Elektrolyse für Spezialisten, Chirurgen und praktische Aertzte. E Morgenstern, Breslau, pp 5–21

Weihe A 1886 Zeitschrift d. Berliner Vereinshomoop. Arzte V, Berlin, pp 206–244

Whytt R 1765 Observations on the nature, causes and cure of those disorders which have previously been called nervous, hypochondriac or hysteric, to which are prefixed some remarks on the sympathy of the nerves. T Becket and P A de Hondt, Edinburgh

Whytt R 1768 The works of R Whytt. T Becket and P A de Hondt, Edinburgh, pp 229–266

2

How does RZT work?

Introduction

Although RZT is known to have been of benefit to many people for a long time, it is only recently that a scientific explanation to account for these good effects has been developed. While therapists have observed pain relief and other responses which were provoked by treatment, *how* they happened was speculated on endlessly. In an age dominated by technology and science, an explanation that involved replication under laboratory conditions was called for. The claims made by therapists and confirmed by patients awaited proofs.

Much Western medicine and research has been shaped and directed over the past century by the germ theory of disease propounded by Virchow and Pasteur. Despite many advances in the treatment of acute illness, chronic illness still accounts for much incapacity and disability, the pathology of which is not satisfactorily explained by the germ theory. This chapter introduces current theories underpinning our present understanding of how RZT and allied therapies, such as acupuncture and neural therapy, effect their healing influence.

Connective tissue is shown to be arranged into highly organised functional units, the sum of which composes the *extracellular matrix* (ECM). Important informative, homeostatic and recuperative mechanisms of the ECM are described, and are termed the *ground regulating system* (GRS). The system depends on the integration of all those factors which affect the cell environment, which will be discussed in detail in this chapter. As mentioned in Chapter 1, recent research into the effects of acupuncture has

shown that the insertion of acupuncture needles tends to increase the release of opioids in cerebrospinal fluid, and elucidated the spino-bulbo-spinal loop pathway through which both segmental and non-segmental analgesia is achieved. Since the effects of acupuncture are also shown to be mediated through the ECM, this may be the means by which pain relief is obtained when RZT is employed.

From yet another field of research is derived the concept of interference fields. An interference field is a circumscribed area of tissue in which the ECM has been degraded by either infective, traumatic or chemical stimuli, and the area of tissue becomes chronically altered. Such an area can cause local or distant functional disturbance via *neural* pathways. This suggests a further pathway through which disorder in one part of the body may give rise to pain in distant reflex zones on the back, feet and hands. Interference fields impose a heavy load on the GRS, impairing both local defences and the maintenance of homeostasis (see below), which if untreated or unresolved leads to increasing debilitation.

Degradation of small compartments of cellular and surrounding tissue in the ECM (the cell environment) throws a load onto the GRS. Once a critical degree of loading occurs, compensatory mechanisms become exhausted, the susceptibility of the individual increases, and illness supervenes. The reflex signs of disease become apparent, and the classical changes of colour, texture, temperature and tissue tonus become visible in the skin. If the disease state progresses, these changes become irreversible, in tandem with failing organ function.

A resilient immune system depends on a healthy ECM. Infections, unless they are overwhelming, are self-limiting. Acute illness necessitates rest and careful treatment. Chronic illness is consequent upon degradation of the ECM, from whatever cause, overloading the ECM, and loss of the resilience of the immune system.

The dynamic processes by which an organism maintains a state of equilibrium of its various functions and tissue chemistry is termed homeostasis. Homeostasis depends on many factors, but there seem to be two major components in its regulation, one is neurovegative, the other a humoral, cell environment system. The second is the one which will be discussed here.

Tissue organisation

The Professor of Histology and Embryology at Vienna University, Professor A. Pischinger, published in 1975 a text based on his researches, called The ground regulation system. He enlarged on the hitherto accepted functions of connective tissue and suggested it was actively involved in healing and inflammatory responses. (This book has been translated into English and published in 1991 under the title Matrix and matrix regulation.)

Connective tissue

Connective tissue is a strong, fibroelastic network which fills all the spaces not occupied by tissues such as bone, liver and muscle. The network extends from head to toe. In fetal life it is formed from mesoderm before the endocrine and neural systems are formed (see Ch. 1, p. 12). Its distribution is general, in the brain, supporting the dermis and epidermis and enveloping all organs. This matrix is the largest to infiltrate all parts of the body, and it is embryologically the basic substance from which all body tissues are formed.

Connective tissue, the framework in which organs are supported, actively helps to maintain the 'milieu interieure', the state in which minutely balanced heat and waste exchange, Po_2 and Pco_2 and endocrine function can continue in a stable state. The nourishment and nerve impulses which sustain parenchymal cells can only reach individual cells by

being transmitted through the extracellular fluid in which they are bathed. Ground regulation activity thus takes place within connective tissue.

The extracellular matrix

Whilst connective tissue forms the basic matrix of the body, this basic matrix is, according to Pischinger, organised into functional units which form the cell–environment system (Fig. 2.1), or ECM, which has elaborate functions.

Each functional unit is composed of:

- parenchymal cells
- the final vascular pathway — an anastomosis of arteriole and venule in the capillary bed
- terminal axon fibres of the sympathetic nervous system (SNS) and parasympathetic nervous system (PNS)
- in some locations, nerve endings of the central nervous system (CNS)
- extracellular fluid, in which they are suspended.

Influences acting on the ECM are derived from:

- the nervous system, primarily the CNS and the brainstem
- the hormonal pole, principally from the pituitary and adrenal glands
- cellular regulating processes, and those from the lymphatic and reticuloendothelial systems.

These functional units are held in a reticulum of connective tissue cells within the extracellular fluid. Electrical and chemical activity at this level can *only* take place in extracellular fluid. This, like lymph, is an ultrafiltrate of blood and moves back into the vascular system.

The ECM is chiefly composed of sugar biopolymers and water, within which are dissolved ions of solid bodies, liquids and gases held within a reticulum of microscopic, connective tissue cellular components such as fibroblasts, mast cells, macrophages and fibres of collagen and fibrin. At molecular level, the ECM is shown to be made up of sugar polymers which are either free or bound to protein or lipids used in the formation of both the cell wall and intercellular substances. The ECM forms a molecular sieve and acts as an intermediary between

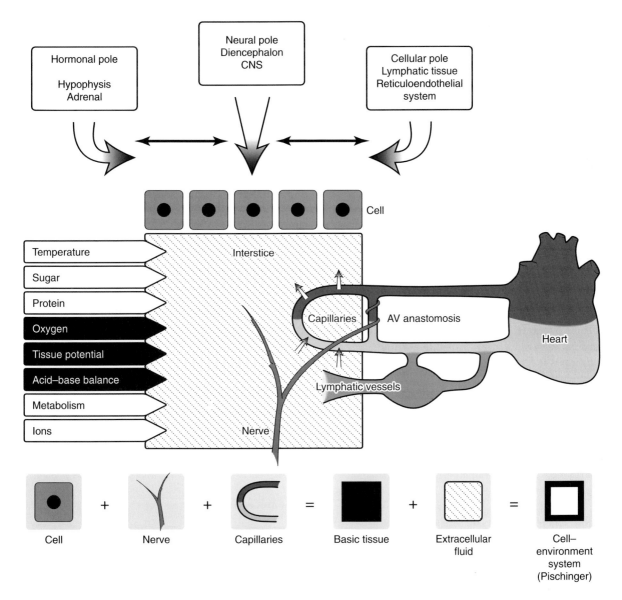

Fig. 2.1 *The basic autonomic system (cell–environment system) according to Pischinger. The relationship of the basic system (connective tissue + nerve + capillaries + extracellular fluid) to the parenchymatous cells, the blood and lymphatic systems is shown diagrammatically, as is its position within the whole of the organism with its relations to the well-known regulating poles (hormonal, neural, cellular). The basic regulating system is a cybernetic bioelectrical energy system with the oxygen-reducing potential at its centre. On this depend the oxygen balance and the acid–base balance on which in turn depend all the other well-known functions (From Dosch 1964, with kind permission of Karl F. Haug Verlag)*

all specific organ cells, the capillary bed and the autonomic nervous system (ANS).

Both defence — *extrusion* of molecules — and nutrition — *inclusion* of molecules — are performed synchronously by adaptation of filter size (the filter being formed by fibroblasts, connective tissue cells, mast cells and polymers in this instance) within each unit — the pattern of all biological economies.

Glycosaminoglycans (GAGs) are unbranched, linear carbohydrate chains and uronic acids forming the structural components of the ECM, of which the most important are hyaluronic acid, chondroitin sulphate, dermatan sulphate, keratan sulphate and heparin. Heparin is the sole polymeric sugar, and is stored in some mast cells or basophilic granulocytes, from where it is released as required to participate in all regulatory processes of the ECM, in the activation of some 50 enzymes, the translation and transcription of DNA and RNA, and promotion of fibrocyte and collagen synthesis (overview in Engelberg 1977). Proteoglycans are formed within the ECM when water–sugar polymers become bound to a protein backbone, which is in turn bound to hyaluronic acid.

Homeostasis and the GRS

It is within the functionally arranged units of this ECM that homeostatic regulatory activities take place. Biological systems, unlike cybernetic systems, have both an integrated direct feedback mechanism and a capacity to override the linear feedback under certain conditions (e.g. fight or flight responses, haemorrhage, shock, infection, trauma). The shutting down of the vascular bed and the immobilisation of the gut are classic examples. 'Information' — electrical and biochemical — is rapidly and effectively disseminated throughout the organism.

Homeostasis is maintained by vital feedback, information dissemination and bioelectrical functions taking place within the entire ECM. These functions are given the new term ground regulating system (GRS), where system means *capacity* and *capability* to have gases and molecules in solution. When the structure and function of the ECM break down, alarm signals are communicated to all other systems of the body. It was shown by Popp in 1984 that a photon emission from traumatised cells was received by surrounding cells within 10^{-7} seconds, and spread throughout the ECM at the speed of sound.

Summary of the functions of the extracellular matrix

Functions include:

- to provide a living, active, framework in which activities of cells can continue at their optimal level

- this is done through:
  - nourishment of cells by distribution through its substance — in solution — of food, oxygen, hormones and heat
  - removal of waste products of cellular metabolism by enabling them to return to the lymphatic or venous trees, in solution
- to act as a shock absorber
- to allow the transmission of nerve impulses from both the ANS and CNS.

The most vital aspect of this activity is the maintenance of the milieu interieure as an intact matrix through which biological information is transmitted and received, so that:

- the pH is maintained (i.e. the balance between acidity and alkalinity of the extracellular fluid)
- isotonia is maintained (i.e. sodium concentrations in extracellular fluid)
- isoosmia is maintained (i.e. osmotic movement of ions).

The compass of these functions is homeostasis.

The ECM and the body's systems

The nervous system

Since there are terminal axon fibres of both the CNS and ANS lying within the ECM, there is a constant feedback from the nervous system to ECM and from ECM to the nervous system (Fig. 2.2).

1. Autonomic nerve fibres in the capillary bed relay information about the maintenance of the 'steady state' to the brainstem. This mechanism is responsible for the peripheral shutdown of vessels when there is a major haemorrhage and blood has to be conserved for vital functions.
2. Autonomic nerve fibres from the periphery convey information to the posterior horn control cells. The gate control system (see p. 9) postulates that neuronal pain impulses carried by thick (mainly somatic) fibres are moderated in the region of the posterior horn at spinal level and

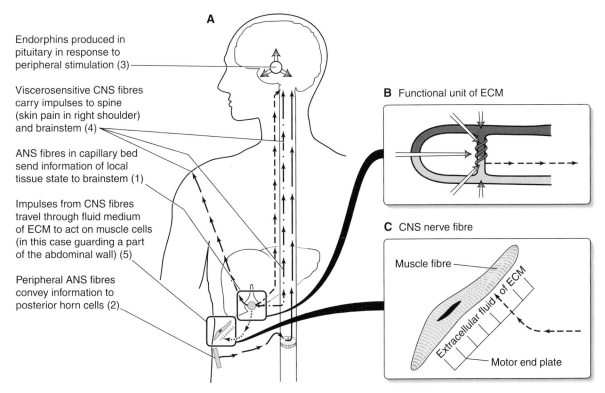

A

Endorphins produced in pituitary in response to peripheral stimulation (3)

Viscerosensitive CNS fibres carry impulses to spine (skin pain in right shoulder) and brainstem (4)

ANS fibres in capillary bed send information of local tissue state to brainstem (1)

Impulses from CNS fibres travel through fluid medium of ECM to act on muscle cells (in this case guarding a part of the abdominal wall) (5)

Peripheral ANS fibres convey information to posterior horn cells (2)

B Functional unit of ECM

C CNS nerve fibre

Muscle fibre

Extracellular fluid of ECM

Motor end plate

Fig. 2.2 *A Diagram to show how information from the ECM is transmitted via the nervous system. (The example is of someone with cholecystitis. The numbers relate to the list in the text.) B Information from ECM feeds ANS capillary bed fibres and thence to the spine and brainstem. C A CNS fibre carries impulse to the motor end plate, then through the ECM to act on the muscle fibre*

can thereby inhibit an unrestricted flow of information. This mechanism reduces the perception of pain. The effect of RZT in reducing pain may be due to the fact that it stimulates these somatic afferent (thick) fibres.

3. The opiate-like substances, endorphins, are found in highest concentration in the pituitary, and are produced in response to peripheral stimulation.
4. Viscerosensitive nerve fibres of the CNS carry impulses to the spine, skin and brainstem. These give a warning notice that 'all is not well within'.
5. Impulses from CNS fibres (such as the efferent motor nerve fibres which act on motor end plates) travel through the fluid medium of the ECM. The impulse goes:

   nerve fibre → extracellular fluid → muscle cell

   This is the conscious pathway used to describe all voluntary movement.

The endocrine system

Similarly, capillaries connect the ECM to the endocrine system. From the ANS to the CNS via spinal ganglia and then on to the brainstem, information is passed between connective tissue cells and autonomic nerve fibres through substances such as prostaglandins, cytokines, lymphokines and proteases released by cells. This interconnecting, intercommunicating feedback mechanism operates within the specialised connective tissues. It is the biological and mechanical framework of psychoneuroimmunology (PNI).

This distinctive arrangement and function of connective tissue allows and facilitates the transmission of information to every part of itself and to every other system, and responds to the information received. This ultrasensitive system strives to maintain homeostasis constantly, in cooperation with the hormonal and all other feedback and regulating systems.

Wurtman Anton-Tay (1969) coined the term 'neuroendocrinological transduction' to describe the recently discovered physiological processes by which neural 'mind' impulses were converted into hormonal 'body' messengers in the hypothalamus. The pathway through which mental states were translated into physical states had begun to be elucidated.

The development of chronic illness

The healthy state

The body is an incomparably well-designed biological system. In health it is *balanced* activity that characterises the organism. Food and oxygen taken in are transformed by biochemical reactions from macroscopic to microscopic levels to provide nutrition. The end point of metabolic activity is the production of waste. These breakdown substances are either transported out of the organism (e.g. carbon dioxide by exhalation) or ultra filtered and, via the lymphatics, returned to the central circulation to be filtered out and excreted via the kidneys. Most of this activity occurs without conscious control. There is an active awareness from the ECM upwards to complex organised structures that monitors neural, chemical and traumatic events constantly. Imperceptible shifts, such as closing down a vascular bed or releasing insulin into the bloodstream after ingestion of glucose, maintain the 'steady state'. Not surprisingly, sudden emotional upheavals, through the same chemical and neural pathways, are also felt within the GRS, which makes the same physical shifts in response. Mental health and well-being are as essential to the 'steady state' as is physical integrity: destructive emotional outbursts are as destructive to the GRS as is chronic ill health. The whole physical organism works in symbiosis. The term 'psychosomatic' correctly expresses the interplay of psyche and soma.

The impaired state

The ECM and the structures it supports can become incapacitated if too heavy a metabolic load is imposed on them (Dosch 1964, Hunecke 1953,

Hunecke & Hunecke 1928). Common examples of overloading (Fig. 2.3) are:

- partial or total failure of the neural alimentary defences, especially after oral antibiotic use, producing a loss of normal gut flora
- ingestion of heavy metals, e.g. lead, cadmium and mercury
- silent and chronic disturbances, i.e. foci and interference fields which are found in dental and faciomaxillary areas (a further explanation of these is given on p. 35)
- chronic appendicitis and cholecystitis
- poorly healed scars including keloid and herniation (see p. 35)
- persistent dietary indiscretions which place too heavy a chemical load on the gut, the liver and the kidneys and impairs their detoxification and filtering functions; in order to maintain as tenaciously as it does the neutrality of the blood, first the ECM and then the other tissues and organs act as buffers to reduce any rise in the acidity of the circulating blood
- malnutrition, vitamin and trace element deficiencies.

If these impaired states are long standing or masked by the use of drugs the following may result:

- oxygen and foodstuffs are absent at cellular level
- waste is not removed at cellular level and accumulates
- vascularisation of the tissue bed is poor, leading to tissue hypoxia and acidosis
- local defence mechanisms cease to function; the connective tissue cell and protein–sugar polymer mesh filter is impaired and becomes less selective.

A GRS that is not functioning perfectly demands more energy because the tissue acidosis which develops leads to:

- an increase in muscle tone
- a rise in temperature
- an increased demand for calcium for biochemical processes
- stimulation of the SNS
- the inflammatory response being raised and prolonged.

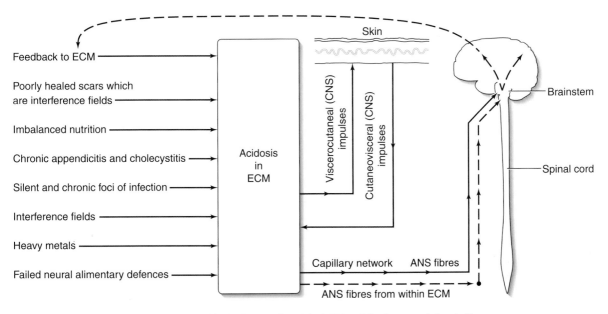

Fig. 2.3 *Diagram to illustrate factors responsible for degeneration of the ECM and development of chronic illness*

Although the SNS and PNS work in tandem with and are complementary to each other, in the normal circadian rhythm of the body the SNS is dominant between the hours of 3 p.m. and 3 a.m. During these hours all metabolic processes, including the inflammatory response, are raised. This is visible in the sick, whose temperatures usually rise during this time. The PNS is dominant between 3 a.m. and 3 p.m., when metabolic processes, including the inflammatory response, are lowered. The result is a fall in body temperature in the morning. Measuring the temperature of a sick person is a simple yet effective method of finding out to what extent the inflammatory process has been raised and extended.

Chronic illness

At this stage chronic illness is established. Symptoms persist and each further acute attack leaves in its train greater debilitation. (In our example, purulent pocketing or the acute emergencies of perforation or gangrenous segment become more likely.) What has hitherto been silent becomes insistent and

various mechanisms have been brought into play:

- the endocrine system is informed via the capillary network, and reorders its functions in response
- the viscerocutaneous nerve fibres carry visceral ECM information to the skin and cutaneovisceral fibres carry information from the surface to the viscera
- the ANS carries impulses from terminal axons within the ECM to the spinal ganglia, from where they travel to the brainstem and onward to the two hemispheres of the brain.

Information in this biological sense provokes a total response of the ECM, and there is a feedback response in reaction, termed 'biocybernetics'. This response is *protective* and *total*, that is, a small segment does not work in isolation. The whole organism seeks to protect itself. If only a small part of the ECM is affected by any of the above conditions, normal activity can continue. But the acute infection that becomes chronic, lead poisoning, or emotional troughs such as depressive illnesses can, if untreated, overwhelm the responsive capacity of the ECM. Even the young can succumb to trauma and infection when there are 'no resources' left. Hans Selye has described (1956, 1974) a series of physiological events in which either physiological or psychological stress is followed by shock, countershock, then convalescence lasting 7–10 days. The physiological pathway of what Selye called the 'general adaptation syndrome' (Fig. 2.4) is effected by hormones of the 'hypothalamic-pituitary-adrenal' (HPA) endocrine axis. The ANS, endocrine and immune systems are simultaneously galvanised by any stressor. But if the shock is repeated many times, then overreaction is followed by exhaustion. Once the body's reserves have been depleted, the vulnerability of the person is greatly increased. Unless care is taken and the ground system allowed to recover, he or she is much more likely to succumb to sickness if any further physical or psychological demands are laid on the exhausted GRS. Acute illness such as meningitis is often seen in the West. Similarly, chronic illness and autoimmune disease are on the increase. Antibiotic abuse and misdiagnosis are a medical challenge. An understanding of the GRS may explain why RZT, which seeks to relieve stresses and strains in *this* system, is so often beneficial.

The reflex signs of disease

Disturbance of the ground system follows a specific pattern. First affected is the quadrant in which disease has occurred within related dermatomes, myotomes and autonomic nervous fibres. Function in the unaffected quadrants is speeded up, using more energy.

Once the extracellular matrix in the affected quadrant is depleted and the infection persists, the second quadrant on the same side becomes similarly affected. If this section is overwhelmed, the whole of the other side of the body succumbs to a generalised deterioration.

Chronic illness is now well established. As the ground system weakens there are changes in the colloid state of the skin and subcutaneous tissue. There is associated hypoxia and acidosis of tissue, with similar changes taking place in smooth muscle. Head in 1896 and Mackenzie in 1909 described these as signs of visceral disease projected onto skin and subcutaneous tissue via the sensory and motor autonomic system. A century later it is known that organs can project their symptoms more widely than this.

In early fetal life, the structures for complex and coordinated movement are developed in the brain and spinal cord (see p. 12). Muscles normally work in groups, forming a kinetic chain (see p. 8), which allows linked, smooth movement. By repetition, patterns are created centrally, often termed 'patterning'. Reflex patterning allows us to talk, play games or a musical instrument, and follow any pursuit in which limb, brain and eye work together. The learning and consolidating of the pathway is forgotten in health, making the actions seem reflex. In stroke patients, it is seen that the relearning of walking and speech becomes labour intensive again.

When a muscle is overstimulated, suffers trauma, or is chronically overloaded, nociceptors lying over trigger points become sensitized (see p. 9). Discomfort or pain is now felt when the trigger point is palpated. Specific patterns of trigger point pain referral are described for each individual muscle (see Fig. 1.4, p. 9) (Baldry 1998, Travell & Simons 1983, 1992). Tone is increased in the affected muscle and in recognisable patterns in the whole kinetic chain. Myofascial trigger points in muscles along the whole kinetic chain in which the tone is raised secondary to the primary insult now become involved and sensitised. This chain may extend beyond the boundaries of the segment. A classic example is found in the patient with a slipped disc, in whom the whole of the anterior abdominal wall almost immediately goes into protective spasm. Muscle tone which remains raised throws unusual strain on all joints, fascia and tendons within the kinetic chain, and soon involves the spine (Fig. 2.5). Spinal information then feeds back into the affected segment and the GRS within that segment. The mechanical strain, from being unilateral, is now also passed to the contralateral side.

Professor Heine (1988a,b) described another change that occurs at the periphery when the GRS is disturbed. At numerous points in the skin, neurovascular bundles penetrate the superficial fascia just under the skin, bringing with them a cylinder of

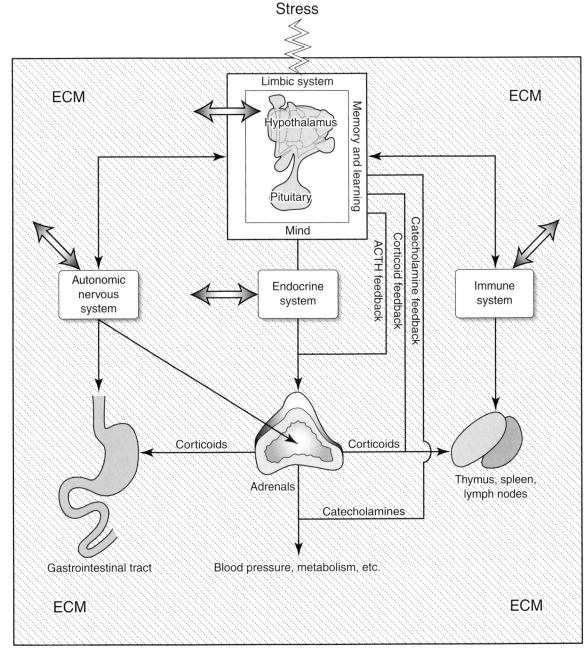

Fig. 2.4 *Selye's general adaptation syndrome (updated) to show feedback mechanisms between limbic, autonomic, endocrine and immune systems — all suspended within the ECM (After Rossi 1993, with kind permission of W W Norton)*

ECM. Professor Heine called these points 'windows to the ground system'. These points have come to be known as Heine cylinders (Fig. 2.6), and are found in the same distribution in all people of every race. All acupuncture points are found over Heine cylinders (but there are innumerably more Heine cylinders or 'windows to the ground system' than there are acupuncture points).

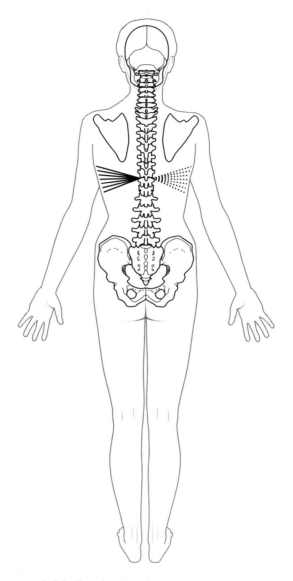

Fig. 2.5 *Persistently raised muscle tone on the left affects the spine, then spreads to the contralateral segment and GRS (on the right)*

Mechanisms underlying the relief of chronic illness or pain

The points described above respond to various stimuli, whether in the form of needle pricking, acupuncture, heat, massage, chemicals, local anaesthesia, or electrical and electromagnetic impulses. The effects of such stimuli are transmitted to and have a regulating effect upon the GRS. These findings are supported by the work of other researchers.

Acupuncture points and trigger points

Bergsmann observed in 1988 that there is a correlation between the location of frequently used acupuncture points and trigger points. Mann had already in 1977 noted the connection between the locus of

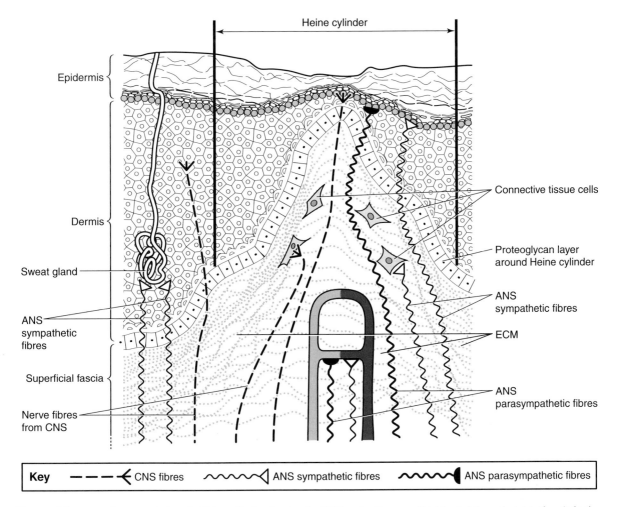

Fig. 2.6 *Diagrammatic representation of a Heine cylinder showing the ECM perforating superficial fascia below a 'point to the window'*

acupuncture points and trigger points so fully described by Travell & Simons (1992), Kellgren (1978), and Sola & Williams (1956). Melzack, Stillwell & Fox (1977) suggested that it was reasonable to assume that, whilst the anatomy of trigger points, along with their relationship to neural and muscular systems could be described, this was not the case with acupuncture points, whose origins were conceptual; however, it was possible that both represented the same phenomenon. A recent addition to the literature which describes the location of acupuncture and trigger points in both East and West has been drawn up in a review by Baldry (1993) (see also p. 9). That the complexity of viscerocutaneal relationships, and

the referral of visceral pain onto the superfices of the body, was recognised thousands of years ago in the Orient is increasingly acknowledged at the end of the 20th century (Lu & Needham 1980).

Physiology of pain relief

The physiological response of the body to injury is to produce pain-relieving substances. This has been experimentally shown by Bing, Villanueva & Le Bars (1991). An acupuncture needle inserted into either a true or false acupuncture point in the hind limb of a rat, and vigorously twisted or manipulated, leads to a threefold rise in opioid and met-enkephalin substances in cervical region cerebrospinal fluid. The widespread analgesia produced by this method is non-selective and not confined to the segment into which the needle is inserted.

The same effect was shown subsequently by Cesselin et al in 1989 who exposed subjects to harmful heat, by Bourgoin et al in 1990 who used exposure to harmful chemical irritation, and by Sjölund, Terenius & Eriksson in 1977 who used electrical stimulation as a harmful stimulus.

The physiological pathways through which relief of pain through acupuncture could be achieved were demonstrated by Bing, Villanueva & Le Bars (1990, 1991). Nerve impulses transmit information about a noxious stimulus from any segment by ascending the spinal cord to the reticular formation lying in the medulla oblongata, from where they are transmitted to higher centres, and pain-inhibiting impulses descend via dorsolateral tracts, terminating in the dorsal horns at all levels within the spine (see Fig. 1.5, p. 10).

DNIC

Le Bars, Dickenson & Besson (1979) had already suggested that diffuse noxious inhibitory controls (DNIC) were situated within the CNS, forming a spino-bulbo-spinal loop pathway. Class 2 (convergent) neurons, responding to both harmful and innocuous stimuli arising in skin, deep soft tissue and viscera are found lying within the dorsal horn. Class 3 (non-convergent) neurons are spinal interneurons responding only to harmful stimuli. Injury to any part of the body involves a greater level of activity in both class 2 neurons and class 3 interneurons in the transmission of pain impulses upward along anterolateral tracts to higher centres, and downward along dorsolateral tracts, the spino-bulbo-spinal loop in the affected segment(s). At the same time class 2 neuronal activity is depressed in all unaffected segments. The resulting anaesthetic pain relief is non-segmental. Le Bars, Willer & de Broucker proposed in 1992 that, by providing a secondary noxious stimulus in the form of acupuncture, a competing DNIC was initiated and had the effect of damping down already stimulated DNIC in someone suffering from the effects of a primary harmful stimulus. (This idea is also in harmony with old and modern concepts of counterirritation in which, to

relieve pain, an irritant is applied at a place or places distant from the primary source of pain.)

Clinical effectiveness of acupuncture

A series of patients suffering from renal colic were treated (by Lee et al in 1992) with acupuncture or Avafortan. Whilst complete pain relief was achieved in 86.4% of patients receiving acupuncture, there were no side-effects, and the calming effects began to be experienced within 1–10 minutes, which was significantly faster than in the Avafortan group. In the latter, whereas 62.3% of patients experienced pain relief within 10–30 minutes, some side-effects (tachycardia, rash, drowsiness) occurred.

The 'puncture phenomenon'

Pischinger described the basic phenomenon of acupuncture as being the result of a puncture which triggers the entire reaction system. He showed in 1975 that venepuncture for the purpose of taking a blood sample triggered major changes in iodine consumption and in leucolysis; this effect was later called by Heine the 'puncture phenomenon' or the 'puncture effect'. In a healthy subject venepucture leads to an immediate fall of at least $50\,\mu g/ml$ in iodine consumption values, with initial values being restored within 3–4 hours. Persons with certain chronic diseases, on the other hand, showed reduced or absent iodine consumption value responses, in accordance with the diminished alarm reaction in a system which had been subject to too many stresses, as previously described by Selye (1956, 1974). In the debilitated state, leucocytic lytic forms are increased by a factor of more than 5.

A needle puncture also brings about bioelectrical changes in the tissues, as described by Kracmar in 1971; a year earlier Kellner & Klenkhart (1970) had used an infrared camera to show the thermoregulatory changes which accompany puncture. These findings further support an understanding of how the effects of therapies such as acupuncture and RZT (where graduated touch is applied to debilitated reflex zones) are rapidly and beneficially spread through the GRS.

The role of point windows

The common features of stressed point windows (see p. 29) are:

- they are always found in the same place
- on palpation, the point lies in a depression with a smoother skin surface
- over the point the skin is less mobile
- the muscle under the skin is felt to be harder.

These features are not present in non-stressed muscles; point windows are also warmer in muscles whose stress is secondary to disease in an internal organ.

Heine described these points as comprising a multifunctional organ:

- with viscoelastic properties
- responsive to electrical, electromagnetic and magnetic stimuli by virtue of the oscillatory capacity of proteoglycan content
- whose electrolabile molecular filaments act as a storage system
- whose electrically labile proteoglycans are immediately responsive to all bioelectrical stimuli, and capable of imparting this information via the GRS
- with the suggestion that changes in muscle tension can be reflected in the point owing to alterations in the muscular vascular bed
- similarly, changes in vasomotor and heat regulation might be reflected in the point owing to the ECM being pulled up into close proximity with body surfaces.

In RZT, when looking at feet, we note the condition of the skin and underlying tissue and all responses to touch and palpation. A healthy reflex zone is not painful to touch anywhere. When the autonomic fibres respond to palpation with pain, cooling or sweating (however slight), this is the distress signal (mediated by the ANS) of disease. It has been suggested that the treatment of disease through these window points provides a stimulus for the ANS, which acts on the surrounding ECM and the rest of the network throughout the body.

The work of Head and Mackenzie has already been mentioned in Chapter 1. Similarly findings elucidating the acupuncture mystery through the Heine cylinder and verifying the physical effects of acupuncture have accumulated. For instance, Bergsmann (1974) showed that, when a point in the region of the seventh thoracic vertebra (acupuncture

point B-17) was stimulated, it produced a relaxation of the diaphragm with an increase in lung expansion; 200 patients were assessed using X-ray control and increased diaphragmatic amplitude was confirmed in all of them. Also, stimulating the skin round the spine of the fifth thoracic vertebra has been observed to cause the pyloric sphincter to relax (Mennel 1940). These and other findings again support the value of RZT, demonstrating that surface palpation at known locations produces improvement in known related organs. (The term 'palpation' covers needling, massage and electrical stimulation, but in daily general practice manual palpation is the most useful method.)

Algotomes

Pain arising as a result of disorder in an internal organ has recently been shown to project symptoms over a wider field than that of dermatomes previously recognised by Head (1896) and Mackenzie (1909). Two broad areas of research have contributed to this broader understanding of how symptoms from visceral organs and deep tissues are projected onto skin, subcutaneous tissues and muscle.

1. Dendritic branching ascending sensory tracts carry information from a particular receptive field at the periphery of the body to the posterior horn. Receptive fields overlap at the borders of the dermatomes, with consequent greater sensitivity over these areas. Melzack, Stillwell & Fox (1977) considered that acupuncture points are found in such areas of increased sensitivity.
2. Pressure on trigger points in muscle both gives rise to pain in the point itself and causes reflex muscular nociceptive hypertonicity along the course of kinetic chains, which cross segmental borders (Bergsmann & Bergsmann 1988, Travell & Simons 1983). Such areas, within which pain is referred in now well-recognised patterns, are called 'algotomes'.

The reflex zones and the GRS

Further reflex signs of disease are found in the 10 zone grid postulated by Fitzgerald & Bowers (see p. 14), in which the body is divided into 10 equal vertical zones: five on the right and five on the left, which traverse the limbs, trunk, neck and head. Zone 1 lies medially and zone 5 is the most lateral on either side. Organs and structures in each single zone are related to one another, and the position of an organ or structure in the body dictates the zone in which it is to be found. Central structures such as the spine, heart, stomach and bladder are represented in zone 1 on both feet. Structures of the left half of the body are found on the left foot, head and hand, while those of the right half of the body lie in the right foot, hand and head, although some crossing over is found.

The body is further divided into three transverse zones at the level of the shoulder girdle, waistline and pelvic floor (see p. 16). These are represented on the feet at the metatarsophalangeal joint line, the metatarsal–cuneiform joint line, and the line of articulation between tibia and talus. Reflex zones to the head and neck occupy the area of the toes; those of the thorax and mediastinum lie over the metatarsal bones; those of the abdomen over the tarsal bones and those of the pelvis are found over the calcaneum.

Any impairment in function or injury to organs and structures within the body is detectably reflected in the corresponding reflex zones. Similarly, when a suitable stimulus is given to abnormal reflex zones, it is transmitted throughout the GRS and has the capacity to affect the whole person. The healing process is an integral part of any biological system. For any treatment to be effective, it must aid the healing process. We are restating Hippocrates (Lloyd 1978).

More recently, in 1859 Florence Nightingale wrote in Notes on nursing 'Shall we begin by taking it as a general principle — that all disease, at some period or other of its course, is more or less a recuperative process, not necessarily accompanied by suffering: an effort of nature to remedy a process of poisoning or decay, which has taken place weeks, months, sometimes years beforehand, unnoticed …'.

Interference fields

A particular instance of the disturbance of the ECM is the appearance of interference fields. Interference fields were first described between 1839 and 1855 at the Royal Society by the English chemist and physicist, Michael Faraday. In early experiments with electricity he postulated that a magnet which attracts has an ionised field around it.

There are widespread fields of electrical activity far from the centre of a thunderstorm. Radio reception sometimes becomes disturbed or distorted. The atmosphere, filled with charged ions, is sensitive to electrical disturbance. Typically this may be caused in the vicinity of electrical or solar storms, or of an electrical apparatus such as a vacuum cleaner or microwave oven when in use. A distorted or spreading reception, in electronics, is called 'interference' and occurs within the electromagnetic field, whose strength depends upon the source of the interference. (Nature is always working against the constraints imposed by the laws of physics, both within and outside of the body.)

The term 'interference field' has been adapted to describe any part of the body in which tissues have become disturbed, and which tissues may themselves in turn be able to create a disturbance (Dosch 1964, Huneke 1953, Huneke & Huneke 1928). In particular, Dr Frederick Huneke, who first described neural therapy in 1925, in 1940 used the term to describe a focus of hyperirritability which could occur anywhere in the body (Dosch 1964). An interference field is an area of tissue which has been injured or infected, and fails to heal completely; such an area was frequently noted by Dr Huneke to be found in the oronasopharynx. As the body responds globally to any change, such interference fields can influence and affect distant organs or systems, and continue to do so until there is a resolution.

In an electronic field, sunspots, microwaves and other electrical apparatus have the capacity to disturb the function of other similar apparatus within their wavelength. Energy which radiates in the form of a wave forms an electrical field, and when this electrical field interacts with a magnetic field the result is electromagnetic (EM) radiation.

This is considered analogous to the way in which the disturbance of acute or chronic foci of infection or scars may give rise to increasingly poor function in a part of the body distant from the site in which the original injury appeared. Such a disturbance forms an 'interference field' whose effects are spread *neurally* throughout the body by means of the GRS and nervous system (particularly the ANS).

The concept of the GRS as an uninterrupted cellular mesh, acting as a channel through which hormonal and electrical messages aid passage throughout the body, should be kept in mind. The same informational response is triggered by either physical or psychological events. The main task of the reticular formation is the maintenance of the internal milieu and its regulating capacity, functioning cooperatively with the ANS centres and the gamma motor system, and participating in a complex, multiple feedback system in which all other known anti-inflammatory, hormonal, neural and humoral defence systems participate.

The primary function of the GRS is protection and damage limitation. An instant and total response means an isolated and walled-off locus of infection or inflammation. This is the commonest response prior to emergency surgery for acute appendicitis, gut perforation, impacted stones or dental decay. The sequence of events, whether visible or not, is always the same, and they are the classical signs of inflammation, rubor, calor, tumor and dolor, as described by Hippocrates over 2000 years ago (Lloyd 1978), or, as we would say today, redness, heat, swelling and pain.

A disturbance field arises when there is any break or damage, however small, and from whatever cause, in the linings, coverings or tissues of the body (Kellner 1966). There are two possible outcomes to the injury. Either a healthy GRS heals the injury completely, or there is imperfect healing. In the latter the GRS is not restored to its faultless function, but an area of 'distress' remains. This may either be contained, even in a small scar such as occurs in peritoneal wrapping, or the disturbed area may remain active. For example, sutures may work their way out of a deep wound site after a period of months or years, and only then does the wound heal and the 'distress' subside.

When the GRS is not functioning well, a disturbance field can spread beyond the confined site of the wound or area of cellular degradation. The effect of the interference field on the GRS is debilitating. Over a shorter or longer period of time the capacity of the GRS is depleted, and tissue acidosis spreads beyond the confines of the immediate vicinity of the interference field. As noted before (p. 28), the spread is from one segment to another on the same side, and then to a contralateral segment. Some distant effects can be traced through the meridians of acupuncture (or along the sensory nerves which overlap at receptive fields on the borders of dermatomes), through which they appear to have spread. It is not uncommon to hear people say that one side of their body is weaker than the other side, or that their pains and aches affect them on either the left or the right side. Frequent small assaults produce adaptation (Selye 1974), an example of this phenomenon being found in people working in noisy conditions who do not notice gradual deafness occurring. Tolerance of and adaptation to noise and pain are often culturally mediated. Any stimulus, whether pleasant, damaging or stressful, whether physical or psychological, initiates the following sequence of events:

- an alarm reaction (which is spread throughout the GRS)
- for a while, exaggeration of all succeeding responses to the stimulus (each stimulus weakening the GRS further) until
- exhaustion of the capacity of the body and mind to respond to the stimulus, so no further response is possible (the GRS has used up all its reserves of oxygen and energy).

Location of interference fields

Disturbance fields which have over time eroded local defences are commonly found in:

1. *The gastrointestinal (GI) tract.* The villi of this tract are filled with connective tissue and the lining is active friable epithelium (renewed every 24 hours) and susceptible to scarring from drugs and bacteria. It is well known that high dosages of aspirin can lead to gastric haemorrhages.
2. *The oronasopharynx.* The mouth, nose and sinuses share a mucous membrane lining through which infection spreads rapidly. The lymphatic system can be overwhelmed by infection which is tightly contained in bony cavities. The pain of tonsillitis, dental abscesses, infected sinuses as well as infection of the ears is well known.
3. *Viscera in the abdominal cavity.*
4. *Poorly healed scars anywhere.* A scar which is an interference field provokes a small but chronic

inflammatory reaction. Since the GRS reacts to inflammation anywhere, and uses energy to do so, some of the total available energy is always used in containing the local but chronic pathology. Any break in the surface of the epidermis or of mucous membrane linings forms a scar, which is potentially an interference field, but only becomes so when local defence mechanisms break down, and the effects of this breakdown are spread to and become apparent in distant sites.

Scars in which a disturbance field is present can be detected by differences in skin resistance. In a scar which has healed well, bioelectrical measurement of skin resistance varies little from that of the surrounding skin, ranging between 100 and 150 kΩ. When an interference field is present, measurements of skin resistance rise to 1400 kΩ over the disturbance field. The resistance is higher only over the area of the imperfectly healed scar. Surrounding tissues, 1 mm away from disturbance fields, have normal skin resistance (Stacher 1966).

All the above can become interference fields. If contained locally the GRS can cope, but new

infection, especially in the poorly nourished, infirm, overburdened or ageing person, leads to less resilience and a breakdown in containment. The so-called silent, chronic infection, because of the surrounding tissue acidosis which is created, places demands on the energy of the whole organism.

Treatment

Interference fields, whose treatment was first described by the French surgeon R. Leriche in 1925 (Leriche 1936) and later elaborated by Huneke & Huneke, can be treated by an injection of procaine, lignocaine, lidocaine or the homeopathic preparation Sensiotin (Atropin sulfuricum Dil D5 0.5 ml and hypericum perforatum Dil D5 0.5 ml). This repolarises the cell membranes, and they cease to be permeable to all ions, becoming selectively permeable again. Normal saline has also been found to be a suitable substance for neural therapy. A variant of neural therapy is more commonly known in the USA as 'nerve block'. After 50 years of research and practice in neural therapy by W. and F. Huneke, their work was collated and published by Dosch in 1964 and translated into English in 1984.

References

Baldry P E 1993 Acupuncture, trigger points and musculoskeletal pain, 2nd edn. Churchill Livingstone, New York

Bergsmann O 1974 Akupunktur als Problem der Regulations — Physiologie. Karl F. Haug Verlag, Heidelberg

Bergsmann O, Bergsmann R 1988 Projektionssymptome. Reflektorische Krankheitszeichen als Grundlage für holistische Diagnose und Therapie. Facultas Universitätsverlag, Vienna

Bing Z, Villanueva L, Le Bars D Z 1990 Acupuncture and diffuse noxious inhibitory controls: naloxone reversible depression of activities of trigeminal convergent neurones. Neuroscience 37:809–818

Bing Z, Villanueva L, Le Bars D 1991 Acupuncture-evoked responses of subnucleus reticularis dorsalis neurons in the rat medulla. Neuroscience 44:693–703

Bourgoin S, Le Bars D, Clot A M, Hamon M, Cesselin F 1990 Subcutaneous formalin induces a segmental release of Met-enkephalin-like material from the rat spinal cord. Pain 41:323–329

Cesselin F, Bourgoin S, Clot A M, Hamon M, Le Bars D 1989 Segmental release of met-enkephalin-like material from

the spinal cord of rats, elicited by noxious thermal stimuli. Brain Research 484:71, 77

Dosch P 1964 Manual of neural therapy according to Huneke. (Regulating therapy with local anaesthetics), 1st English edn tr. Lindsay 1984. Karl F. Haug Verlag, Heidelberg, pp 12, 27, 74–77

Engelberg H 1977 Probable physiological functions of heparin. Federation Proceedings 1:36

Faraday M 1839, 1844, 1855 Experimental researches in electricity. Royal Society, London

Fitzgerald W H, Bowers E 1917 Reflex zone therapy. I W Long, Columbus, Ohio

Head H 1896 On disturbance of sensation with especial reference to the pain of visceral disease, Part 3. Brain 19:153–276

Heine H 1988a Anatomische Struktur der Akupunkturpunkte. Deutsche Zschrift Akupunktur 3:26–30

Heine H 1988b Akupunkturtherapie — Perforation der öberflachlichen Körperfaszie durch kutane Gefas-Nervenbundeln. Therapeutikon 4:238–244

Huneke F, Huneke W 1928 Unbekannte Fernwirkung der Lokalanästhesie. Medizinische Welt 27:1013–1014. Nachdruck 1957 Hippokrates 28:251–253

Huneke W 1953 Krankheit und Heilung anders gesehen. Staufen Verlag, Köln (Cologne)

Kellgren J H 1978 Observations on referred pain arising from muscle. Clinical Science 3:175–190

Kellner G 1966 Funktionelle Morphologie der Haut und der Narbe. Arztliche Praxis 18:89, 105

Kellner G, Klenkhart E, 1970 Zur Differenzierung der Serumiodometrie nach A. Pischinger (Elektro-metrische Titration) Österreiche Zeitschrift für Erforschung und Bekämpfung der Krebskrankheit 25:81–88

Kracmar F 1971 Zur Biophysik des vegetative Grundsystems. Physik. Medizin und Rehabilitation. Zeitschrift allgemeine Medizin 12:120–122

Le Bars D, Dickenson A H, Besson J-M 1979 Diffuse noxious inhibitory controls (DNIC) 1. Effects on dorsal horn convergent neurones in the rat. Pain 6:283–304

Le Bars D, Willer J C, de Broucker T, Villaneuva L 1992 Neurophysiological mechanisms involved in the pain-relieving effects of counterirritation and related techniques including acupuncture. In: Pomeranz B, Stux G (eds) Scientific bases of acupuncture. Springer-Verlag, Berlin, p 79–112

Lee Y-H, Lee W-C, Chen M-T, Huang J-K, Chung C, Chang L S 1992 Acupuncture in the treatment of renal colic. Journal of Urology 147:16–18

Leriche R 1936 Die Stellatumanästhesie bei der Hirnembolie, bei Gefässpasmen, nach Hirnoperationen und bei Hemiplegien. Revue Chirurgie (Paris) 55:755

Lloyd G E R (ed) 1978 Hippocratic writings. Penguin, Harmondsworth, pp 70–75. First published 1950, Blackwell, Oxford

Lu G D, Needham J 1980 Celestial lancets: a history and rationale of acupuncture and moxa. Cambridge University Press, Cambridge

Mackenzie J 1909 Symptoms and their interpretation. Shaw, London, p 68

Mann F 1977 Scientific aspects of acupuncture. William Heinemann, London, pp 63–73

Melzack R, Stillwell D M, Fox E J 1977 Trigger points and acupuncture points for pain correlation and implications. Pain 3:3–23

Mennell J B 1940 Physical treatment by movement, manipulation and massage. J & A Churchill, London, p 13

Nightingale F 1859 Notes on nursing. Harrison & Sons, London, p 1

Pischinger A 1975 Matrix and matrix regulation. Basis for a holistic theory in medicine, ed. Hartmut Heine (1st English edn Haug International, Bruxelles, 1991). Haug Verlag, Heidelberg

Popp F A 1984 Biophotonen. Schriftenreihe Krebsgeschehen. Bildung 6, 2 Auflage Verlag für Medizin. Dr Ewald Fischer, Heidelberg

Rossi E L 1993 The psychobiology of mind-body healing. W W Norton, New York, p 29

Selye H 1956 The stress of life. McGraw Hill, New York

Selye H 1974 Stress without distress. The New American Library, New York

Sjölund B H, Terenius L, Eriksson M B E 1977 Increased cerebrospinal fluid levels of endorphins after electroacupuncture. Acta Physiologica Scandinavia 100:382–384

Sola A E, Williams R L 1956 Myofascial pain syndromes. Neurology 6:91–95

Stacher A 1966 Zur Wirkung der Herde auf dem Gesamtorganismus. Österreiche Zietschrift für Stomat 63:294–303

Travell J G, Simons D G 1983 Myofascial pain and dysfunction: the trigger point manual, vol 1. Williams & Wilkins, Baltimore

Travell J G, Simons D G 1992 Myofascial pain and dysfunctions: the trigger point manual, vol 2, the lower extremities. Williams & Wilkins, Baltimore

Wurtman R, Anton-Tay F 1969 The mammalian pineal as a neuroendocrine transducer. Recent Progress in Hormone Research 25:493–513

The basics of RZT practice

3

Planning treatment: practical issues

Equipment

Before treatment the therapist needs to prepare the following:

- the room
- the couch
- the chair or stool
- towels, sheets and other covers
- pillows and pads
- record cards
- other accessories.

The room

The ambience of the room where treatment is given should convey both privacy and attention to detail. A quiet and restful room where the patient and therapist will be undistracted needs to be set aside for the purposes of treatment.

The room should be adequately ventilated and clean, warm and large enough for the purpose. Coathangers and space to hang coats, with room for outdoor shoes, should be provided. Toilet and washing facilities must be available.

The lighting should be warm and bright, illuminating the room, without harsh or direct light shining onto the patient's face. A source of light (natural if possible) is needed under which the feet can be examined.

As organisms are carried on the skin, breath and clothes, from where they can be transmitted to others, there should be no unnecessary furnishings. Fabrics in the room should be laundered regularly.

The couch

A bed, couch or plinth for the patient is needed which is sufficiently high, long, broad and firm (Fig. 3.1). It should not be too high for the patient, so that transferring on to and off it is not difficult, and at a comfortable working height for the therapist. After some practice, it will be found that the most convenient working height of the bed is no higher than just below the waist of the therapist. Although to the beginner this may seem low, as practice increases and more dependence is placed on palpation and less on watching the way the hands work and on locating the reflex zones, then a height of about 60 cm (2 feet) will be found by most therapists to be both comfortable and practical. It allows the breathing, colour, expression and body language of the patient to be monitored constantly so that, when the need arises, touch and depth of palpation can be adapted immediately.

In all cases the couch should also be long enough and broad enough so that anyone who is elderly or infirm will feel secure on it, and so that it will accommodate people of all heights, weights and ages. A couch length of 2m (6 feet 6 inches), a breadth of 0.9 m (3 feet) and a height of 0.6 m (2 feet) suits most people.

Finally, it should have a firm base, and coverings which can be removed and washed with ease.

The chair or stool

A chair or stool (preferably without arms) is needed for the therapist to sit on. It should be the same height as are the therapist's legs from heel to knee, so

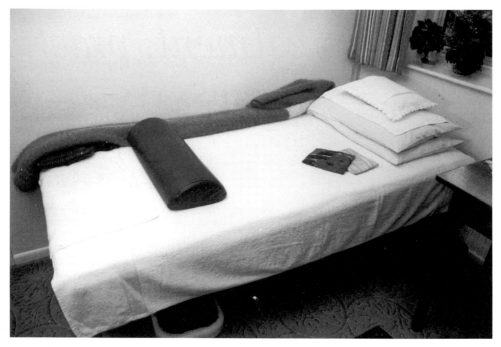

Fig. 3.1 *Couch for the comfortable positioning of the patient*

that he is able to sit comfortably with both feet on the ground with knees and hips at a right angle to each other (see also working posture, Ch. 6, p. 96).

Towels, sheets and other covers

Clean and fresh cotton sheets, towels or paper towels are used to cover the bed and should be changed regularly.

A fresh, clean cotton or paper towel is also needed to place under the feet of each patient, since sweating sometimes occurs, and another under the head to protect the pillow from hair creams and sprays.

A light towel or blanket is needed to cover the patient in all but the hottest weather, and even then if she feels cool. Extra, light but warm coverings should be to hand in case they are needed.

Tissues, paper towels and water should all be within reach of the patient.

Pillows and pads

One or two pillows are used under the head and neck. These should be carefully positioned so that the patient's head is comfortable, without undue flexion of the neck. More pillows should be available for those with breathing difficulties.

A number of small pads and pillows, each some 16×20 cm (6×8 inches) in size, are useful for placing in the small of the back if the patient has backache (although a rolled-up towel does equally well), or for supporting painful hips, knees, elbows and/or neck.

A support for the knees should be carefully positioned so that it lies underneath the knees and lower thighs, and does not rest against the calves, where it is both uncomfortable and obstructs the venous return of the lower legs.

Record cards

A supply of record cards should be available (of the feet, face, hands and back), pen and pencils for notes (record cards are dealt with in more detail below).

Other accessories

A sphygmomanometer is useful to record the blood pressure of all new patients, and to allow comparisons to be made at the end of a series of treatments.

Scar cream and sterilised needle (boiled, flamed or placed in alcohol) are needed for the treatment of scars. Appropriate oils are needed for back treatment. Cream can be applied to the feet at the end of treatment (never the beginning) if the skin is very dry.

A nail file or emery boards to keep the nails short and a pair of nail scissors should be to hand.

If essential oils are used in the room, they should be used discreetly. The pungent and heavy smell of excessive fragrances is often nauseating to the sick.

Radios, music machines and the like have no place in the treatment room, and are a nuisance to most patients. Many people prefer, when they are listening to music, to do so intently, without other distractions. Most people have their own preferences in music, and the prevalence of the distorted sound of music in most public places and spaces harries many people. The room should be as quiet and restful as possible.

There should be a surface on which the patient can put keys, bag and pocket contents, and a second comfortable chair in which she can sit whilst talking and putting on socks and shoes. A long-handled shoehorn with which to ease on shoes is useful for those who have difficulty in bending down, and should be available.

A hotwater bottle and a large bowl for footbaths make up the complement of requirements in the treatment room.

For children a few soft toys always give pleasure. A few wooden and clay whistles fashioned into birds and animals which the children can blow should treatment be uncomfortable can be a useful device for allowing even small children to let the therapist know when he has palpated a painful reflex zone.

A plastic jug in the toilet allows for the collection of urine specimens, enabling their volume, colour and odour to be checked.

Checklist

- A quiet and private room; pay attention to the heating, lighting and ventilation.
- Couch, pillows, small pillows.
- Supplies of towels, both large to cover the bed and small for feet and head.
- Washing and toilet facilities.
- Record cards, recording materials.
- Tissues, paper towels.
- Chair and table for the patient, therapist's chair.

Records

Every patient should have her own record of history, assessment and treatment, which is confidential. Patients who are being treated in a hospital setting should have all treatment and its effects recorded in the hospital notes. Therapists working independently need to keep a complete and accurate record of treatment and its outcome after each visit.

All observations, together with the findings on palpation at assessment, are recorded most easily on a diagram of the feet which shows all its surfaces (Fig. 3.2). A body chart to record painful areas is also useful (Fig. 3.3).

If a distinction is made on the record card between the symptom for which the patient has sought treatment and the underlying disorders which are found on palpation (Fig. 3.4), the relationship between cause, treatment and reactions becomes more apparent.

The card should have space to note any reactions, whether of relaxation, pain relief or those deriving from the ANS at each session, as well as the zones palpated at each session, and finally any reactions which have occurred between one visit and the next. Any advice which has been given about exercise, relaxation, breathing or nutrition also needs to be recorded.

Attention to detail and care with record keeping alerts the therapist to the possibility that RZT is inappropriate treatment for this person, or that the illness is worsening, or there is some serious underlying illness, indicating that the patient should be referred to her general practitioner. If, on the other

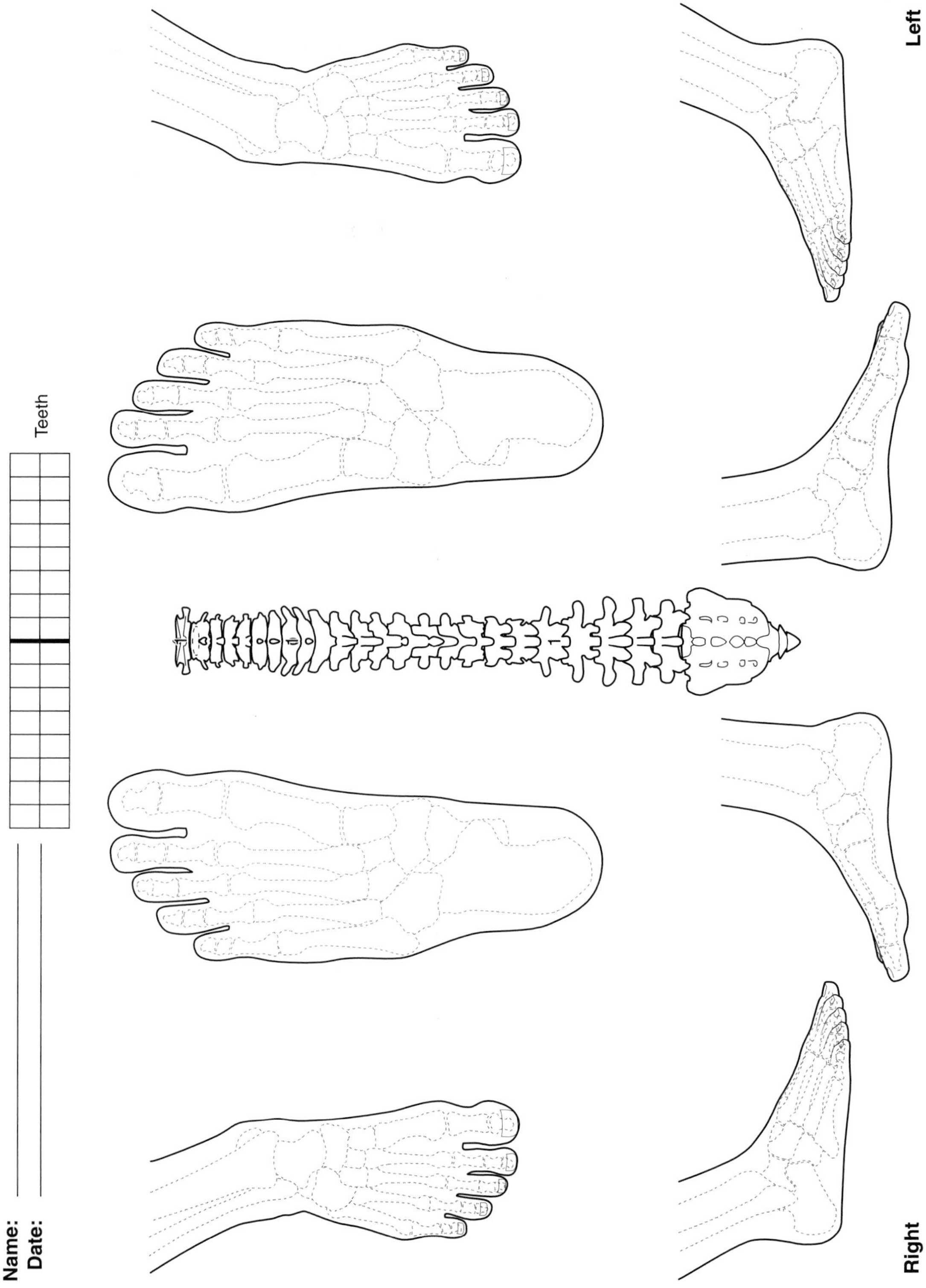

Left

Right

Name:
Date:

Teeth

Fig. 3.2 *Example of a treatment card*

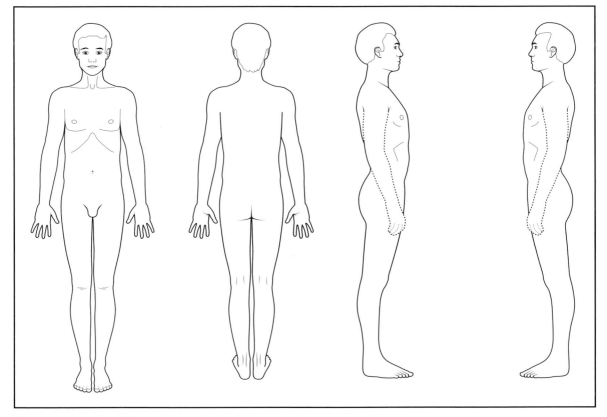

Fig. 3.3 *Body chart on which to record pain*

hand, treatment is beneficial, records build up a valuable profile of circumstances and conditions in which RZT is most likely to be useful, and similarly define when it is either contraindicated or inappropriate. In the UK it is a legal requirement that nurses, midwives and physiotherapists keep records of all treatment given. Written consent for therapy is required from the parent or legal guardian of children under the age of 16.

Records should be kept in a place of safety, and not shown to anyone other than a member of the medical team caring for the patient.

Legal issues

The practice of RZT in the United Kingdom is governed by legislation enshrined in the two branches of English law.

One branch is criminal law, which governs the actions of the community vis-à-vis the state. A person who contravenes criminal law is prosecuted by the authority of the state and, if found guilty, is fined or imprisoned for the offence. Criminal law is, for the most part, contained in Acts of Parliament.

The second branch is that of civil law, first encoded by King Alfred the Great (*c* AD893) in the words: 'what ye will that other men should *not* do to you, that do ye not to other men'. Later, in the 14th century, local traditions of self-government in boroughs and shires dating back to Anglo-Saxon times were confirmed by the Crown and have survived to this day in the form of case law.

Civil law governs the duties and rights of members of a community towards each other. If one community member has a grievance against another community member, she may take out a law suit against the offender who, if found guilty, is ordered

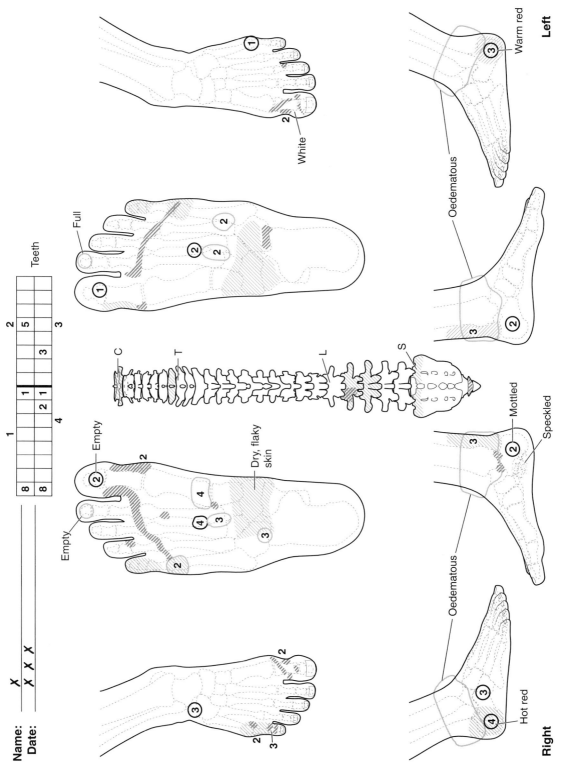

Fig. 3.4 *Example of a completed record card after the first visit of a patient complaining of right shoulder pain (areas of discomfort or changed tissue tonus which are experienced by the patient as painful are shaded)*

to pay damages to the plaintiff as monetary redress for the injury sustained. This injury may be physical, due to negligence, or against one's good name, as in libel and calumny.

Therapists should also be aware of the vast volume of subsidiary legislation promulgated in Orders in Council, statutory instruments, local authority by-laws and other instruments. Although these subsidiary laws derive, ultimately, from Acts of Parliament they are not popularly considered to be criminal law but may, nevertheless, lead to fines or imprisonment. Health and Safety Regulations are particularly important in the present context and there may be local requirements with the force of law. Some local authorities, for example, require premises where massage is carried out to be licensed.

Statutory restrictions

Specific Acts of Parliament lay down statutory restrictions to protect the public from the unscrupulous activities of quacks and charlatans, and it is a criminal offence to infringe any of these statutory restrictions. The following paragraphs briefly outline those statutory restrictions which are relevant to the practice of any therapy.

1. Unqualified persons are prohibited by law from using one of the following titles unless they hold the necessary qualification:
    chemist, chiropodist, dental practitioner, dental surgeon, dentist, dietitian, general practitioner, midwife, nurse, occupational therapist, orthoptist, physiotherapist, radiographer, remedial gymnast, surgeon, veterinary practitioner or veterinary surgeon.
2. The practice of dentistry, midwifery or veterinary surgery can only be conducted by an appropriately qualified person.
3. Patients presenting with dental problems must be referred to a dentist.
4. Pregnant or parturient women must be under the care of a registered midwife.
5. It is an offence for anyone except a registered general practitioner to treat for direct or indirect reward a person presenting with venereal disease, to try to prescribe any remedy for such a

person, or to offer advice for the treatment of venereal disease.

Venereal disease is defined by the Venereal Diseases Act (1917) as syphilis, gonorrhoea or soft chancre. Treatment of any of these renders the unqualified practitioner liable for prosecution. Therapists should not undertake to treat anyone with a venereal disease until the patient has received the necessary medical care.

Acquired immune deficiency syndrome (AIDS) is not covered by the 1917 Act, and is therefore not legally classified as a venereal disease. It is left to the individual therapist to decide for himself whether or not he should undertake treatment in any given situation.

6. While first aid may be given to animals in an emergency, it is an offence liable to prosecution to make a diagnosis of disease in any animal, to treat an animal medically or surgically, to operate on an animal, or to advise on any of the above.
7. It is an offence liable to prosecution to advertise any treatment or remedy, or to give advice for any of the following specific conditions: Bright's disease, glaucoma or cataract; locomotor ataxia; diabetes; paralysis, epilepsy or fits; tuberculosis or cancer.
8. It is an offence for a parent or guardian to fail to provide medical aid for any child under 16 years of age. It is not prohibited for them to receive any particular therapy, but it can only be given after adequate medical care has been provided.

Professional standards

A person who holds himself out as ready to give medical treatment or advice implies thereby that he is possessed of skill and knowledge for such a purpose, whether or not he is a registered practitioner. The duties are a duty of care, including a duty of care in deciding whether or not to undertake the case and in deciding what treatment to give, a duty of care in administration of the treatment, and a duty of care in answering a question put by a patient in circumstances in which it is known that the patient intends to rely on that answer. A breach of any of these actions will support an action for negligence by the patient.

The law recognises the right and duty of the therapist not to accept a patient for treatment when he does not have the requisite skills to treat that patient in a competent manner. Therapists working within the National Health Service (NHS) must agree the practice of all therapies that they use with their employing authority as well as with their medical colleagues. Many local and regional health authorities have drafted guidelines for the practice for all therapies outside of present mainstream medicine and these apply to all their staff. Many hospitals have a nominated, or elected, standards group through which all new therapies have to be filtered, as well as through the ethics committee.

Referrals, recording and evaluation of collected data are required by some employing authorities.

Accountability

UKCC Guidelines for professional practice (which govern the conduct of nurses, midwives and health visitors) state in the 1996 edition (p. 7):

■ *"As a registered practitioner, you hold a position of responsibility and other people rely on you. You are professionally accountable to the UKCC, as well as having a contractual accountability to your employer and accountability in law for your actions. The Code of Professional Conduct sets out your professional accountability — to whom you must answer and how."*

The Code of professional conduct drawn up by the same body in 1992 states that:

■ *"Each registered nurse, midwife and health visitor shall act, at all times, in such a manner as to:*

- *safeguard and promote the interests of individual patients and clients;*
- *serve the interests of society;*
- *justify public trust and confidence and*

- *uphold and enhance the good standing and reputation of the profession."*

In its regulation Professional conduct and discipline: fitness to practice (1991) the General Medical Council laid down in paragraphs 42 and 43 the conditions under which treatment or other procedures could be delegated to non-medical staff. These regulations state that any doctor who delegates care to anyone who is not a registered medical practitioner must be satisfied that the person carrying out the treatment, or other procedure, is competent in their execution. Overall responsibility for the care of his or her patients is retained by the doctor, whose training has been undertaken with this responsibility in mind.

Most professional organisations require certain standards to be met by their members at all levels of practice, and these must be adhered to. For example, in the Rules of professional conduct laid down by the Chartered Society of Physiotherapy rule 1 was elaborated in January 1992 to state that:

■ *"Chartered physiotherapists shall confine themselves to clinical diagnosis and practice in those fields of physiotherapy in which they have been trained and which are recognised by the profession to be beneficial."*

Within their scope of practice:

■ *"Chartered physiotherapists shall only practise to the extent that they have established and maintained their ability to work safely and competently, and shall ensure that they have appropriate professional liability cover for such practice."*

In 1998 the Chartered Society of Physiotherapy published a booklet, Standards and guidance for good practice in reflex therapy, to cover all aspects of professional responsibility. In their standards and guidance for good practice it is recommended that assessment, verbal questioning, informed consent and treatment be recorded and audited, and that therapists should continue to develop their knowledge and skill.

All registered practitioners must be convinced of the relevance and accountability of the therapy which they are using, and must be able to justify its use in particular circumstances, especially when using the therapy as part of professional practice.

On the subject of accountability the UKCC Guidelines for professional practice in 1996 (p. 8) state:

■ *"Accountability is an integral part of professional practice, as in the course of practice you have to make judgements in a wide variety of circumstances. Professional accountability is fundamentally concerned with weighing up the interests of patients and clients in complex situations, using professional knowledge, judgment and skills to make a decision enabling you to account for the decision made."*

The same document takes cognisance of the growing interest in complementary therapies (p. 33), requiring also that:

■ *"The registered practitioner therefore must be convinced of the relevance and accountability of the therapy being used and must be able to justify using it in a particular circumstance, especially when using the therapy as part of professional practice. It should also be part of professional team work to discuss the therapy being used with medical and other members of the health care team caring for the particular patient or client."*

The UKCC believes that courses undertaken by its registered members should be valid and credible, and should not need to be supported by registered status with the UKCC.

In the latest Guidelines for records and record keeping distributed to its members by the UKCC (1998), the following recommendations are included:

■ *"There are a number of factors which contribute to effective record keeping. Patient and client records should:*

- *be factual, consistent and accurate*
- *be written as soon as possible after an event has occurred, providing current information on the care and condition of the patient or client*
- *be written clearly and in such a manner that the text cannot be erased*
- *be written in such a manner that any alterations or additions are dated, timed and signed in such a way that the original entry can still be read clearly*
- *be accurately dated, timed and signed, with the signature printed alongside the first entry*
- *not include abbreviations, jargons, meaningless phrases, irrelevant speculation and offensive subjective statements*
- *be readable on any photocopies*
  ...
- *be consecutive*
- *identify problems that have arisen and the action taken to rectify them*
- *provide clear evidence of the care planned, the decisions made, the care delivered and the information shared."*

The guidelines were drawn up with the safety of both the patient or client and that of the practitioner or carer in mind. It is a professional and common law offence to mislead the public or to misrepresent oneself.

Code of conduct

Therapists must adhere to the Code of conduct of their professional organisation. Responsible training schools also have a Code of conduct which should be part of the induction into training.

Therapists should not give a medical diagnosis to the patient, nor should they countermand instructions or prescriptions given by a doctor.

All communication between the patient and the therapist is confidential. It may not be divulged, except to medical colleagues when necessary.

Selling, endorsing and promoting the sale of goods in clinical practice is not allowed.

Fees should accord with those of professional colleagues. Therapists may not promise to 'cure' a patient, nor to guarantee any specific recovery. It is not in the gift of any practitioner to know the outcome of any particular course of treatment. All that can be described to persons wishing for treatment is to outline the possible therapeutic benefits which may follow from therapy.

If, in the judgement of the therapist, there is no benefit to be gained from a particular form of treatment, this should be clearly and kindly explained to the patient and/or her family, and a more appropriate alternative sought.

Because it is difficult, if not impossible, to maintain emotional objectivity when treating family, intimates and friends, giving RZT within this circle should be confined to first aid or to treatment over a very short term.

If the therapist finds that personal feelings over and above those which must be present for the giving of any true care and treatment begin to intrude on RZT sessions, the therapeutic relationship should be brought to an end, and the patient should attend another therapist. The red mist of emotion can obscure the finest judgement.

Insight into one's own motives for choosing to become a therapist should be developed early on in training. These include compassion, a desire to help and care for the sick as well as the need for approval and a sense of worth. However, any unresolved personal difficulties accompany the therapist wherever he goes and, for as long as they are not perceived and taken cognisance of, he is unlikely to become an impartial and balanced practitioner.

Professional negligence and insurance

Therapists who work privately must comply with the conditions of their professional organisation and should be appropriately insured against claims for professional negligence. They should also be insured against public liability in their professional capacity; the public liability provisions of an ordinary household will not usually be sufficient to cover a professional practice.

Employing authorities carry insurance to cover their staff against public liability and professional indemnity. Professional organisations similarly insure their members when certain conditions are met. However, neither employing authorities nor professional organisations cover the therapist in private practice unless specific insurance has been taken out. The therapist in private practice should remember that all insurance arrangements must reflect the fact that a business is being carried out. Failure to declare this may vitiate a policy.

Post mortems

A post mortem has to be carried out before a death certificate can be issued in any case where the deceased has not been seen by a doctor during the 4 weeks preceding the death, or if the coroner thinks it necessary. A post mortem can lead to a coroner's inquest.

Therapists should be aware that they can be called upon to give evidence at an inquest and should ensure that adequate medical care is sought for all their patients.

Premises

Premises used for therapy must comply with legislation which requires them to be suitable for the purpose for which they are used. Local authorities have by-laws governing practice in clinics or at home which differ widely throughout the country.

Therapists working at home should pay attention to the terms of their lease or other title deeds, and any other local authority regulations limiting such practice. Local authorities are empowered to levy business rates on all premises in which therapy is conducted.

Taxation

Therapists in private practice should be aware that their fees attract taxation under different conditions to employed people and that they will be classified as self-employed. Under the recently introduced self-assessment of income tax scheme they are required to keep detailed records of income and expenditure and to retain receipts, vouchers, etc. for at least 6 years.

Therapists who are partly publicly employed and partly in private practice will be taxed under different schedules for their employment and for their private practice and they may require professional advice to help complete their tax returns. Pay slips, etc. received from employers should be carefully retained.

Expenses wholly incurred in connection with private practice may be set off against fees received but some difficulty may arise with marginal items: expenses such as rent, insurance, telephone and electricity may have to be apportioned. The purchase of furniture and equipment is classed as capital expenditure and cannot be set off against income. Capital allowances are, however, available in certain circumstances.

Regulations in other countries

Each European country has its own legislation governing the practice of individual therapies. Therapists are advised to familiarise themselves with local regulations when working abroad.

In the United States of America a statutory prohibition against the unlicensed practice of medicine (which is widely defined) exists. Medical licensing statutes have been enacted by each state and these also vary widely.

Therapists should acquaint themselves with local, national and state legislature before starting their practice.

Working alone — issues of risk

Issues of safety and risk for the therapist when working alone are of increasing importance. A number of areas of potential vulnerability should be addressed before beginning practice, in order to minimise if not eliminate such risks. These include avoidance of potential legal liability arising from the physical nature of the therapy, as well as measures to ensure physical safety. In this respect, the RZT therapist is in a broadly similar position to that of bodywork practitioners such as physiotherapists. Box 3.1 details some advice given to physiotherapists, much of which is equally pertinent to RZT working practice.

References

Alfred the Great (King of the English) *c* AD893 Dômbôc (Doom or Judgement Book). Prologue. Quoted in: Hodgkin 1952 History of the Anglo Saxons, 3rd edn. Oxford University Press, Oxford, pp 59, 67

CSP (Chartered Society of Physiotherapy) 1990 (October) Working alone — advice to members. Physiotherapy 76(10):621

CSP (Chartered Society of Physiotherapy) 1992 (January) Rules of professional conduct. CSP, London

CSP (Chartered Society of Physiotherapy) 1998 Standards and guidance for good practice in reflex therapy. CSP, London

GMC (General Medical Council) 1991 (February) Professional conduct and discipline: fitness to practice. GMC, London, paras 42, 43

UKCC (United Kingdom Central Council) 1996 (June) Guidelines for professional practice. United Kingdom

Central Council for Nursing, Midwifery and Health Visiting, London, pp 6, 8, 33

UKCC (United Kingdom Central Council) 1992 (June) Code of professional conduct. United Kingdom Central Council for Nursing, Midwifery and Health Visiting, London

UKCC (United Kingdom Central Council) 1998 (October) Guidelines for records and record keeping. United Kingdom Central Council for Nursing, Midwifery and Health Visiting, London

Venereal Diseases Act 1917 24th May In the Public General Acts passed in the 7th and 8th years of the Reign of H M King George V Being the 7th Session of the 13th Parliament of the United Kingdom of Great Britain and Ireland Eyre and Spottiswoode London for Sir Frederick Atterbury. KCB, Kings Printer of Act of Parliament, London, Ch 21, pp 34–36

BOX 3.1 WORKING ALONE — ADVICE TO MEMBERS *(From CSP 1990, with kind permission)*

… With the increase in violence seen in our society and the development of a more litigious ethos, physiotherapists working alone need to consider carefully their working practices. This need is not unique to physiotherapists; the increase in the number of attacks on social workers, for example, should indicate the need for physiotherapists to be vigilant and circumspect. Added to this is the nature of the practice of physiotherapy which is primarily a handling profession … This handling and contact must be carefully explained, and patients adequately prepared, otherwise our practice is open to misunderstanding and misinterpretation, which can lay a member open to allegations of assault or even indecent assault.

Physiotherapists are also vulnerable to attack. This may come from patients or from relatives or carers of patients. There may be many reasons for this: patients and families under stress following injury or disease, the effects of drugs, or other abuse. Physiotherapists need to be aware of the family situation to judge, if possible, their vulnerability to attack, verbal or physical.

In private practice — … private practitioners should always be on their guard. Remember the contract to treat is between the private practitioner and the patient, no third party is involved as in the NHS, and physiotherapists can *refuse* to treat if they are unhappy in any way.

In the community — primarily domiciliary work — members are reminded of the few simple rules that are observed and practised by health visitors and social workers, such as, let your colleagues know where you are going and when you are expected back, do not make an appointment to see a new patient when it is dark, and avoid difficult urban areas or remote villages. Keep the doors of your car locked when driving and try to park your car safely when visiting patients. Try to make joint visits with other professionals to patients who you feel may pose problems if this is possible.

… So again, these members are open to untrue allegations regarding their practice, and to physical or verbal attack. Most members over the years develop warning systems that certain patients or their relatives could be a problem. When such a patient attends it is wise to alert other staff in the unit or, if possible, 'borrow' another professional to act as chaperone and/or assistant.

… All members are advised to look carefully at their working practices to ensure that so far as possible they are not put in a position where unfair allegations of professional misconduct can be brought against them, or an attack, either physical or verbal, could be made.

The results of such actions by patients are extremely disturbing, and unpleasant; they may also be costly for the employing authority or the individual practitioner — members are urged to do all they can to avoid these situations.

4

Assessment

An assessment of all the reflex zones, whether of feet, hands or back, is made at the first visit, unless the patient

- is too ill, and palliative or symptomatic relief is called for
- is in the acute phase of illness, such as rheumatoid arthritis
- has strong SNS reactions which preclude completion of the assessment at the first visit
- is in need of first aid only at this time — for example, is unable to pass urine postoperatively, in which case the bladder needs to be stimulated and the solar plexus sedated.

Initial assessment

Treatment is usually sought when pain, debility or increasing weakness in an organ, joint or limb interferes with daily tasks and living. These presenting symptoms are generally easily identified. However, except in the case of trauma, they rarely give a full picture of the patient's ailments. Taking a short history precedes the assessment, in which all the reflex zones are palpated.

The history

A history provides the therapist with information having a bearing on the patient's present ailments. However, it should never obscure the important personal interchange which takes place between patient and therapist at each treatment. Nearly all the information necessary to give good treatment can be found by the therapist on the feet as she examines the reflex zones. It should be established at the outset whether there are any contraindications for treatment.

Learning to ask questions about how people live and how their bodies function without being intrusive is an art and a skill. The more skilled and observant one becomes, the more refined questioning becomes. A pleasant manner on the part of the therapist helps to put the patient at ease. It is helpful for the therapist to have a 'confidential' file in her mind, into which all such information goes. The only occasion for opening that file outside of the treatment room occurs if information has to be given to another health professional (e.g. the general practitioner).

The purpose of taking a history is to provide the therapist with relevant information about the patient's:

- present complaint
- present health or otherwise
- past health or otherwise
- lifestyle factors having a bearing on his complaint and general health
- familial factors.

There are advantages to using a questionnaire and asking the patient to fill it in and bring it to the first visit. This allows time for unhurried recall of sickness and accidents which may or may not be related to the present complaint, and the format of a questionnaire ensures that all important areas are included. It is, however, an impersonal way of collecting information at a time of personal need, and does not give an impression of the vitality, bearing and presence of the person. For this reason a verbal history may be preferred, or a combination of both may be used. In either case, the therapist must not be submerged under a wealth of detail, and must learn to record precisely and concisely what is found on examination.

The purpose of taking a history is to learn:

- the present complaint and the limitations it imposes
- the general health of the patient, both past and present
- the background to both of the above (i.e. lifestyle and whether and in what way it contributes to the general health or illness and present complaint)
- the salient features of the patient's personality, and the therapeutic approach which would be most helpful.

The following information is useful at the first visit.

General history

Important items to include are:

- name, address, age, sex
- occupation
- name and address of the general practitioner
- any drugs or medicines which are currently being taken.
- What has brought the patient to you for treatment now?
- if pain is present:
  — when was it first noticed
  — where precisely is it (the patient should indicate with finger tip where the pain is at its worst)
  — its nature
  — for how long it usually lasts
  — whether the pain is predictable or random
  — what eases and what aggravates it
  — to what extent it interferes with function (e.g. does it make sitting down, getting up, standing or walking difficult?)

  — whether the function of a limb, joint, spine or body function is affected
  — whether the pain wakes him at night.

It is helpful if the patient can locate problem areas on the body map (see Fig. 3.3, p. 45).

It should be asked what treatment has been given to date, with what effect, and whether there is any concurrent treatment. The therapist should have as clear a picture as possible of the complaint and the limitations which it imposes, so that progress, or lack of it, can duly be assessed.

The therapist should not forget to enquire also about the person's social situation — whether he is living alone, supported by family and friends, or supporting dependants, and whether or not this is by preference.

General health

Important items to include are:

- family illnesses
- past illnesses, operations and injuries
- past hospitalisation
- appetite, and any food preferences, dislikes or intolerances
- usual weight and any recent fluctuations (any unexplained and rapid recent weight loss is a potentially serious sign, and should be further investigated)
- whether sleep is restful, light, deep or interrupted
- whether the person is energetic, or tired for most of the day
- how the bowels usually function — e.g. whether bowel action is normally once or twice each day
- how many times a day the person normally passes urine — as bladder tone and capacity diminish with age, the elderly often have to pass urine during the night, otherwise it is normal not to have to do so
- whether there are any discharges from the skin, eyes, ears or genitourinary tract
- whether there are any breathing difficulties.

Women should also be asked about the nature of their menstrual cycle, and whether it is regular, also about the circumstances surrounding any past pregnancies, childbirth and miscarriage.

Lifestyle

Important items to include are:

- how much time is spent at work and under what working conditions
- whether there is time for regular recreation
- the nature and frequency of exercise (too much exercise is as harmful as too little)
- the amount of fluid, including alcohol, tea, coffee, water, etc., drunk daily
- the amount of tobacco consumed each day, if appropriate
- the content of the usual diet
- whether there have been any recent stressful events such as bereavement, separation, moving home, promotion, studying, exams, unemployment, etc.
- any other information which the person would like to give.

While it is important to fill in this broad canvas, history taking should not overshadow treatment. Many details emerge at subsequent visits to give a more complete picture.

Informing the patient

The patient is given a description of what he may expect from and during the sessions. Specific treatment is not given at the first visit, although it is usually accompanied by a sense of well-being. If the patient is in severe pain, use only sedating movements, and carry out or complete the assessment only when the acute episode is over. The purpose of the first visit is to sift out what is significant from the complaint, history and physical findings.

Depending on her interpretation of the assessment findings (see Ch. 5), the experienced therapist will be able to tell the patient whether RZT is an appropriate therapy for his complaint, and:

- what the possible outcome might be
- approximately how many sessions will be needed
- what measures the patient can take to reinforce therapy and hasten recovery.

A sense of relaxation is the most commonly experienced reaction during and after the

first session. However, there may be others, usually:

- a feeling of tiredness (often described as welcome)
- a headache
- worsening of the symptom for a short time
- in women, menstruation may be earlier than expected.

The patient should be told of these normal and usually mild responses so that he knows what to expect and does not become needlessly alarmed. He is, however, asked to let the therapist know of any reactions or changes in his normal habits and pattern of bodily functions at the next visit.

A *simple* information sheet or booklet noting the important points about therapy or reactions can be given to anyone who has not had RZT before or who, knowing little about it, wishes for more information.

Assessment procedure

Preparing the patient

The patient lies in a comfortable position on the bed, his heels level with the edge of the couch (Fig. 4.1). His head should be supported with one or more pillows, which should have been well positioned so that they do not cause undue flexion or extension of the neck, and be covered with a clean paper towel for each patient. As the patient does not know what to expect and may be anxious when deciding to be treated with RZT, he should always be able to see the therapist's face during a treatment session on the feet, and more especially so at the first visit.

It is common for people to be nursed on low beds in their own homes, and the therapist who regularly finds herself in the position of treating bedfast people at home might care to carry a low stool with her on such visits. If no low chair is available, the therapist should raise the patient's feet on two foam wedges or pillows, so that they are at a comfortable height for treatment for both the patient and herself.

If the patient is unable to lie in the supine position, any position in which he is most comfortable can be adopted. Extra pillows should be used to support

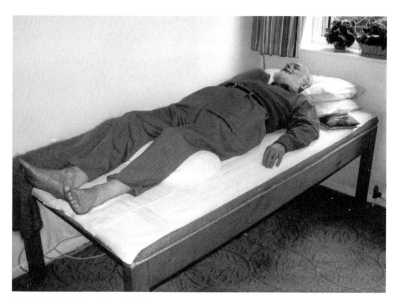

Fig. 4.1 *Positioning the patient*

him, with small cushions or pads being placed under shoulders, hips or knees if they are painful, and to support a limb in a desired position. The therapist adapts herself accordingly.

All patients need a warm, light covering, even on warm days and in hot climates. Many people feel cool during treatment, particularly if they have been active before lying down, and a covering provides comfort, privacy and security.

All constricting clothes, such as tie, belt and any tight jeans fastenings should be loosened, so that deep breathing is not inhibited, and treatment is able to encourage a good expansion of the lungs and concomitant relaxation of the abdominal wall.

The patient should be asked not to wash his feet immediately before treatment. Any enhanced and uniform warmth and moisture can be misleading for the therapist at assessment and subsequent sessions.

He should also be asked not to apply any creams, oils or perfumed sprays before the visit. Any of these make palpation difficult and mask the appearance of SNS reactions such as cooling or sweating. The feet often give off specific odours during treatment; these are usually related to the customary food and fluids which make up the patient's daily diet, but may also relate to the illness. (Ketotic and all other odours should be noted and recorded, as they provide

important information about the patient's illness.) Both assessment and treatment are done on the bare skin, so as not to mask any SNS reactions. If the patient is very nervous or ticklish, or has marked reactions to light palpation, treatment can be given over a light pair of socks, muslin cloth or towel. It does not usually take very long before the patient is able to tolerate normal touch on his uncovered feet, possibly four sessions. (If normal touch and palpation are still intolerable after this time, either the therapist's technique or the suitability of RZT for this person should be questioned.)

The hands of the therapist should be warm, and her nails shorter than the pads of her thumbs and fingers so that they do not provoke any discomfort (which could be mistaken for disorder) in the reflex zones. At no time should the fingernails of the therapist come into contact with the skin of the patient. The therapist should learn to rely principally on the information derived from the reflex zones, so that any disorders presenting there can be correctly interpreted and treatment adapted accordingly.

It is a good idea for the therapist to demonstrate to the patient on his hand what she will be doing on his feet, and to show him that her nails are short. Many patients are surprised by the sensations which they experience during treatment and, while these are often pleasant and relaxing, they will also often remark that they are experiencing sharp or pricking sensations, and ask if the therapist is working with her nails, or comment that it feels as though needles are being used. It is important for the patient to understand that it is only the pads of the fingers and thumbs which are used in treatment, that normal touch and pressure without any great variation is used, that different sensations may be experienced in different reflex zones, and that the aim of treatment is to restore normal sensation to areas where it is perceived by patient and therapist to be abnormal.

Note: No oil, cream or talcum powder should be applied during treatment. As mentioned above, they interfere with the immediate recognition of any autonomic nervous system reactions. Such reactions should be perceived by the therapist before the patient becomes aware of them, and treatment adapted accordingly.

Visual inspection

The following general observations are made, and will be referred to as treatment progresses in order to determine improvement:

- the general mien of the patient whilst lying on the bed
- the facial expression and colour
- the respiratory rate and rhythm.

The patient's tone of voice and manner of speaking, whether slow, rushed, hesitant, or clear and to the point, are valuable indicators of his present state of mind and feelings. His facial expression and gestures likewise indicate the extent to which he is at ease with the situation.

Any difficulties with walking and movement should also be noted.

As what is normal for one person may not be normal for another, teasing out the dividing line between function that is normal and function that is on the borderline of abnormality requires skill.

The first step in the assessment of the feet is to make a thorough general visual inspection. Their general appearance is noted, including the:

- temperature
- bony structure and blood supply
- colour and texture of the skin

- any change in the shape and structure of the toenails
- any change in the contour of the tissues.

From this can be seen in which organs, structures or systems any disorder is reflected. Visual inspection does not and cannot give the full picture of the illness — palpation yields far more information about which zones are disordered — but it does provide important clues as to where disorders are to be found, as do the small but detectable changes which take place from one visit to another.

Temperature

Both feet may be uniform in temperature, one may differ from the other, or there may be variations over distinct parts of the feet. Temperature changes ranging between cold, cool, warm and hot are often found on one or both feet on the same person.

These changes may reflect local disorders on the feet; a condition affecting the whole body; or external factors such as weather, constrictive nylon shoes, socks or stockings, recent exercise or immersion in hot water.

The use of an alternate stroking method called Yin-Yang strokes (see Ch. 6, p. 99) gives the therapist a clear impression of any temperature variations over the whole foot and lower leg.

The bony structure and blood supply of the feet

Structure. The feet are a marvel of architecture and engineering. The curving and arched bony structure gives a firm, rigid yet shock absorbent platform for all body movements, and the complex arrangement of the small, long and irregularly shaped bones, with their attachment of ligaments, tendons and muscles, allow for such diverse activities as standing on the toes of one foot, walking, running, jumping, climbing and heavy weight bearing, whilst all the time the load is distributed in such a way as to maintain the erect posture and balance of the whole.

While it is not possible to identify the outline of each individual bone on either the sole or the dorsum of the foot, familiarity with their position, shape and arrangement allows the therapist to find anatomical landmarks on the feet and, with the help of these

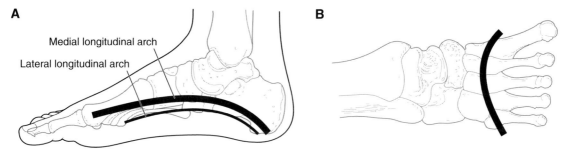

Fig. 4.2 *A Longitudinal arches of the foot. B Transverse arch in the tarsal and metatarsal region of the right foot (phalanges removed) (From Anthony & Thibodeau 1983, with kind permission of C V Mosby)*

landmarks, to locate and chart the reflex zones of each system with a high degree of accuracy. Twenty-six bones, either long, short or irregular in shape, form each foot and are arranged in such a way as to form both longitudinal and transverse arches (Fig. 4.2). That part of the *longitudinal arches* (medial and lateral) which is formed by the os calcis (calcaneum) and the talus is about 50 mm in length, and their forward part, underneath the tarsal and metatarsal bones, is about 70 mm in length in a normal-sized adult. The highest point of the longitudinal arches is the superior articulating surface of the talus, and weight is borne posteriorly on the tubercles on the under surface of the os calcis posteriorly, and the heads of the metatarsal bones anteriorly.

The *transverse arch* (which is not a true arch but more a half dome), is formed by the distal portion of the tarsal bones and the proximal portion of the five metatarsal bones, and looks somewhat like a bridge.

The individual bones of the foot are as follows:

- the os calcis is the large irregularly shaped bone which bears the weight of the body at the heel (Fig. 4.3)
- the irregularly shaped talus articulates (joins and moves) with the os calcis on its superior middle third, with the tibia and fibula, and with the navicular
- the smaller, wedge-shaped navicular articulates with the talus, the three cuneiform and the cuboid bones
- the irregular but flatter cuboid bone on the outer margin of the foot articulates with the os calcis, the navicular and the third cuneiform
- the first, second and third cuneiform bones form the transverse arch where they articulate

with the bases of the first, second and third metatarsal bones; they articulate with the navicular posteriorly, and the third cuneiform articulates with the cuboid at its lateral border
- the five long metatarsal bones are numbered from one in the midline to five on the lateral aspect of the foot; they articulate with the cuneiform bones and the cuboid proximally and the phalanges of the toes distally
- the toes are formed by the phalanges, of which there are two in the first or big toe, and three in each of the other toes.

Before beginning any practice, it is a useful exercise to explore the structure, appearance and function of one's own feet, and to familiarise oneself with the anatomical landmarks of the feet.

The sole of the foot is formed by a bed of soft tissues forming the shock absorbent cushion on which we walk. However, the joints where the heads of the metatarsal bones articulate with the proximal phalanges of the toes can be readily identified, since these are the joints with the most movement in the feet. Articulation takes place here with each step — as the heel lifts off the ground, weight passes to the ball of the foot and the toes until it is taken by the heel of the other foot as it meets the ground.

Certain landmarks are easy to find on the upper surfaces of the foot (Fig. 4.4). These are chiefly, as stated beforehand, the heads of the metatarsal bones where they meet the phalanges of the toes. To find this joint line, plantar flex the toes slightly, and the heads of the metatarsal bones usually become prominent.

The base of the first metatarsal is usually slightly elevated on the dorsum. The smooth line of the bone

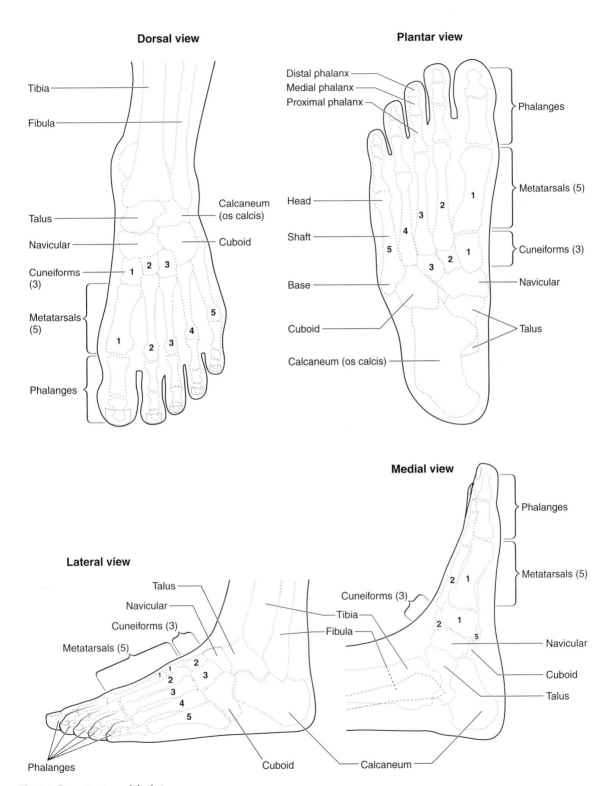

Fig. 4.3 *Bony structure of the feet*

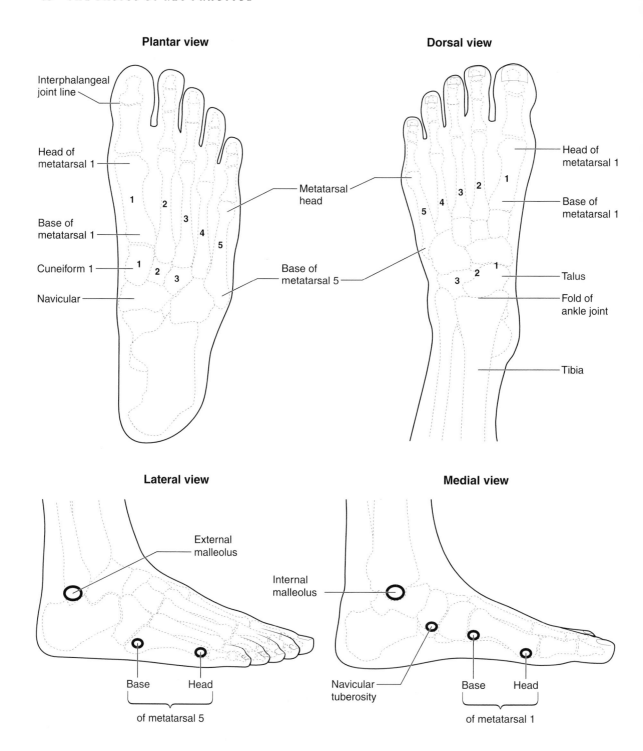

Fig. 4.4 *Bony prominences palpable on the feet*

shaft is interrupted by a thickening of the base on its medial surface. The head of the fifth metatarsal is usually quite easy to find on the lateral border of the foot where it articulates with the proximal joint of the fifth toe. The base of the fifth metatarsal is the prominence which in general is readily felt just distal to the halfway mark on the lateral border of the feet.

Along the midline, the navicular projects slightly (or sometimes greatly) into the midline, and can be found by running your index finger down the midline until this bony projection is felt.

Landmarks which need to be identified are:

- on the dorsum:
  — the head of metatarsal 1
  — the head of metatarsal 5
  — the base of metatarsal 1
  — the highest point of the transverse arch, which is usually the first cuneiform, but which may be the navicular, the fold of the ankle joint on the dorsum, where the talus articulates with the tibia
- in the midline:
  — the head of metatarsal bone 1
  — the base of metatarsal bone 1
  — the tuberosity of the navicular as it projects into the midline
  — the internal malleolus
- on the lateral border of the foot:
  — the head of metatarsal bone 5
  — the base of metatarsal bone 5
  — the external malleolus.

Once the position of these landmarks are readily identifiable, and the therapist knows what she is looking for and where, and has become familiar with the feel of the tissues, the wide variations in shape, texture and colour which are encountered take on a new significance. The bony structure of the feet provides a graphed map which enables the therapist to be quite specific about the areas in which pain or discomfort are found, and to relate these areas to particular reflex zones. An easy competence in holding, exploring and palpating the feet is a prerequisite for any therapist.

Observation procedure. First both feet should be observed together. Consistently following the same sequence when looking at the feet is helpful, as it establishes a structure and pattern for purposeful observation. Moreover, it is unlikely that any feature will be overlooked or forgotten when observation is so structured.

The following should be included:

1. The external malleolus is checked to see if it is normal in shape and size. Common causes of change are generalised bone disease, the rheumatoid group of diseases, and renal malfunction in the later stages.
2. The medial and lateral longitudinal arches are compared from heel to toes, with both feet held together (Fig. 4.5). The concavity may be the same in both feet, but where the spine is out of alignment the arch becomes flattened. The arches of the feet are checked to see whether they high, low or absent, and whether they are similar in both feet.
3. The metatarsophalangeal joint 1 (mtp joint 1) is checked for any irregularities, most commonly a hallux valgus.
4. The outline of the lateral border is compared on both feet to note their similarity or differences.
5. The outline of the heels is examined, noting any irregularities of shape, or the presence of any exostoses.

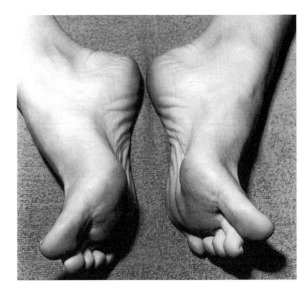

Fig. 4.5 *Comparing the longitudinal and transverse arches in each foot*

6. On the dorsal arch formed by the tarsal bones, a note is made of whether the same smooth bony outline to both arches exists on both feet.
7. The dorsal surfaces of the feet are checked where the metatarsal bones articulate with the phalanges of the toes (the mtp joints) to see whether they are prominent or depressed.
8. All the toes are examined to compare their structure, shape and size.
9. On the plantar aspect, both feet are examined together to gain an impression of the underlying bony structure. It is helpful for the therapist to imagine that she is looking at the feet as though they were standing on fresh, soft sea sand and looking at the imprint the feet would make. One foot may bear more weight than another; the

musculature and tendons of one part of the foot may be more taut or flaccid than in another part. While the same weight-bearing pattern may be reflected in both, it may be evident that weight is borne more heavily on one foot than another, and there may be subtle differences from one to another.

The blood supply to the feet. The dorsalis pedis artery gives rise to the medial and lateral plantar arteries, from which the dorsum of the foot receives its blood supply (Fig. 4.6). A pulse can be felt where these arteries overlie bone, either over the transverse arch or on the medial and lateral aspects of the calcaneum.

The presence and volume of these pulses should be ascertained at the first assessment and at every

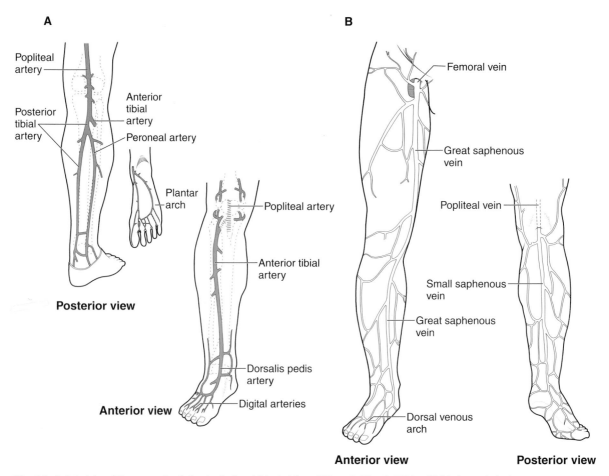

Fig. 4.6 *A* Arterial and *B* venous circulation in the legs (Adapted from Wilson & Waugh 1996, with kind permission)

subsequent visit. If the pulses remain absent and the feet cold, and if the feet do not become significantly warmer during a series of treatments, the diminishment in blood supply may be caused by peripherovascular disease, diabetes, or some other generalised illness or an obstruction to the blood supply which requires further investigation.

The arteries from the plantar arch supply the sole of the foot. The venous drainage is by means of the long saphenous vein, which begins on the medial side of the foot and passes upward in front of the medial malleolus. There is also the short saphenous vein, which begins on the lateral side of the foot and passes behind the lateral malleolus. These veins become engorged if the valves of the leg veins are weakened and become incompetent, allowing blood to pool in the lower extremities, and their pathway is then easily visible.

The texture and colour of the skin

The colour, texture and condition of the skin are general indicators of the nutrition, hydration and present health of the person, and may be changed as well by climatic exposure, occupation and local wear and tear. The therapist should note the natural skin tone, which may be ivory, white, porcelain, olive, sallow or dark. Any variations in this tone, such as yellow, blue, pink, red, mauve, grey or orange tinges are significant in relation to the reflex zones which they overlie, as they denote disorder in that zone.

A note should also be made of the elasticity of the skin, and whether it springs back to normal when picked up between thumb and finger.

Changes in the texture of the skin are also important. Even small areas of transparency, shininess, thickening (as in callus formation), roughness, dryness, moisture, folds, furrowing or fissuring (Fig. 4.7) and flaking are significant. The presence of any corns, warts, fungal infections or patches of eczema or dermatitis, and their location over any particular reflex zone, should also be noted.

The state of the tissue turgor

Both feet should be examined together in order to compare them better. A check is made of the contour of the lower legs, ankles, dorsum of the feet, toes,

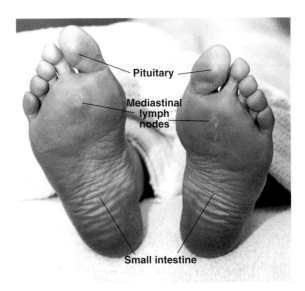

Fig. 4.7 *Fissuring and furrowing over the reflex zones to the small intestine and callus formation over the mediastinal lymph nodes. The reflex zone to the pituitary is prominent*

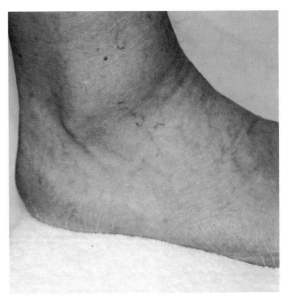

Fig. 4.8 *Fluid retention (not yet pitting oedema) over the cuboid and above the external malleolus*

plantar view, heels and the medial aspect of both feet to see whether or not they are similar, and, if not, where they differ from one another. Areas of irregular puffiness, swelling (Fig. 4.8), oedema or depression are all recorded.

Palpation

Palpation is described as the method of physical examination in which the hands are applied to the surface of the body, so that, by the sense of touch, information is obtained about the condition of the skin, the underlying tissues and organs.

Fingertip palpation is the method in which only the tips of the fingers are used to appreciate the sense of resistance, which varies according to the nature of the underlying tissues, whether air containing, solid or fluid (Butterworth's medical dictionary, 1990). At the initial assessment, the thumb or fingers move millimetre by millimetre over the whole surface of both feet, and by means of fingertip palpation the therapist seeks to determine the state of the underlying tissues and any accompanying changes in skin texture, and to detect any abnormalities of sensation which accompany normal touch.

The movement which is used for palpation is a regular, active intrusion of one or more thumbs or fingers into the tissues (Fig. 4.9). This is immediately followed by a passive extrusion, during which time the therapist observes the way in which the tissues, previously compressed under her fingertips, resurge to resume their normal contour before the next active movement is begun.

To do this, the therapist sits a forearm's distance away from the feet of the patient, whose heels should reach to lie flush with the end of the couch. The correct hand position is that formed when the relaxed hand is rested, palm down, on any flat surface and falls into an unforced position. Whilst the tips of the fingers rest on the flat surface, the thumb is rotated medially and lies to a greater or lesser degree somewhat on its side. As the tips of the fingers and the medial tip of the thumb touch the keys when playing the piano, so in RZT the tips of the fingers and the medial tip of the thumb are used for palpation.

All movement is possible through the action of muscular tissue. As muscles contract they shorten, utilising food and oxygen to do so. As they relax they lengthen again, the metabolites produced as a result of their activity are removed, and food and oxygen stores are replenished. Muscle fibres become fatigued after sustained contractions owing to a build-up of metabolites and oxygen deficit, and are then no longer able to contract. This oxygen debt is relevant to everyone using their muscles in the performance of any activity. For this reason it is valuable for the therapist to learn to use her hands correctly when palpating, and to pay due attention to both the active phase, during which all the muscles of the hand, wrist and forearm contract, and the passive phase, during which all the muscle groups are allowed to relax, permitting the increased demand for food and oxygen of muscular activity to be met. If therapists fail to grasp this principle they are likely to develop muscular cramp or pain at metacarpophalangeal joint 1, the wrist, elbow, shoulder or neck; at the same time the sensitive awareness of the fingertips is jeopardised.

The active phase

In the active phase:

- the shoulders are relaxed
- the arms are held about 10° from the body
- the elbows are loosely bent
- the wrists are straight
- the interphalangeal joint of the thumb does not flex more than 90°
- no joint should be hyperextended (as this weakens them with use over time)
- a wide arc should be present between the thumb and the index finger
- the wrists should not be pronated or supinated, and the working tip of the thumb remains always level with the wrist.

Next, the extended fingers are laid supportively on the dorsum of the foot, without applying any pressure (Fig. 4.10A).

The medial tip of the thumb is applied to the sole of the foot and probes gently into the tissues, keeping

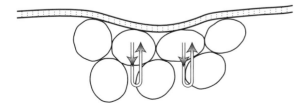

Fig. 4.9 *Normal tissues are displaced downwards and return with elasticity to resume their normal contour on palpation. (The arrows indicate the normal resilience which is felt when the thumb probes into tissue)*

A

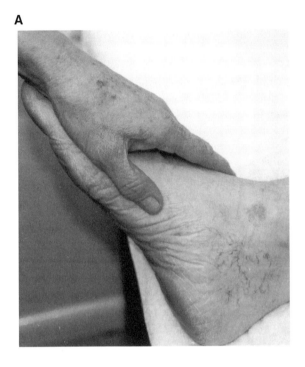

B

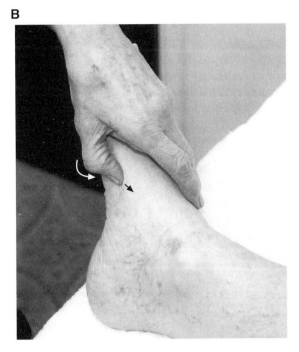

C

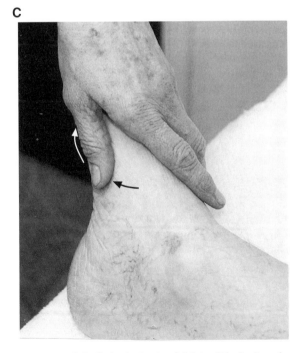

slight flexion in both the base and interphalangeal joints of the thumb (Fig. 4.10B).

As the tissues are probed the following are noted:

- the condition of the skin
- the resistance or flaccidity of the tissues
- any change in normal sensation (discomfort diminished or absent) which is registered by the patient
- any feeling of excess fluid or inelasticity of the tissues
- the evenness or otherwise of the tissues beneath thumb and finger (see p. 69, Fig. 4.12).

The passive phase

Next follows the passive phase (Fig. 4.10C), in which the muscles at the base joint of the thumb relax. Correspondingly the muscles of the forearm relax as the tip of the thumb is gradually retracted from the tissues and comes to lie on the surface of the skin in a resting position, with the wrist straight, the interphalangeal joint slightly flexed and the tip of the thumb lying level with the wrist.

Fig. 4.10 *A Slight flexion in the thumb joint as it begins to probe the tissues in the active phase. **B** Note that the skin is not displaced as the thumb palpates deeper into the tissues. The thumb reaches maximum flexion at 45°. **C** The thumb returns to the resting passive phase*

The 'springiness' (or otherwise) of the tissues is noted as the thumb tip slowly returns to its resting position (see p. 69). It should also be noted whether the tissues are quickly or slowly restored to their normal contour, or whether the retracting thumb leaves behind it a depression.

The therapist should furthermore see whether the tissues are so full that the thumb is almost ejected, or so empty that they offer no resistance and no elastic rebound to the probing thumb.

The passive phase lasts just as long as does the active phase, allowing the muscle fibrils to relax and the blood supply (which has been constricted during muscular contraction) to be restored.

As the medial tip of the thumb is retracted the following are noted:

- the colour of the skin after palpation
- if it is changed, how long it takes before the previous colour returns
- whether the tissues remain indented and, if so, for how long.

If the thumb, forearm, elbow, shoulder or neck of the therapist become painful, either the wrist or the thumb is being held in an incorrect position (which may be pronated, supinated, hyperextended or overflexed) or the passive phase is too short and there is insufficient muscular relaxation. When the thumb is being used for palpation, one should take care that the fingers remain at rest on a surface of the foot and on another plane. Pressure should never be applied to the tissues by fingers and thumbs working in apposition.

The pain nerves of bone are for the most part situated in the periosteum. Any bone lying close to the surface of the body which is accidentally knocked or hit is sharply painful, and there is often a tingling sensation. Any injury, infection, or stretching of periosteum is exquisitely tender, and pressure applied to the periosteum also causes pain. The therapist should avoid any possible confusion between periosteal irritation and a painful reflex zone, and at no time should she probe so deeply over a bony surface that she causes periosteal pain and tingling sensations.

The patient's feet should always be allowed to adopt the position in which they lie most comfortably. Any position into which the therapist puts the feet in which joints are stretched should not last for longer than is necessary to work on a disordered reflex zone.

From the start, the student therapist who is learning the technique should aim to acquire equal competence with left and right thumb and to use them in equal measure during assessment and treatment. Once the therapist achieves the essential skill in recruiting hand, wrist and forearm muscles whilst actively probing — however gently — followed by relaxation of all muscle groups during the passive phase, individual fingers on each hand are introduced, first singly and then working in concert. In time, any one thumb or finger or all together can be used, depending on the size of the therapist's hands, the size of the patient's feet, the area which is to be treated and its requirements.

Whether thumbs or fingers are being used singly or together, the same principles apply:

- during palpation, the position of all joints of the fingers and thumbs is that of slight flexion at all times
- the wrist joint remains straight, and is neither flexed nor extended at any time, while the tip(s) of the working thumbs and fingers are kept at the same level as the wrist (Fig. 4.11A)
- a wide arc is maintained between the thumb and forefinger (see Fig. 4.10A)
- no counter-pressure is applied to the feet by fingers or thumbs which are not being used to give treatment (Fig. 4.11B)
- the periosteum is protected during palpation
- care is taken never to pinch the tissues nor to cause a painful friction erythema on the skin
- the patient's foot may be supported by the other hand, the fingers (if the thumb is used), or the thumb under the metatarsal head (if the fingers are used) (Fig. 4.11C, see also Fig. 6.2, p. 100), and must always be comfortably positioned
- the sequence of therapeutic movements is an active (probing) phase succeeded by a passive (relaxed) phase
- the movement by thumb and fingers is always directed away from the body of the therapist (in other words, the thumb joints move towards the thumbnail, and the nail should not move towards the base of the thumb) (Fig. 4.11D)

A

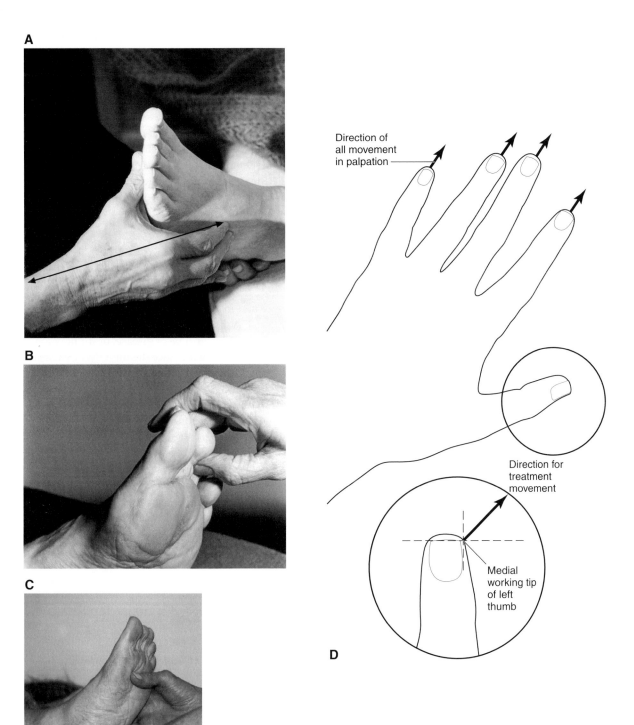

Direction of
all movement
in palpation

B

Direction for
treatment
movement

C

Medial
working tip
of left
thumb

D

Fig. 4.11 *A The tips of the fingers should be kept at the same level as the wrist when one or more fingers are being used. **B** Palpating the plantar aspect of the toes. No pressure should fall onto the foot from the weight of the therapist's hand. **C** Supporting the metatarsal heads with one thumb. **D** The movement by thumb and fingers is always directed away from the body of the therapist*

- this basic movement of thumbs or fingers is used for palpation on any surface of the feet, that is, over the toes, on the plantar and dorsal aspects, the medial and lateral aspects of the heel, and over the lower third of the tibia and fibula.

As she will be making the same movements many times a day, the therapist must be careful not to develop a repetitive strain injury. Rotating the thumb, fingers, wrists or elbows during palpation places a heavy strain on these joints, particularly the interphalangeal and metacarpophalangeal joints of the thumbs. Some people have stronger joint structures than others, and they may be able to use their hands in ways which are not possible for everyone. But all treatment movements should be carried out with the aim of preserving the integrity of the therapist's joints and avoiding any disruption of essential joint structures such as ligaments and tendons. If strain or pain are noticed in the thumbs or fingers, only the basic active/passive movement should be used as, performed properly, palpation carried out in this manner is not detrimental to any system.

Tissue alterations on palpation

The following alterations in tissue tone are commonly felt:

1. Minute particles which feel like sand or grit are distributed thickly or sparsely, evenly or in small aggregations within the tissues (Fig. 4.12A). In a variant of this particulate impression there is a sensation of small bubbles of air distributed throughout the tissues, which produces a 'bouncy' sensation on palpation.
2. A 'knot' with a discrete margin is palpable, and the surrounding tissues usually feel dense (Fig. 4.12B). This indicates an area of muscle spasm, usually found in the spine or abdominal wall, but which may be found in any muscular tissue. In treating such an area the medial tip of the thumb covers the 'knot', then rhythmically flows into and is allowed to retract from the disordered reflex zone. (If the pain in the reflex zone is so severe that palpation is not tolerated,

the medial tip of the thumb is held steadily in the same place in the tissues and over the surface of the 'knot' until the knot and the pain disperse.)
3. The tissues beneath the palpating finger are dense and full (Fig. 4.12C).
4. Excess fluid is felt in the tissues (Fig. 4.12D).
5. A superficial resistance to the palpating finger covers a reflex zone which is perceived to be hollow underneath (Fig. 4.12E)
6. The tissues are perceived to be 'empty' (Fig. 4.12F).

Palpation procedure

All reflex zones have to be palpated in the assessment. Each reflex zone is palpated but once. The touch which is used should be even, flowing and penetrate the tissues only deeply enough to establish whether and in what manner the reflex zones are disordered. A disordered reflex zone reveals nothing of the cause, form or type of disease, or for how long the patient has been ill. Since the underlying cause of the symptoms is as yet unknown, it is wise to use only that sensitive touch which begins to stimulate the regulatory processes of the GRS in the patient and which is sufficient to provide the therapist with the information she needs.

The term 'disordered reflex zone' is used throughout to denote reflex zones in which there is:

- any alteration in the texture of the skin (see Fig. 4.7)
- any change in the tissues, such as altered texture, fluid retention or dehydration (see Figs 4.8, 4.12)
- discomfort
- pain
- diminished sensation
- absence of sensation.

Scale to determine the level of discomfort

The patient is asked to tell the therapist whenever palpation gives rise to discomfort. If this is graduated on a scale of 1–5, a clearer picture of the most painfully disordered reflex zones will emerge.

- at level 1 the discomfort is minor, but palpable
- at level 2 the discomfort is marked
- at level 3 there is pain

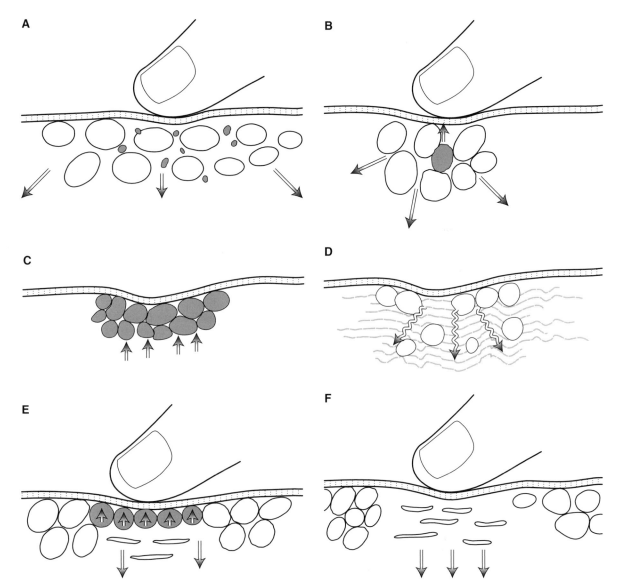

Fig. 4.12 *Alterations in tissue tonus which can be felt on palpation.* **A** *Normal fluid quality of the tissues is lost, becoming gritty to touch.* **B** *A 'knot' offers resistance to palpation, while surrounding normal tissue is displaced downwards.* **C** *Tissues are inelastic and the tone is full. There is resistance to the palpating finger. (In extreme cases the impression is of touching a wooden surface.)* **D** *Boggy, fluid-filled tissues offer little resistance to palpation. Tissues are hollow.* **E** *Penetrating resistance which is superficial reveals flattened, toneless interior, which has lost its resilience.* **F** *Tissues fall away tonelessly and without resistance or resilience to the palpating finger. Elasticity is lost, and indentation in the skin remains*

- at level 4 the pain is severe
- at level 5 the pain is intolerable.

Almost everyone is able to distinguish between these levels but, if the patient is unable to do so, the therapist has to assess the degree of disorder, one important indicator being the ANS responses (see Ch. 6, p. 112) to treatment.

Although the therapist depends initially on the patient's response to palpation as he tells her which zones are painful, the therapist who is experienced will have developed a sensitive and skilful touch which enables her to detect any palpable abnormality within the reflex zones, whether or not the patient is able to describe the sensations he is experiencing in his feet and body. Honing these skills develops confidence in the ability to distinguish between a healthy and a disordered reflex zone which grows with practice. But it should not be forgotten that therapy is a cooperative endeavour between patient and therapist, and what is detected by the therapist on palpation should be verified against the patient's perception of discomfort or pain in any affected reflex zone.

In those who have impaired sensation because they have suffered a stroke, paralysis, diabetes, peripherovascular disease or any of the neuropathies, sensations of discomfort and pain are muted or absent. The therapist should note carefully for future reference and comparison in which areas of the feet sensation is distorted. With small children and some other patient groups who are likewise unable to give verbal feedback, the therapist is reliant on her immediate perceptions during palpation and the ANS reactions.

Although the degree of pain in the reflex zones and the number of zones which are disordered are a valuable indicator of the current state of health or illness of the patient, it must not be assumed that the greater the number of painful reflex zones, or the more intense the pain, the sicker is the person or the worse the likely outcome. Diminished and absent sensation in a reflex zone is in general a more serious indication of advanced generalised disease than is pain.

Reflex zones in which sensation is diminished are graded as follows:

- at level 3 there is diminished sensation
- at level 4 there is marked diminution
- at level 5 sensation is absent.

Order of assessment. The therapist needs to palpate and note the response in each of the reflex zones in a consistent manner. Unless circumstances preclude it, the initial assessment is always done in the same order on the zones of the feet. These are detailed under RZT of the foot (Ch. 8, pp. 137–177), starting with the reflex zones to the head over the toes.

It is recommended that therapists follow the given order for each assessment, starting with the head zones on first one foot then on the other, and assessing each system on both feet before progressing to the next system. Whether the left or right foot is chosen first depends on the history and what the therapist observed during her first inspection of the feet. The foot which bears least evidence of disorder is the best one on which to begin.

In certain circumstances, the recommended order of assessment may need to be varied. For example, if the person coming for treatment has epilepsy, has suffered a stroke or head injury, the pattern given on pages 137–167 should not be followed by the beginner. Instead the therapist should start by assessing the gastrointestinal tract or urinary system and leave the assessment of head zones until the following session when, from what she has found on the feet, she is in a better position to evaluate the response to therapy and any reactions which might occur.

To begin with, the therapist palpates with the thumb of one hand, using left and right hands alternately according to the way in which they rest most comfortably on the feet. With practice, both hands come into play, enabling the therapist to compare subtle changes between the temperature and tissues of left and right feet, as well as to be economical with time. Patients also prefer the two-handed contact as the treatment acquires a rhythm which cannot be attained in the same way when just one thumb or finger is used. Chapter 8 gives details of using both hands for the assessment (p. 167).

If the patient shows any signs of distress or signs of ANS overstimulation which do not respond to harmonising measures (sedating the adrenals and solar plexus, and stroking and holding the feet, see Ch. 6, p. 99) the treatment is brought to an end, and the assessment continued at the following session. An example of such a reaction is shown in Case study 4.1.

Concluding the assessment

The assessment should take no longer than 45 minutes, particularly once the therapist is using both

CASE STUDY 4.1

A 19-year-old university student was experiencing pain in his right hip joint. The pain was sufficient to interfere with walking, had developed over the past 3 months, and he had had to give up all sporting activities. When he came for treatment he gave no history of past illness or injury. Within 2 minutes of starting the assessment, whilst still palpating the reflex zones of the head, his feet began to perspire and he commented that he was starting to feel cold. He was given another blanket, and left to rest for half an hour, by which time he was well enough to leave. On inspection the skin over the thyroid gland was pale and cool, and there were small patches of dry flaky skin over the adrenal reflex. On palpation the reflex zone to the pituitary was markedly painful. These findings suggested that the predominant weakness lay in the endocrine system.

At the second visit the whole of this system was sedated before continuing with the assessment. After 5 minutes, when the reflex zones to the musculoskeletal system had been palpated, he again developed cool and clammy feet. He was given breathing exercises and asked to avoid stimulating foods and drinks.

At the third visit the endocrine system was again sedated, and he was able to tolerate 10 minutes of treatment. Painful reflex zones were found to the appendix, gall bladder and right kidney. He became

somewhat tired for a few days, had a diuresis and lost his appetite.

By the fourth visit the pain in his hip had lessened slightly, palpation to the reflex zones of the endocrine system continued to provoke SNS reactions and all were painful to level 4.

At subsequent visits the endocrine system was repeatedly sedated and, in view of his reactions, the spleen, stomach and kidneys stimulated. He began to visibly relax and breathe more efficiently. After eight sessions he was once again moving freely without pain. All the reflex zones could be palpated without discomfort, and the temperature, colour and texture of the skin on both feet were uniform.

This young man had been studying hard for many hours each day, exercising whenever possible, and eating and drinking mainly convenient 'fast' foods with a high caffeine content. His adrenals, stomach and spleen were visually and palpably depleted on the feet, and he was persistently sympathetically overstimulated because of forthcoming examinations and an inappropriately stimulating diet. His youth, vitality and basic good constitution enabled him to respond quickly to a more sensible way of eating and treatment to counteract the overstimulated adrenal glands.

Seventeen years later he has had no recurrence.

hands simultaneously and able to incorporate the use of all the fingers in treatment. If, for any reason, it is not possible to conclude the assesment of all the systems in this time, either because the patient is frail or because the therapist is still learning, it is better not to overrun the allotted time but rather to complete the examination at the next visit.

As the assessment draws to a close, an increasingly light and effortless touch is used. The strokes used at the end of the assessment should be barely perceptible for either patient or therapist.

The therapist should ensure that the patient is warmly covered afterwards, as patients should feel warm and comfortable after a treatment and this heat is best preserved, thereby allowing neural regulating capacities strengthened from treatment to have their full effect. Also heat is quickly lost in the sick, who

are vulnerable to the cold anyway, partly due to their inactivity and partly as a reaction in the early stages of treatment, when they are more labile.

When the assessment has been completed, the patient's colour, breathing and general position on the couch should be observed.

The patient is then left to rest quietly for 20 minutes — a period which most people come to value greatly. During the rest period there should be as little disturbance and noise as possible around the patient. Meanwhile the therapist makes a note of the following on the record card (see Ch. 3, p. 44):

- the *visual* findings —
  colour and condition of the skin, changes in the skin and nails, bony structure and other tissues
- the *palpable* findings —
  temperature of the feet, any disordered zones,

showing which had heightened and which had diminished or absent senstion, which were painful and to what level — pain in a reflex zone being assessed by the patient on a scale of 1–5

- the *general effect* of the treatment on the patient, and how this has affected his movements and the way in which he lies on the couch
- any *reactions* which have been observed or on which he has commented, principally pallor, cooling of the feet, sweating, dry mouth or changes in respiration.

If it is not possible to complete the assessment, a record should be made of the stage of assessment at which treatment was stopped, and for what reason. At the end of the rest period, the therapist should check the patient's feet again to see whether they are warm and whether there are any further colour changes, or whether those changes which arose as a result of treatment have persisted.

If the feet are cold, the patient should be given a warm footbath. The water should be warm but not too hot, and the patient keeps his feet in the water up to the ankles until they feel thoroughly warmed. Giving a warm footbath ameliorates any severe reactions (which, although they are rare, do appear from time to time). It occasionally happens that after a treatment the patient feels cold when he gets home, but usually warms up satisfactorily if he is able to soak his feet in warm water. Although this is a simple remedy, it should be used before giving sedatives to elderly people or to children, as more often than not it helps them to sleep. Many elderly people do not respond well to drugs and, whilst they may be sedated, this does not mean that they either rest or sleep. The patient will usually comment on the effect of the assessment; if not, the therapist can ask for some feedback.

Before leaving the treatment room the patient should be oriented in time and space, and able to walk or drive safely. On the rare occasions that he is not, he should sit quietly and comfortably under observation until he feels ready to leave. Although disorientation is rare, it can occur — usually if a meal has been missed, as a side-effect of some medicines, or if he is taking several medicines and they are interacting with one another.

Assessment to be made at the second and all subsequent visits

1. The patient should be observed generally when he arrives. In particular a note is made at each visit of any changes in the voice, expression or movement. Changes are most marked in the face, where there may be subtle alterations of colour and texture in the skin. Reflex and other zones of the face mirror from day to day the delicate balance in which all physical and emotional functions are held. Slight daily changes are easily missed and accepted as normal, but as they are recorded on the skin they indicate which systems have reacted to the last treatment.

   The patient should be asked whether his symptoms have improved, worsened, or are the same. It is advisable to check his range of movements if they were limited when he first arrived. He should also be asked whether there have been any reactions to the previous treatments.

   A record needs to be kept of both the patient's assessment of his progress or otherwise and the therapist's evaluation of any improvement in symptoms, bearing and manner, voice, mood, sleep, energy, appetite, bowel and urinary function, etc., as well as any changes in the menstrual cycle for women patients.

2. Once the patient is lying down, the appearance (skin, tissue, tone) and temperature of the feet are compared with observations made at previous visits. Many of the changes which take place are small and subtle, therefore an accurate record to which the therapist can refer is invaluable.

   Changes in the colour and texture of the skin over any of the surfaces of the foot, whether plantar, dorsal, medial or lateral, should be noted.

   There may be more or less obvious changes in skin colour, most notably hues of pink, red, blue, yellow, green, grey or white which become visible over smaller or larger areas.

   Changes in the texture of the skin may be those of increased fragility, hardness, the presence of small white blisters or tiny raised round or irregularly shaped areas, often seen on the medial surface of the heel or on the dorsum of the feet over the metatarsal bones. A note is made of any fissures (see Fig. 4.7, p. 63), particularly the zones over which they begin and those over which they end.

An assessment is needed of any increase or diminution of pain in the affected zones. For example, if the reflex zone to the right kidney was previously graduated at pain level 4, and falls to 2, the change should be noted. Likewise, if the reflex zones to the tonsils have been graded at 2, and at the next visit are perceived as a sharp 4, the change should be shown on the card.

Assessment at the last visit

The therapist needs to note and record changes in colour, temperature and tissues; also a record should be made of those reflex zones which have responded to treatment and are no longer painful, and those which are still abnormal.

References

Anthony C P, Thibodeau G A 1983 Textbook of anatomy and physiology, 11th edn. C V Mosby, St Louis, p 121

Butterworth's medical dictionary 1990, 2nd edn. Butterworth, London

Wilson K J W, Waugh A 1996 Anatomy and physiology in health and illness, 8th edn. Churchill Livingstone, New York, p 111

5

Interpreting assessment and deciding upon treatment

Introduction

Once the assessment has been completed and the observations recorded, the therapist has to interpret his findings and decide how or whether treatment should proceed.

First of all, he must decide whether treatment is fitting, and within his sphere of competence. RZT does not offer a cure for specific illnesses or conditions, but its regulatory and supportive effect on the GRS leads to improved functioning of all systems, giving rise to a sense of ease and relaxation. Inappropriate treatment in any form is ineffective, however, and may even be harmful. So the therapist's first responsibility is to decide whether RZT is a suitable treatment for the person and the presenting condition.

It is important to remember also that RZT assessment is not a diagnostic tool except in the hands of someone who has been trained to make a diagnosis. Doctors, acupuncturists, naturopathic and osteopathic practitioners and physiotherapists are qualified by virtue of their training to make diagnoses within their field of competence. The doctor may require further physical investigations (such as X-rays or blood tests) before he is able to establish a diagnosis. Yet a working hypothesis about which of the patient's organs and structures are malfunctioning can be fashioned by a therapist with skill, knowledge and experience once he has made a careful assessment of the reflex zones. He can undertake to give the patient appropriate treatment and a reasonable appraisal of what can be expected from a course of RZT.

A therapist who is trained and competent develops a reasonable confidence in his capacity and judgement and will not hold out unreasonable hope of improvement to any patient whose illness is unlikely to be ameliorated by the treatment. He is able to truthfully describe reasonable expectations of improvement.

Practitioners who are still students are advised to be in contact with an experienced therapist to whom they can turn for advice whenever puzzled by any aspect of therapy.

Uses and limitations of RZT

Present theory and empirical experience provide for safe and effective practice. Impairment of systemic functions can be assessed, and the therapeutic stimulus which carefully directed treatment imparts to the GRS is strengthening and healing. However, it must be reiterated that a medical diagnosis cannot be made on the feet, except by a doctor.

For example, at assessment painful and disordered reflex zones are found to the stomach. Palpation does not reveal whether the patient is:

- suffering from an infection
- suffering from the side-effects of either prescription or non-prescription medicines
- suffering because the medicines are not taken as prescribed (soluble aspirin being a common offender; it should be dissolved in water before being swallowed, and should not be taken on

an empty stomach) — the times at which medicines are prescribed to be taken, either before or after meals, should be adhered to, otherwise they are likely to cause discomfort and may not act in the expected manner

- digesting an unaccustomedly heavy or spicy meal some hours ago
- eating too fast, or on the move
- not chewing food properly
- taking too much liquid with meals
- producing too much gastric acid
- not producing sufficient vitamin B12.

Therapists rely on their training, experience and professional accountability to help them decide when RZT is appropriate and when it should be withheld.

There are circumstances in which RZT of the feet is unsuitable and should not be used. A capable and experienced practitioner will have learned to recognise these limitations in the early stages of treatment, while the novice should avoid giving treatment where he is unsure of the outcome, when special precautions are necessary, or when there are definite contraindications.

Uses

RZT:

- is not invasive
- can be repeated at regular intervals
- involves no machinery
- can be done in the patient's own home
- has a psychological dimension:
  - there is a one-to-one relationship
  - the same person always gives therapy
  - privacy is assured
  - there is a routine with which the patient becomes familiar (very important to the sick)
  - the patient can unburden herself by talking to a known and attentive therapist before and after each treatment.

RZT is particularly appropriate for the treatment of people suffering with:

- acute or chronic disorders of the locomotor system, including postural disorders
- headaches, including those due to trauma
- sinusitis

- chronic respiratory disease
- stress-related gastrointestinal disorders
- dysmenorrhoea and other disorders of the menstrual cycle
- lethargy and malaise
- lowered resistance to infection
- disturbed sleep patterns.

Whilst all sickness is accompanied by a stress overlay, unrelieved stress on its own can, and does, contribute to the development of many illnesses (see Ch. 2, p. 28). Stressed people respond well to RZT, the effect of which is not limited to the body alone, its calming effects extending to both mind and emotions. The common manifestations of stress include anxiety, affective depression, fatigue, poor sleep or concentration, and muscular tension, which may seat itself in the jaw, neck, shoulder girdle, knees or indeed anywhere in the body. Stress is an inevitable and necessary part of many inbuilt physiological responses on which life depends, but it becomes damaging to the person when impossible physical, mental or emotional demands are imposed, either by the person herself or by others. It is a common observation that more people are sick because they are unhappy than unhappy because they are sick.

Doctors familiar with RZT find it a useful additional technique for clarifying a diagnosis. It is difficult to palpate the taut, drum-like abdominal musculature when there is an acute infection in the abdomen. The pain and ANS reactions which are provoked by touching the reflex zone to an acutely infected organ aids the differential diagnosis between, for example, a ruptured appendix and an ectopic pregnancy. Similarly, assessment of the reflex zones in a person presenting with severe backache can distinguish pain emanating from a kidney, from that coming from an ovary, the small intestine or muscular spasm.

Patients often complain at assessment of generalised abdominal discomfort without being able to pinpoint any other specific symptoms. After two or three treatments, it is usual for the pain to localise to the epigastrium, hypochondrium or iliac fossa on one side or another, becoming at the same time more focused, and suggesting the diagnosis of, for example, an inguinal hernia.

Limitations of RZT

RZT is at times:

- inappropriate
- to be given with caution
- contraindicated.

Circumstances in which RZT is inappropriate

These include the following situations.

1. When it does not prove beneficial.
2. When privacy for the patient needs to be assured unless first aid is being given, and is best performed without an audience.
3. When there is no reasonable expectation of benefit for the patient.
4. When the patient, or the family, have unrealistic expectations of the therapy or the therapist.
5. When recovery is not complete, but a plateau of partial recovery has been reached and is maintained, then it is inappropriate to continue. Further sessions can be arranged subsequently to maintain the plateau, to treat any new condition, or to counteract times of high stress.
6. Certain peoples have cultural restrictions on who may or may not touch whom, and at which times. Caste, religion and custom govern what is permitted or disallowed. Peoples will generally seek treatment within their own cultural communities, but in cross-cultural encounters the therapist should always enquire of his patient what her customs dictate.
7. During the flare-up of any chronic disease (such as rheumatoid arthritis) first aid can be given by sedating the reflex zones to the solar plexus and adrenals (see Ch. 6, p. 98), but no stimulating treatment of any kind should be given. When the acute attack is over, an assessment can be made and treatment started or continued.
8. When RZT provokes an attack of biliary colic on two successive occasions in a patient who has gall stones. No further treatment should be given.

Circumstances when precautions should be taken

Certain precautions are necessary when treating people with the following conditions.

1. *Any illness whose course is labile and unpredictable.* When starting treatment, more especially on a child, a responsible adult or companion should be present to monitor any change in the patient's condition, at least during and after the first few sessions. If no such person is available, it is advisable to postpone treatment until suitable care arrangements can be made. For example, a young child or elderly person who is an unstable diabetic should be supervised by a responsible adult after treatment.
2. *Epilepsy.* Individual responses to epilepsy are many and varied. Some children and adults will, in the early stages of treatment, have a fit during or shortly after each treatment. This does not mean that RZT is contraindicated. If the intervals between each fit grow longer, and if each fit lasts for a shorter time and is less intense, RZT is appropriate and should be continued. If there is no change in intensity or duration after six to eight sessions, RZT should be discontinued. The patient should carry her usual medicines with her, and the therapist should have the means within reach to maintain a clear airway.
3. *Diabetes mellitus.* As the incidence of this condition is growing and the onset insidious, it is not uncommon for patients seeking treatment to have as yet unrecognised diabetes. The classical symptoms of thirst, polyuria, polydipsia and nocturia, unexplained weight loss, pruritus and increased susceptibility to infection, especially in someone over the age of 60, should raise the therapist's index of suspicion.

    All diabetics must check their blood sugar and/or glycosuria before treatment begins. As mild hypoglycaemia lasting 24–48 hours is a fairly common reaction, the patient should carry extra carbohydrate on her person for 48 hours after each session. Blood sugar and urine should be tested regularly, since the need for insulin and other drugs is often reduced as treatment progresses. This should be carefully monitored.
4. *Arthritis.* When osteoarthritis of the hip, knee, shoulder or spine is advanced, RZT is useful in so far as it relieves pain, strengthens the GRS, stimulates the circulation, venous and lymphatic drainage in those whose mobility is reduced and encourages proper full use of the lungs. It is

therefore beneficial before surgery for joint replacement, but it cannot repair already damaged joints and their linings.

5. *Shoulder pain*. There are a variety of causes for pain in the shoulder joints. Those arising when pain is referred as a result of dysfunction in an organ such as the liver, gall bladder or small intestine respond well to RZT. Those due to trauma or a mechanical defect of the joint or any of its components do not. A common injury is a tear of the rotator cuff group of muscles of the shoulder joint. RZT is inappropriate in this instance, and surgery is the only guarantee of repair. When treating someone with a painful shoulder joint which does not respond after four sessions, the advice and help of a physiotherapist or orthopaedic surgeon should be sought.

6. *Tuberculosis*. This rapidly debilitating, notifiable disease is considered to be the most important communicable disease in the world. While it may involve any organ, the lungs are most commonly the first to become affected. The individual drug regime must be adhered to for the 1–2 years for which it is prescribed. RZT can be given, with care, once the acute infective phase is over, starting with very short sessions and slow measured palpation. Treatment is directed at strengthening all systems.

Contraindications

RZT is contraindicated in the following situations:

- when the patient does not wish to have RZT
- when the treatment of the patient's illness is beyond your scope of practice.

As an example of the latter, a person seeks treatment for an apparently minor complaint, but fear causes her to withhold mentioning those signs and symptoms which affect her most acutely. If, from careful history taking allied to observation and findings on assessment, you suspect that she has a serious illness, she should be referred for the medical or specialist care which is necessary.

Or you may be asked to give treatment to someone who complains of a physical problem, and may indeed have one, but who is found more urgently to be suffering from a psychiatric

disturbance. Unless this is your field of expertise she should also be referred for the specialist help which is needed.

Treatment should not be given by a therapist who is overtired or ill. Rest and receiving treatment are more appropriate to his situation than is the giving of RZT, and therapists must follow the same advice they give their patients.

A number of specific medical conditions are also contraindications for RZT. They include the following.

Hyperpyrexia. RZT should not be given to anyone whose temperature is raised above 39°C. If it is suspected that a child's temperature is elevated, a thermometer can be used to check it before starting the session. A raised temperature is a sign of a raised basal metabolic rate (BMR). Since one effect of treatment is to increase the BMR, the effect would be to raise the temperature even higher. Calming stroking movements may be made if they are comforting, and first aid in the form of gentle, sustained pressure to a particular zone (such as the tonsils or the middle ear) to relieve pain may be attempted. Patients with high temperatures are best kept at rest in bed, and given sufficient fluids, especially water. If desired some light food such as diluted vegetable soups, fruit and steamed or lightly boiled vegetables will not increase the load on the alimentary tract, liver, kidneys or endocrine system.

Deep vein thrombosis. Anyone who has had a deep vein thrombosis in the past 6 months is not a candidate for RZT. The local venous return is stimulated during treatment and this increased circulation may be sufficient to dislodge small or micro emboli in the veins of the calf, with potentially fatal consequences.

Once the blood-clotting picture has been restored to normal, with or without the use of blood-thinning agents, RZT is safe to use as a treatment. Neither is it contraindicated to treat someone who has had a recent coronary or other thrombosis, but the first session should be short and only gentle pressure should be used initially. The therapist can increase the amount of time spent at each treatment noting whether the patient is able to tolerate and benefit from each session.

People who are receiving warfarin or other blood-thinning agents may be given RZT, but it should be remembered that they often bleed easily from capillary or corpuscular fragility, at least in the early stages, and a very light touch is required on the hands, feet or back (whichever is being treated).

Acute fevers and infectious diseases. In acute tonsillitis, otitis media, appendicitis, glandular fever or similar conditions in which there is a high temperature, treatment is contraindicated, and will not influence the course of the illness.

Treating someone with an infectious disease in a private practice brings with it the necessities of disinfection and the need to exclude all chances of cross-infection to other patients; it is probably best avoided where possible. Symptomatic treatment may be given to relieve any local pain, itchiness, restlessness, etc. once the disease has passed its peak.

Local disorder or inflammation of the venous system. No treatment should be given over the area of varicose veins of the feet and lower legs. The attendant thinning of venous walls causes the skin and tissues to be friable and liable to break down. If there is an area of broken-down skin, the lesion plus a wide margin are to be avoided. The therapist should treat only those areas where the skin and underlying tissues are intact, and local pressure will not cause further tissue deterioration. If there are any signs of inflammation (classically redness, heat, swelling or pain) any treatment involving local pressure on the feet, back or hands must be avoided until all signs of inflammation have disappeared.

Local or generalised inflammation of the lymphatic system. If there are signs of inflammation of the lymphatic system in the feet or legs, or if the glands behind the knees, in the groin or under the armpits are swollen, RZT is contraindicated. Since one of the effects of treatment is to bring about an increase in the local venous and lymphatic return, the mechanical pressure on already overloaded and inflamed fluid-filled vessels will be detrimental.

Cellulitis of the feet or legs. When there is local infection of the interstitial cells, usually as a result of a break in the skin and subsequent bacterial invasion, the tissues swell and are painful to touch. The skin is shiny and becomes thinned with increased swelling. This condition is aggravated by RZT, and it is therefore contraindicated.

If there is a wound it should be kept clean, and the foot kept elevated and at rest.

Surgical emergencies. Any life-threatening situation needs immediate medical care. The diagnosis of a ruptured appendix, ectopic pregnancy, or a subphrenic abscess can be made only by a doctor. Anyone who is visibly collapsing and ill, or who has a fracture, large wound, burns or any other such emergency needs treatment in hospital.

Medical emergencies. These need the same immediate care.

Malignant melanoma. Any mole or darkening area of skin (usually on a surface intermittently exposed to sunlight) which changes in size, shape or colour, becomes inflamed, bleeds or forms a crust, undergoes sensory change or has a diameter larger than 7 mm should be properly investigated and treated before RZT is given. Other suspicious features are an irregular border or colour, asymmetric shape, or elevation of the surface. Since the incidence is rising rapidly and, once beyond a certain stage of development, the spread is so wide and swift and the prognosis so poor, it is considered wiser not to start RZT or any other physical treatment until a diagnosis has been established. If the patient wishes and the doctor sanctions it, RZT may be given postoperatively or during convalescence, but the usual monitoring mechanisms must be in place.

Psychoses. People with complex pyschological disturbances need to be in the care and supervision of appropriately trained medical personnel. Treatment can be given for physical complaints such as, for example, backache, and should be given as part of the all-round care, with responses carefully monitored.

RZT can neither palliate nor relieve any truly psychotic state.

Fainting. This is rare but always significant. If the patient complains of dizziness, blurring or darkening of vision, or feels faint (usually within the first 2 minutes of the session), the feet should be held quietly and the therapist should wait for a few minutes before proceeding. A note should be made of the reflex zone which has responded so sensitively, and therapy resumed at a point and system distant from that which gave so marked a response.

If the sensations recede, the session is continued. If there is another attack of giddiness the session should be brought to a close, with a few stroking movements if they are tolerated. Otherwise the therapist should stop straight away, and the patient reassured and asked whether she knows what may have been the cause, whether she often feels faint, or whether she has a complaint in the corresponding area.

Fainting may occur when a reflex zone which corresponds to a congenital abnormality is palpated. This is not a bar to further treatment, but palpating that reflex zone will probably always provoke the same response. If a normal treatment can be given but avoiding that part of the foot, and if there are no other adverse reactions, there is no contraindication to completing the series of treatments. (Case study 5.1 is an example of this situation.)

Another cause of fainting may be past or present heavy use of or dependence on mood-altering drugs, and it may be appropriate to ask if the patient has taken any substances recently or in the past. If so, the therapist may get the same response even if he moves to treat another part of the foot. In this case RZT is unlikely to be helpful, and if the patient becomes giddy whichever reflex zone is palpated, another therapy should be chosen.

Not everyone who is taking or has taken addictive substances reacts in this way, however. If there are no adverse reactions a normal course of RZT can be given.

Depressed immune system. RZT has no effect on an immune system so depressed that it is unable to respond to any stimulus. All the harmonising and stroking movements are beneficial, but treatment should not be attempted.

During pregnancy. The following situations are particularly to be avoided:

1. *Pregnancies which are unstable or at risk.* The first 3 months are the period of greatest instability in any pregnancy. If the woman has had a previous miscarriage or miscarriages, has a Shirodkhar suture, or has had an episode of bleeding or lower abdominal pain, she should be treated only by a midwife who is experienced in the use of RZT. Whatever treatment is given at this stage will be designed to calm and relax the woman. As pregnancy is a time of intense hormonal activity, any inadvertent stimulation of the endocrine system should be avoided.
2. *Placenta praevia.* Here, instead of the placenta occupying the fundus of the uterus, it lies over

---

CASE STUDY 5.1

Having had a difficult labour, Mrs A. came for RZT as she was lethargic and not sleeping well. At the first visit an assessment of the reflex zones of her feet was carried out. Soon after commencing the session, whilst still assessing the reflex zone to the ears, Mrs A. complained that the room was beginning to spin around, and she became very pale. Palpation was immediately stopped, and her feet, which had become very cold, were quietly held under the blanket. She was reassured and asked about any past infection or trauma to her ears (the reflex zone to the left ear had been responsible for the reaction). She disclosed that she had a congenital deficiency of the pinna of her left ear (which was hidden from view by her long hairstyle). When she felt less dizzy and her feet were warmer, it was possible to continue treating her and to complete the assessment. The remaining 11 sessions covered all areas of her feet except for the reflex zone to the left ear. Two further attempts to palpate this reflex zone gave rise to a similar reaction and it was therefore omitted in all further treatments. By the time the course was completed she was sleeping well again, had enough energy to see her through the demands of the day, and the ailments of which she had not complained (cystitis and persistent lochia) had resolved.

the cervix and the baby must be delivered by Caesarean section, usually before term. RZT is contraindicated.

3. *Antepartum haemorrhage.* Bleeding before the baby is due to be born is an obstetric emergency. The mother should be put quietly to bed and remain there while the midwife is sent for.

4. *Postpartum haemorrhage.* Haemorrhage after the birth of a baby is likewise an obstetric emergency. The mother needs quiet bed rest and an unruffled presence while waiting for the midwife if she is not already there.

(Pregnancy is more fully discussed in Chapter 12.)

Local abnormalities of the feet

Abnormalities of shape or structure

The purpose of assessment is to discover any disordered or painful reflex zones reflecting systemic disorder in the feet, hands or back. The therapist must be able to distinguish between local trauma or inflammation in the area over which she is working and disordered reflex zones which mirror organic disease. Both are painful on palpation.

Local disorders on the foot can and do reflect changes taking place in other parts of the body. However, treatment is contraindicated in certain local inflammatory conditions. No treatment should be given over or near any inflamed area. General healing times for injuries to joints and tendons are known. When a joint which is not subject to undue strain becomes persistently weak, painful, or both, the therapist should question whether this pain or weakness is being referred from an internal organ. RZT is an appropriate treatment in such instances.

The following abnormalities of the feet are commonly seen.

Structural abnormalities

Hallux valgus. Here there is a fixed displacement of the big toe toward the other toes. The mtp joint enlarges and becomes painful. The joint may become inflamed, and is then red and pain is exacerbated.

Painting the enlarged joint daily with tincture of iodine is a simple and effective naturopathic remedy. The iodine should be applied every 24 hours for as long as the iodine is absorbed within that time, and may be continued for 8–12 months.

If, when the joint comes to be painted, it is still discoloured then no further applications are necessary. Pain is relieved to a greater or lesser degree, and further joint enlargement may be prevented.

Hallux rigidus. Here there is loss of movement at the mtp joint of the big toe, which loses its normal joint flexion and causes pain on walking.

Exostosis. This bony outgrowth on the surface of the bone is commonly seen in rheumatoid arthritis and is, in general, painful. Many exostoses may develop.

Calcaneal spur. Here a spur-shaped bony outgrowth develops as a result of continual overstrain of the plantar fascia. It is usually seen on the plantar aspect of the calcaneum of the foot. It may cause pain on walking which can become severe and so inhibit mobility.

Dropped metatarsal heads. This condition commonly affects the second and third metatarsal heads and gives rise to pain on walking at the moment when weight is transferred from the heel to the metatarsal heads.

Clubbed foot. This congenital abnormality (now rarely seen in the West, although a mild uncorrected form is sometimes seen in older people) is an alteration in the size, structure and arrangement of the tarsal bones, which become displaced.

Fallen arches. Undue strain on or laxity of the ligaments supporting the arch of the foot combined with gravitational pull and the loss of support cause the navicular and talus bones to collapse groundward. The longitudinal arch of the foot (see Fig. 4.2A, p. 58) is lost, walking becomes arduous, and sooner or later most people with fallen arches complain of low backache.

If the fallen arches are congenital, good foot exercises started early in childhood are helpful. In order to gain and maintain the necessary muscle tone to support the arches, the exercises need to be practised daily. Should the arches give way in adult life a physiotherapist or osteopathic practitioner is able to prescribe appropriate remedial exercises. An orthotist or podiatrist can prescribe supports to wear inside the shoes.

Whilst not being curative, RZT can help to improve the muscle tone of the feet, and to relieve the associated backache. The musculature of the abdomen is frequently concomitantly weakened, either as a result of the altered posture and consequent abnormal strain borne by the muscles inserted into the lower spine, or as a result of childbearing, surgery or carrying heavy loads. Treatment of the reflex zones to these muscles is given to either reduce raised muscle tone or to restore muscles which have become lax.

Inflammation

Inflammation of a tendon sheath. This is usually seen in the plantar tendons, and presents as tenosynovitis. Walking is painful, and heat and pain are felt (usually along a traceable and direct pathway) in the feet, even at rest. The inflammation may take about 8 weeks to resolve, and treatment around the inflamed tendon should be avoided during this time.

Athritic changes. Here the periarticular tissue and synovial membranes of small joints become swollen. The (mainly peripheral) joints are painful at rest as well as in activity, and show classical flexion deformities.

RZT should not be given during a 'flare-up' and, as the feet are usually very painful, they should be held and treated gently at all times. The therapist should not flex or extend any joint beyond its range of movement, however limited this is.

Gout. In this condition there is acute pain and swelling in the mtp joint of the big toe. Men over the age of 40 years are more commonly affected than are women, but it may occur at an earlier age, and there is a familial tendency. In an acute phase the joint becomes hot, red and tender, the pain can be excruciating, and pyrexia is usual. RZT is inappropriate at this time. As the pain subsides the skin over the joint becomes scaly and itchy. The disease may continue into a chronic form (though this is now rarely seen in the West) in which case the joint becomes deformed, stiff and constantly painful. Tophi, which are chalky white urate deposits, may form in the tissues around the joint (and may also be found in ear cartilage). Once the patient is over the acute phase, treatment may be initiated. Attention should be paid to all disordered reflex zones, which always include the metabolic and excretory systems.

Pseudogout closely resembles attacks of true gout, but in this condition calcium pyrophosphate is deposited in the joint tissues, and there is no generalised metabolic disturbance.

Oedema

There are many possible causes of oedema, some common and some rare. Gravitational pull is constantly exerted on the body, whether sitting, standing or walking. Any excess fluid which accumulates in the body is subjected to this force, and is usually first noticed in the feet and ankles, particularly after being upright for an extended period.

Common causes of oedema include the following.

1. *A rise in venous hydrostatic pressure.* This causes fluid to leak out from the blood vessels into the surrounding tissue spaces. Failing heart or kidney function usually has this effect, but it is not seen in all such circumstances.
2. *Drugs.* It may be a side-effect of some drugs, principally cortisone, some hypotensive agents and oral contraceptives with a high oestrogen content.
3. *Premenstrual pelvic congestion.* This is followed by a physiological diuresis once menstruation begins, and is a common and normal phenomenon. Usually there is tissue swelling in the area below and around the internal and external malleoli for a few days before menstruation. This swelling subsides as soon as the diuresis begins.
4. *Pregnancy.* Small amounts of water retention are normal. Abnormal water retention demands investigation.

5. *Nutritional deficiencies*. Thiamine and protein lack are the commonest form and kwashiorkor is the most severe form.
6. *Obstruction to the lymphatic system*. This may be congenital, as in Millroy's disease, or result from trauma, radiation or surgery.
7. *Infection from tropical parasites*. These may progress to the liver where they form cysts and later ascites.
8. *Flying*. This may cause immobility for long periods with the legs in a cramped position.

EXAMPLE 5.1

The feet of an elderly woman who came for treatment for her varicose veins were well shaped and cared for. The only visual abnormality was a corn over the left medial proximal phalangeal joint space of the fourth toe. Despite the methodical and routine care of a chiropodist, the corn had returned regularly to the same place over a period of 40 years, corresponding to the reflex zone of tooth 36. This tooth relates to the venous system (see Ch. 11).

Skin disorders

Skin disorders can be persistent, and if so, they indicate a weakness in the underlying reflex zone or the corresponding body zone. Mechanical irritation from shoes which do not fit well is best avoided. The skin responds to regular attention, and washing, soaping, scrubbing, the use of a pumice stone or loofah, and visits to a chiropodist are recommended. A pumice stone should be used only on dry skin as it is ineffective on damp tissues.

Corns

These most often occur over the toes and may be hard or soft. If they recur over the same place despite well-fitting shoes and good foot care they signify weakness in a related system (see Example 5.1).

Callus formation

This occurs most commonly around the outer rim of the foot and over the mtp joint line. It is noteworthy that in the West women have many more callosities on their feet than do men.

People admitted in emergency to intensive care units often have healthy skin on their feet. Within a short while (7–10 days) most have developed callus on the heels. The injury, immobility and effect of medicines on the GRS are here reflected in the liver and lymphatic system. Deep, painful cracks developing over the heels which fail to respond to creams and general footcare indicate that the liver function is becoming impaired, owing to the demands being laid on that organ, involvement of the lymphatic system soon follows, and this is readily seen over the pelvic reflex areas.

It is always worthwhile to examine the feet of bedfast patients regularly as they are likely to develop bedsores. Fullness of the tissues over the internal and external malleoli and the medial and lateral aspects of the heels becomes apparent whenever the lymphatic system is weakened, and the reflex zones are painful. Treatment of these areas (as well as regular turning and all other preventative measures) has the effect of strengthening the skin and underlying tissues in related areas.

Warts and veruccae

Verruccae are caused by a virus. They are best treated by a chiropodist. They can be painful and it is not advisable to work directly over any such infected area. The therapist should avoid treating the surrounding tissue if it is painful.

Eczema, dermatitis and psoriasis

As before, the areas where the skin breaks down are significant. Careful palpation around these areas, and not over them, allied to a careful history, should indicate which reflex zones of the feet need treatment.

Fungal infections

The most common sites of infection are the webs between the toes. 'Athlete's foot' between the toes is painful and frequently becomes bacterially infected. Infection is often long standing and resistant to treatment. As these areas on the feet mirror lymphatic drainage of the head and neck such infections are common in those with chronic throat infections.

Treatment is directed toward encouraging a good blood supply to the surrounding areas while avoiding any areas where the skin is broken, too painful, or has fungoid growth. The blood supply to the webs between the toes can be improved by the fingers directing small sweeping movements of the skin and subcutaneous tissues toward the infected webs. If the affected area is small and the surrounding skin appears healthy, treatment may be given to the unaffected areas. The areas should heal after a few sessions. Soaking the feet for 5 minutes twice a day in a warm footbath, adding either a tablespoon of cider vinegar to a pint of warm water, or the recommended dosage of an antifungal shampoo to a bowl of warm water is suggested.

If more than a third of the surface of the skin is affected by fungus, the effects of RZT will be limited, and it may be preferable and more effective to work on the hands or the back (or to choose another therapy).

Ingrown toenails

The nails of the big toe are those most commonly affected in this painful condition. RZT can be given on the big toe provided that palpation is not too painful. The thumb on the same side of the body should also be treated (see cross/reciprocal reflexes in Ch. 7). The services of a good chiropodist should be sought.

Varicosities

Touch and treatment which is light can be given around the area of delicate and friable skin. The patient should be encouraged to elevate the feet above the level of the hips (taking care to avoid drawing the thighs up to the trunk at an acute angle, which further obstructs the venous return) for at least 10 minutes twice a day to encourage passive venous drainage. The remaining patency of the valves is thus spared as the overload in the veins is reduced.

Support stockings should be put on while still in bed, before putting the feet to the ground, otherwise the veins will already have become distended and engorged. If the stockings are taken off for any reason during the day, the feet should always be elevated before putting them on again.

Ulcers

Anyone who has developed an ulcer of the leg (of which the causes may be numerous) should have their care supervised by their general practitioner. For varicose ulcers a radical change of nutrition with adequate rest is the treatment of choice. RZT assists the venous and lymphatic return but is not adequate to heal a varicose ulcer on its own.

Excessive sweating of the feet

This is associated with unrelieved adrenal sympathetic overstimulation.

Burns

All burns, small and large, heal best if they are kept scrupulously clean. If the area is large, the foot should be kept elevated and at rest. As well as any prescribed care, RZT can be given to reciprocal zones on the other foot and the hand on the same side until the wound has healed. Once a healthy skin has formed the therapist should treat the scar tissue and resume treatment as normal.

Gangrene

The only treatment for gangrene is surgery.

Sudeck's atrophy of the feet

This rare and extremely painful condition looks very like gangrene, except that the skin and underlying tissues are white. It is usually seen on either the hands or the feet, and may follow a penetrating injury, a fractured olecranon process or the application of a plaster cast. Sudeck's atrophy is difficult to treat by any method.

Deciding on treatment when there is more than one complaint

When a patient seeking treatment has numerous complaints, of which one (such as hernia) requires operative treatment, and another, such as headache, is amenable to therapy, the limitations of RZT with regards to the hernia should be discussed at the first visit. Although treatment is a vital exchange between the therapist and the patient, and is influenced at each visit by any visual or palpable changes in the reflex zones, the therapist has to decide which link in the chain of illness should be treated first.

Healing always follows the same pattern during a course of RZT. Recent and minor ailments are the first to improve, whether or not these ailments give rise to reactions. This is followed by a functional improvement in one or more of those systems in which there had been functional deterioration. Finally, providing that disease has not overwhelmed the capacity of the GRS to respond fully (see Ch. 2, p. 26), the system which is or has been most weakened is strengthened. This is rarely accomplished without one or more reactions, whose purpose is to reduce the acid overload of tissues.

The gastrointestinal tract is the body's first line of defence against harmful or improper foods, which it seeks to eliminate as soon as possible. When the defences of the lymph nodes which are so abundantly provided in the gut lining are overcome, substances which would not normally be absorbed filter through the absorptive mucous membranes and are carried to the liver for detoxification.

The liver is the 'body's master chemist, also the fuel storage and supply office, housekeeper and poison control centre' (Miller & Goode 1961). Its astonishing powers of regeneration make it almost immortal. As well as its own functions it now has to take over those of the lymphatics of the intestinal lining, and limit the damage arising from the harmful substances which have been absorbed. Many complex metabolic processes are involved but, provided the kidneys are functioning well, an intact liver function maintains the pH of circulating blood at its optimal level of 7.4.

When liver function is impaired, acidosis results. This leads to overstimulation of first the adrenal glands and then the whole endocrine system. The blood reservoir of the spleen, in which is also stored a large number of red blood corpuscles, contracts rhythmically about twice a minute, releasing small quantities of its reserve blood into the circulation. Heat, physical exertion and strong emotional excitement increase the demand for oxygen, and the spleen responds by increased rhythmical contraction.

This pattern of disorder is found repeatedly on the feet, and treatment is directed at the whole complex. The integrity of the intestinal defences must be restored, the liver must be relieved of any unnecessary metabolic challenges and the already overstimulated adrenals must not be aroused any further. Until the spleen is able to build up its reserves once more, the immune system and essential reservoir remain depleted.

Case study 5.2 shows how RZT can yoke the recuperative energies.

Procedure for deciding on treatment

1. Studying the record card

First of all, before starting treatment, the therapist should study the record card and decide which reflex zones are the most disordered — that is, either uncomfortable, painful, or where sensation is diminished or absent. More than one sensation may be present in any reflex zone. For example, in the uterus both pelvic inflammatory disease and loss of muscle tone may coexist. The absent, diminished or heightened sensation which is felt by someone who receives RZT gives an indication of the cause of the ailment (see points 4 and 5 below).

A note is made of the visual changes to skin, bony structure and tissues. One or more systems, such as the gastrointestinal tract or the urinary system, may be the most visually and palpably abnormal. Or it may be that the disorders, visual and palpable, are concentrated in (for example) the right shoulder, the neck and the small intestine.

CASE STUDY 5.2

A 15-year-old boy had been born with meningitis and hydrocephalus, was diagnosed as having chronic hydrocephalus and he had a severe kyphoscoliosis. A shunt was in situ. Six months previously he had been playing football, but recently his condition had deteriorated, and he presented as a tetraplegia. Investigations showed a narrowing of the cervical cord and no subarachnoid layer.

The boy was very depressed, had difficulty maintaining a sitting balance, suffered with chronic constipation and had no appetite. The physiotherapist decided to treat him with RZT. At assessment he was able to tolerate only 15 minutes of palpation on the feet, which showed pain over the ascending colon and spine.

At the second visit the pain in the ascending colon and spine reflex zones had increased, and these were treated; only 15 minutes treatment time was tolerated.

At the third visit painful reflex zones to the spine, ascending colon, ileocaecal valve and the whole of the digestive tract were noted, also the shoulder girdle, which was worse on the right than the left; only 15 minutes of treatment were tolerated. After this session the boy had his bowels opened and vomited on two consecutive days.

Over the fourth and fifth sessions he developed urinary retention, and the feet became very hot and dry. The spine, especially the cervical spine on the left foot, and the stomach on the right were painful, along with tenderness over both heels. He complained of neck pain.

During the sixth treatment the right foot was cold and the left foot very hot; the patient complained of severe abdominal pain and he remained very depressed. The spine and digestive system were highly sensitive to touch, and only a short treatment was tolerated. The patient's mother had meanwhile noticed that 'his back was stronger, and his sitting posture had greatly improved'.

At the seventh treatment both feet were warm; however, there was acute pain over reflex zones to the left kidney, pancreas and duodenum, and the lad withdrew his feet. Harmonising grips were used. Later that day the patient's mother reported a remarkable change; her son was very happy, joking, and the happiest she had seen him in a long time. He began to pass urine normally, and catheterisation was avoided. An improved sitting posture was maintained, and his appetite returned.

2. Deciding on primary treatment areas

The therapist should then decide which are the primary areas most in need of treatment (stages 4–5). Then the secondarily disordered zones (stages 2–3) and finally zones showing mild discomfort (1–2) are noted; they usually require less treatment and reflect recent or less established disorder.

3. Changes in primary treatment areas

The areas of the feet needing treatment alter as therapy progresses. Those which remain painful or become more so need to be treated at each session, and any system which reacts to RZT must also be included in treatment at the next session. Any such reflex zones will be sensitive during the reactive phase, even if they were not at assessment (see Ch. 6, p. 111 for reactions). The therapist often sees a process of an 'unfolding' of past illness, generally through reactions, during a course of treatment.

4. Dysfunctional reflex zones

Discomfort or pain in the reflex zones reflects dysfunction. The sensation may be heightened owing to: injury; present, recent or past unresolved infection; irritation or allergy. The patient commonly describes prickling, heat, pain, needling or a burning sensation in these reflex zones. They are frequently described when treating conditions such as chronic tonsillar, dental and sinus inflammations over the head zones.

A dull, spreading and aching sensation reflects muscle spasm.

A dull, contained sensation, often described as stony, is found in depleted endocrine glands.

Examples of the above include the following.

Injury

Injury is reflected in the corresponding zone within 1 minute.

Tiredness

A mother who has sat up all night with a sick child will have more discomfort on palpation than if she has had a restful sleep.

Strain

A person who has spent many hours looking at a VDU screen is more likely to have painful reflex zones to the eyes than if she had less eyestrain before her visit.

Infection

If a throat infection is developing, the reflex zones to the throat area are likely to become painful 3 or 4 days before the patient is aware of any infection. Thus prodromal stages of illness can often be detected in the feet.

Past trauma

The reflex zone to an old injury which has healed imperfectly may be painful to touch for decades after the event.

Surgery

The same is true for past surgery.

Constitutional weakness

Many people have an inherent weakness of one system or another (e.g. stomach, bladder or lungs), and this is reflected in the reflex zones, either in small visual changes or in a slightly heightened sensitivity to touch.

Disease which is developing

A person may say and feel that she is fit and well, yet there are evidently painful reflex zones on the feet. For example, painful reflex zones are often found to the prostate gland in men of middle age, without their having any symptoms of frequency or nocturia. Similarly, painful reflex zones to the uterus may be found in young women who do not complain of gynaecological problems. Painful reflex zones to the gall bladder are found in young adults of both sexes, although they do not always complain of fat intolerance.

5. Factors that influence sensation in reflex zones

When the therapist has completed an assessment on a patient, and the findings in terms of discomfort and response are at variance with the history, the symptoms and his own observation, he should consider whether one of the following causes may be responsible for the variation.

Diminished or absent sensation

Diminished or *absent* sensation in the reflex zones is usually evidence of degeneration, exhaustion (which may be systemic or general), or regulatory blockade in the GRS. Sensitivity in the reflex zones may be impaired, and is usually diminished, by one (or more) of the following:

- drugs — these may be medically prescribed, principally: hypnotics and narcotics (to induce sleep), hypotensive agents (to reduce blood pressure), especially beta blockers, drugs to relieve pain, steroids, hormone replacement therapy, tranquillisers, chemotherapy; or non-prescription drugs, particularly heroin, cocaine, LSD, and their like, alcohol, or any mood-changing drugs
- radiotherapy
- peripherovascular disease such as arteriosclerosis, diabetes, Buerger's or Raynaud's disease, polyarteritis
- in any disease causing peripheroneuropathy, such as multiple sclerosis, Parkinson's, disorders, stroke, CNS tumours
- in nutritional deficiency of whatever cause; in later stages of 'burning feet syndrome' (commonly associated with a lack of the B group vitamins) the soles of the feet feel hot and burning, particularly at night (in this case there is usually a heightened sensitivity to touch)
- after long journeys, particularly long aircraft flights

- in paralysed patients
- in psychoses
- in the terminal stages of illness.

Heightened sensitivity

Sensitivity is usually *heightened* in:

- extreme anxiety or fear
- burning feet syndrome (early stages)
- severe and acute illnesses
- hysteria.

Sensations may be combined in one reflex zone. For example, in the uterus both pelvic inflammatory disease and loss of muscle tone may exist. Patients often describe an 'old', dense type of pain combined with a sharp prickling sensation over the tonsillar area when they are suffering from infection. The sharp pain reflects the current infection and the 'old' pain is the consequence of repeated infections in the past.

6. Considering the possible causes of illness

The complaints and findings need to be considered against the possible causes of disease. They are:

Genetic

Some diseases, such as cystic fibrosis and Down's syndrome, have simple genetic causation.

Infective

The majority of these are either bacterial or viral.

Chemical

Chemicals may enter the body by inhalation (e.g. the fumes of carbon tetrachloride, used in dry cleaning), ingestion of, or through skin exposure.

Burns

Tissues which have suffered a partial or full thickness burn often remain sensitive long after the injury, influenced in part by the amount of nerve damage sustained. The possibility of an

interference field (see Ch. 2, p. 34) should be borne in mind.

Mechanical

This may be due to poor posture; poorly considered carrying, lifting or moving methods; or having to carry loads which are too heavy. In repetitive strain injury the strain is caused by the same small movement repeated over and over. There are also sporting injuries, such as tennis elbow.

Trauma

This includes any injury in which the integrity of the body is breached, such as a wound or a fracture, bringing with it the possibility of infection. If the injury does not heal by primary intention the scar may become an interference field, with its negative impact on the GRS (see Ch. 2, p. 34).

Nutritional excess or deficiency

Both of these may be present in the same person.

■ *"Every careful observer of the sick will agree in this, that thousands of patients are annually starved in the midst of plenty, from want of attention to the ways which alone make it possible for them to take food …*
Defect in cooking, or of preparation,
Defect in choice of diet,
Defect in choice of hours of taking diet,
Defect of appetite in patient"

observed Florence Nightingale in 1859 (Nightingale commemorative edition 1980). Since people nowadays spend much shorter periods in hospital than they did some 50 years ago, many sick people are nursed in the community, and one does not have to be lying in a hospital ward to be a patient. Malnourishment is all too often seen and is the cause of much debility. In the West, the young, the frail, the elderly, the sick, the vulnerable, new immigrants and consumers of a monodiet are particularly at risk of deficiency.

Choosing the correct foods to eat in health is never simple, and is even less so in illness (Bieler 1966). Prescribing which foods help and which hinder recovery for each individual person and different disease is a decision best made by someone with informed knowledge of the subject. Some general principles of good nutrition are given in Appendix I, but therapists should seek out a competent colleague to whom they can refer their patients when they do not have the proper expertise. Trained practitioners of naturopathy, herbalism and TCM have a wide knowledge of diet in health and illness.

Emotional life

As usual, the poets have expressed this best. In Epistle to a young friend (1786) Robert Burns wrote:

■ *"I waive the quantum o' the sin,*
The hazard of concealing,
But och, it hardens a' within,
And petrifies the feeling."

The effect of feelings on the endocrine, digestive, nervous and lymphatic systems are well documented. A sense of well-being or listlessness can spread in a remarkably short time throughout the body to affect every part via the GRS. RZT supports the whole person at times of emotional lability and stress, and is directed at ameliorating their debilitating effects.

Illness can be caused by *shock*, as in 'shock diabetes', also by unrelieved stress and weariness, with consequent erosion of the natural defence mechanisms of the body.

The mind

'Whenever God prepares evil for a man, He first damages his mind, with which he deliberates' (anon). The concept of *mens sana in corpore sano* (a healthy mind in a healthy body) has been known more than 2000 years ago. Hippocrates prescribed:

- isolation
- bedrest
- being away from home, in quiet temples of healing.

He made a relationship between the psyche and the immune system whose physiological intricacies are just now being unravelled (Lloyd 1978). Excess of any sort impairs physical, mental and emotional health.

Climatic factors

Diseases found in one climate may be specific to that region. Rheumatoid arthritis is more common in cold and damp climates than in hot and dry ones. Angina is often exacerbated by a cold wind. Death from a stroke is more common at the beginning of winter when the coagulability of the blood is greater than it is in summer.

Central heating and air conditioning provide a milieu in which Legionnaire's disease thrives if the *Legionella* bacteria is present in the water of the cooling system. Air and temperature control are difficult to adjust to suit all individuals.

Hypothermia in cold climates and heatstroke in the tropics are complicating factors in illness. In all parts of the world climatic conditions have given rise to prescribed forms of eating, drinking, clothing and working habits which are suited to local conditions.

Occupational factors

Loss of salt during excessive sweating leads to muscular cramp, and is a well-known hazard amongst miners. Neck and shoulder problems are common in drivers of large buses and pantechnicons, as is back pain in nurses, varicose veins in shop assistants and sports injuries for athletes. Some hazard is associated with all occupations and activities, and likewise with inactivity.

Poisons

The spectrum of poisons includes alcohol, drugs, cigarettes, mushrooms, rhubarb, shellfish and spoiled foods. The effects may range from mild diarrhoea and vomiting to death from botulism.

Environmental

Although there is an overlap with the above category, the known and unknown consequences of certain substances found in air, food and water can be damaging. These may be natural substances emitted by earth or sea (e.g. radiation from a volcanic eruption, radon from the rocks) or from human activities, producing toxic compounds combining with each other which are then inhaled, ingested or absorbed through the skin. Radiation from the sun, nuclear fission, medical and chemical establishments are likewise environmental factors producing potential hazard.

Parasitic infestations

Parasites include head lice, hook worms, thread worms, tape worms, bilharzia amongst others and are ever present. They may be held in check by good public health measures, but reappear rapidly if these break down. Such infestations are debilitating and can be fatal.

Disease caused by vectors

Malaria, from which more people die worldwide every year than from any other disease, is the prime example. Its incidence is again spreading, and it is now seen in areas where it was unknown a decade or two ago. Plague, typhus and tick bite fever are rarely seen in Europe today, but reappear in unexpected locations with increasing movements of populations and in travellers.

Periods of increased vulnerability to illness

At times of physiological, biological and social change there is an increased vulnerability to illness. Birth, puberty, marriage, promotion, separation, divorce, childbearing, bereavement, unemployment, the menopause and moving home are, amongst others, recognised periods of increased vulnerability. The accompanying stresses depress the person's immunity to an illness which in less difficult different circumstances would be withstood, or which would affect her less severely.

7. Evaluation of appropriateness of RZT

Reflex zone therapy can now be evaluated for its appropriateness in the light of the person's illness.

In some of the circumstances described above, it is clearly inappropriate as the first line of treatment. Burns, poisoning, fractures and infestation require medical intervention. RZT may be given in support, to promote rest, relaxation, healing, elimination, pain relief, circulation and, when given by the same therapist, continuity of care. The therapist must consult with his colleagues in the clinical situation to decide when RZT is the best available or additional treatment.

In other circumstances, RZT can be given by itself, or in conjunction with changes in diet, working practices, exercise or recreation.

In trying to identify which combination of the above factors are responsible, the therapist's awareness of the complexity of those factors which affect health and disease should be kept constantly in the foreground.

Where RZT is inappropriate, the patient should be be referred to someone with the necessary expertise, and an explanation given for the referral. For example, a young man with habitually poor posture who presents with chronic low backache would be better advised to have Alexander or Feldenkreis lessons for postural re-education. Musicians with chronic musculoskeletal problems also benefit from such lessons because of the long hours which are spent in one position while practising and playing.

On occasion headaches can be relieved by simple changes in habits or the way in which the working environment is arranged, such as moving a VDU screen to the correct height and distance from the eyes, or having a table which is the right height for work.

The patient should be encouraged to persist with any changes which are recommended in order to relieve the immediate overload on the GRS and impaired systems or structures. The body takes time to heal — the skin is renewed every 28 days, the life of a red blood corpuscle is some 100 days and the bones are constantly being remodelled so that the whole skeleton is renewed every 7 years. The therapist has to find appropriate ways of motivating the patient to persevere with her new regime. Quiet encouragement and monitoring her progress at regular visits in the early weeks of treatment are in this respect helpful for her. Case study 5.3 gives an example of this situation.

CASE STUDY 5.3

A successful, professional man of 56 years came for RZT. His blood pressure was low at 90/60 mmHg, and he complained of extreme tiredness. His history revealed that during his busy office days he did not eat any food. On assessment his feet were cold, and the significant finding was of very painful (level 5) reflex zones to the adrenals, which produced SNS reaction on the lightest palpation.

Having been asked to keep a diary of what he ate and drank, he was surprised to realise that he was drinking about 16 cups of strong black coffee between 8 a.m. and 5 p.m. for the 5 working days of the week.

It had become habitual for him to have a cup of coffee on the desk, and it gave him 'a lift'. Soon afterwards, as he stopped drinking coffee and started to eat more balanced meals, his sleep began to improve. After a few weeks he had more energy, and the palpitations of which he had been complaining ceased.

During a course of RZT, the adrenal glands were regularly and repeatedly sedated at each session, and the disordered endocrine and urinary systems treated. Over some months his blood pressure returned to a previously normal reading of 120/90 mmHg.

Discrepancies between the patient's complaint and assessment findings

Apparent discrepancies between what the patient complains of and what is found on the feet amplify the picture of dysfunction. The therapist may find the following.

1. The pain of which the patient complains does not register as painful or disordered in the corresponding reflex zones. Other zones may, however, be disordered. This usually indicates that the root of the problem lies elsewhere, and that the pain is being referred; the shoulder is a classic example of referred pain from gall stones.
2. In some instances, only the referred pain of which the patient complains registers as a disordered reflex zone at the first visit. This picture may remain constant throughout, or may change as treatment progresses.
3. Usually there are areas of discomfort and others of decreased sensitivity, with some zones being more painful than others. This picture can also change with further treatment.
4. Disordered reflex zones may become less painful once treatment begins, whilst some become more painful during the first few sessions before the hurt begins to subside.

While it is important to note and be aware of the patient's complaint, and to treat the related areas if they are disordered, it is equally important to note which are the most visibly and palpably disordered areas on the feet, and for treatment to be concentrated in these zones.

For example, the therapist may be asked to treat someone complaining of pain in the right lower lumbar region. The pain has been present for some weeks, and is progressively worsening. On examination and palpation of the feet the musculature of the left lumbar spine is found to be more painful than that of the right. The possibilities are: an injury to the spine or musculature on the left side to which the patient has accommodated (usually by guarding the left, and bearing more weight on the right side), or pain has been referred from an abdominal organ (affecting originally the segment on the left side, subsequently spreading to involve the spine, and now experienced contralaterally and over many segments). The resulting strain on the joints and muscles of the right cannot at this point be accommodated by increased weight bearing on the left, and treatment is sought. An episode of back pain on the left side months or years ago may be recalled by the patient on questioning, and if the pain is referred from an abdominal organ, the corresponding reflex zones will show disorder.

Likewise, many people come for treatment complaining of neck pain. Findings on the feet may show greater disorder in the reflex zones of the lower

---

CASE STUDY 5.4

A 52-year-old woman had been suffering from migraine headaches for 22 years. They had become worse over the past 7 years, occurring three or four times a week, and lasting for 6–8 hours. She had classical migraine symptoms, including aura, vomiting and photophobia. There was a family history of headaches.

Fifteen years previously she had had meningitis, and 10 years previously had suffered a whiplash injury to her neck. She was presently suffering pins and needles in her right arm (suggesting nerve compression), which were probably but not necessarily related to the whiplash. Eight to ten pain-relieving drugs every 24 hours offered variable relief.

At the first visit she expressed anxiety about the worsening nature of her headaches despite taking more analgesia. Assessment revealed painful reflex zones to the diaphragm, adrenals, kidneys, stomach and neck.

Treatment included relaxed abdominal breathing exercises three times a day started at the second visit, and practised at each subsequent session until she was able to do them easily. All disordered reflex zones were treated at twice-weekly visits. During the first few sessions palpation of the reflex zones corresponding to the site of the whiplash injury threatened to provoke a headache. Reflex zones to the liver, spleen, vocal chords, small intestine and shoulder girdle became painful for three sessions, but then subsided. The adrenals were sedated several times at each visit, and gradually became less painful.

After 12 sessions the headaches had virtually disappeared. Yet the reflex zones on the neck remained painful, though her neck was by then only occasionally painful, and she still had minimal tingling in the right arm. All other previously disordered zones had become normal on palpation. She was referred to a physiotherapist specialising in neck injuries, and after four sessions at weekly intervals the pain and tingling had subsided and reflex zones to the neck were pain free.

---

spine, with mild discomfort over those of the neck areas. This indicates the original strain or injury was to the lower back, and has been compensated for by holding the neck in a rigid position. Usually the musculature of the shoulder girdle and the temporomandibular joint have been recruited to stabilise the spine, and are all painful on palpation.

The same process may also be seen in reverse, when someone presents with lower back pain but the problem really lies in the neck. Examples are given in Case studies 5.4 and 5.5.

CASE STUDY 5.5

A physiotherapist was attending a course. During a practice session she was found to have disordered reflex zones to the bladder, but said that she had had no urinary symptoms in the past, and had none at present. On mentioning the incident to her mother that evening, she was told that at the age of 1 year she had had a urinary tract infection, and had been prescribed a 6 month course of antibiotics. She also mentioned that it was her custom to empty her bladder only two or three times a day, which she considered quite normal.

Deciding upon the amount of treatment

It is difficult to be precise when asked how many sessions will be needed. Some people need three and some 20 sessions. The amount of treatment needed by any one person varies with age, the chronicity of the illness, constitution, temperament, state of nutrition, workload and any other pressures or demands which fall upon the person at the time.

It should be noted that a person's physique and appearance is not a guide to the depth of palpation nor the length of time which is needed for any one treatment session. Each patient has to be individually assessed, and it is the ANS reactions that are the unfailingly reliable indicators of what is tolerable for this particular person on this particular occasion. Someone with a small physique may need longer treatment than another who is taller, or has a larger frame. A person who needed 30 minutes a week ago may need only 20 minutes of treatment on the present occasion. When the tissues have become uniformly warm and are elastic, and do not feel too dense or too flaccid, and the reflex zones have become less painful, sufficient treatment has been given on this occasion, provided always that the patient is relaxed and comfortable.

In general, when disease has been present for some time, 10–12 sessions are necessary to relieve the imbalances in function which have gradually built up, and to allow for improvement to be consolidated. A longer period of treatment is necessary in anyone who is much debilitated, and when the illness is chronic. As a general rule, two or three treatments should be given over the first week, then two sessions a week for 6 weeks. This gives sufficient stimulus to the patient's recuperative capacities, and is the most effective delivery of RZT. If the intervals between treatments are too long the effects are vitiated, and if the intervals are too short one stimulus falls too hard on the heels of its predecessor. The GRS needs time to respond to any new therapeutic stimulus, and to adapt to the resulting changes in biochemical balance. If one stimulus follows another too quickly, the demands laid on the GRS are increased, and instead of being strengthened it is further weakened. Any treatment can be overdone, and all that this brings about is the opposite effect to that which was desired. Should more than the usual 10–12 sessions be needed, the twice-weekly sessions can be reduced to three in 15 days, and then to once weekly, according to the patient's reactions and progress.

It is not advisable for patients to have more than one physical treatment in 24 hours, otherwise the effect of one diffuses with the other and the benefits of both may be lost. As the therapist becomes more proficient he is able to adapt the treatment pattern according to the patient's reactions and progress in the light of his experience.

Summary

The case studies in this chapter illustrate:

- the need for careful history taking
- the need for careful assessment, during which all the zones of the feet are palpated
- the need to establish what is 'normal' and
- the need to be able to rely on palpation.

The wider picture that is revealed during assessment enables the therapist to tailor a personal treatment to the individual needs and complaints of the patient over the whole course of treatment.

References

Bieler H G 1966 Food is your best medicine. Random House, New York
Burns R 1786 Epistle to a young friend. In Wallace W (ed) 1990 poetical works of Robert Burns. Chambers, Edinburgh
Lloyd G E R 1978 Hippocratic writings. Penguin, Harmondsworth. First published 1950, Blackwell, Oxford

Miller B F, Goode R 1961 Man and his body. Victor Gollancz, London
Nightingale F 1980 Notes on nursing, commemorative edn. Churchill Livingstone, New York

6

Treatment: basic principles, techniques and procedures

Introduction

At the second visit it is explained to the patient that treatment will be given to those reflex zones which were found on assessment to be disordered, and he is asked to:

- direct the therapist to the centre of discomfort if he feels that the touch is only at the margin of discomfort
- to tell the therapist once the area which is being treated is no longer uncomfortable and
- to tell the therapist if the treatment is too painful.

For many people it is a curious fact that treatment of the painful areas is relieving, and they will often ask the therapist to stay on a painful reflex zone until the tautness which is felt in the foot beneath her fingers disperses. While the student therapist is as yet unable to detect when there is a lightening in the tension beneath her finger, the patient will readily volunteer this information. With experience, the therapist learns to feel the release of tension in congested tissues. One needs to distinguish at each treatment between those areas where touch gives rise to a normal sensation (which do not need treatment), and those where normal touch is not well perceived, or those where sensation is heightened (which do need treatment) (see Ch. 5, p. 87).

The therapist also has to distinguish between those zones which are painful and those which give rise to autonomic nervous system sensations (see p. 112). For example, reflex zones to the kidneys and those to the adrenals lie very close to one another, and their functions are closely intertwined. If disorder is present in one of them, it will be reflected in the other also. However, one may be painful on palpation, while palpation of the other causes sweating or cooling of the feet. The therapist should avoid the impression that 'pain' is the only sensation of importance on the feet, or that a reflex zone must be palpated until it is painful. Reflex zones which are painful when they are subjected to normal touch indicate dysfunction, and are in need of treatment, but treatment should not be conducted only on the premise of pain.

A safer guide to treatment is given by the ANS. People may be embarrassed to say that the treatment hurts, and so say nothing, but the SNS is not so shy, and responds immediately to a stimulus which is too strong, long or deep.

Treatment of those reflex zones which are abnormal to touch leads to relaxation, the relief of pain and symptoms, and imparts healing impulses which are then spread throughout the GRS. Although RZT is an adaptable form of treatment, and can be given to a subject who is sitting, standing or lying down as first aid, or in a series of treatments, both patient and therapist derive the maximum benefit when the following conditions are met in learning the technique. The treatment should be restful for the patient and the therapist should work with economy of effort.

Treatment technique

Maintaining the correct posture

An erect, supple posture is graceful and attractive and has become a casualty in the West in the recent past. It may seem difficult to accomplish initially, but if the therapist makes it part of her practice to sit well, in time it becomes effortless. Since the body functions best in this position, she will be rewarded with an increase in concentration and energy. The line of the spine and of the bones of the lower limb lie close to the centre of gravity in humans, so that relatively little muscular effort is required to maintain erect posture. When sitting or standing upright, gravity exerts its pull on the smallest base, and consequently there is less demand for oxygen from muscles which are in axial alignment. The most comfortable and energy efficient position for this work is to sit with both feet placed firmly on the floor, the weight of the body being borne by the two ischial tuberosities, and with the trunk some 30 cm (12 inches) distant from the patient's feet. Both plantar surfaces of the feet lie directly under the knees, which are 30 cm (about a foot) apart, and remain on the floor throughout the session. The thighs should be at right angles to the trunk, with the knees lying in line with the hips and bent at a right angle.

Holding the spine erect (Fig. 6.1) and at the same time maintaining the normal lumbar and cervical curves also permit the therapist's breathing to be deeper and more effective than if she slumps. Shallow breathing (with inadequate oxygenation) is a common cause of tiredness during and after treatment. Quiet, regular, abdominal diaphragmatic breathing should be learned by the therapist to prepare her for the task in hand. (In diaphragmatic breathing the abdominal muscles as well as the intercostal muscles are recruited during inspiration, and relax during expiration.) This is the most efficient way to breathe, providing an adequate oxygen supply for the body.

The body is said to be in stable equilibrium when a vertical line through its centre of gravity falls within its base of support. Adopting this position allows the therapist to move around the centre of equilibrium while giving treatment without putting any unnecessary strain on any of her own joints or body structures. The head should remain erect and not be allowed to droop forwards, which also allows the therapist a constant view of the patient lying on the bed. The shoulders fall into a relaxed and natural position, and should not be raised at any time during

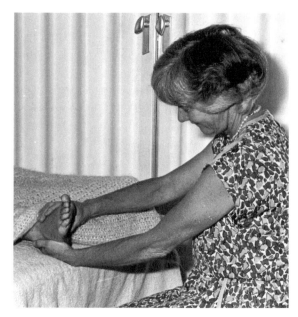

Fig. 6.1 *To maintain a correct working posture, the therapist should keep the length of a forearm's distance between the end of the bed and her chair, hold her spine and head erect, and keep her shoulders relaxed*

treatment. All movement is concentrated in the hands, wrists, forearms and elbows.

On sitting down before starting treatment, the therapist should let the body relax and the mind become clear as she focuses on what she is doing. Since the senses are essential informants, harnessing the eyes, ears, smell, touch and perception will fill in all the details which form her impressions. The therapist should practise noticing as much as possible about the person in front of her.

The basic treatment movement

The same palpation technique as used in the assessment is the basis of all subsequent treatments (see Ch. 4, p. 64). However, during treatment only those areas of the feet which were found to be abnormal on palpation are probed (see Ch. 8, p. 137 for general order of treatment on the foot). The following points should also be noted:

1. The movements made by thumbs or fingers should always be directed away from the body of the therapist, and not towards her trunk.

Movement toward the body results in a cramped and less fluent rhythm, since one or more joints must be hyperextended or overflexed in order to achieve this direction.

2. Effective treatment does not depend on pressure, weight or strength. It is more a question of probing into the tissues, and feeling the 'give' or 'resistance' which is met, followed by the resilience or otherwise of the tissues as perceived by the sensory receptors in the therapist's retracting thumb.

   Neither is good treatment a simple repetition of pressure on reflex zones. Lightening and relaxing respites from treatment of painful zones or after a reaction are woven into each session, and play as important a part in the whole as does palpation.

3. Treatment movements should at all times be rhythmical, flowing and without hesitation. They are experienced by the patient as a 'wave-like' movement inducing relaxation and a sense of well-being.

4. One hand should remain in contact with the feet at all times, so that unbroken contact with the patient is maintained throughout the treatment session.

5. When working on one foot only, the other foot should be kept amply and warmly covered. It is surprising how quickly the patient begins to feel the cold in a foot which is temporarily untended.

Varying the degree of touch

While there are great differences in the depth of touch which people prefer and to which they respond, some liking a firmer and others a lighter touch, too much pressure applied to the feet is as counterproductive as is too little. The therapist crafts her touch to deliver an appropriate stimulus to the GRS, dispersing any underlying tissue tension, equalising imbalances throughout the tissues of the feet, and stimulating 'empty' tissues.

Too heavy or too prolonged a pressure may:

- cause a prolonged paralytic dilatation of the arterioles
- damage already weakened tissues
- cause the patient to wince; wincing is accompanied by contraction of the voluntary muscles, physiologically reducing the lumen of veins, and impeding venous return; instead of aiding circulation, an extra load is now placed on cardiac function
- breach the patient's pain threshold
- obstruct the circulation if it is already poor.

This nullifies any benefits the treatment may have otherwise.

Too little pressure is barely perceived by the patient, may be experienced as irritating, and may fail to have its proper effect.

If the therapist's touch invokes a reponse of muscular contraction, then either:

- this is protective on the part of the patient
- a skin muscle reflex has been stimulated or
- advanced nerve disorder (such as spasticity, epilepsy or the like) is present.

Treatment is most effective when the thumb or fingers apply appropriate pressure to the centre of the painful reflex zone on the foot. The patient will often be able to direct the therapist to this point, and in time she will be able to feel it for herself, as an apparent change in pressure within the tissues. Unless the area is too painful to touch, the therapist should gradually increase the pressure as her thumb flows into the tissues for as long as the patient tolerates her touch there.

The therapist may need to begin with very light pressure, remaining on this area for a few seconds, and must move away whenever the patient has reactions (see p. 111) then returning to it 3 or 4 times during the session. As she learns to give appropriate treatment she will be able to apply more consistent pressure to the area and the pain in the reflex zone diminishes over one or several sessions.

Treatment is administered through the wave-like impulses passing through the skin to subcutaneous tissues and transmitted via the GRS to nervous, endocrine and all other tissues.

At times the basic rhythmic movement is:

- speeded up as a more stimulating impulse (see below) is passed to the (usually empty) tissues
- slowed down (usually because the reflex zones are too painful for normal treatment)
- held unwaveringly without movement in acutely painful reflex zones until the pain disperses.

During RZT the therapist maintains a still awareness of the impulse which passes through her hands, and the effect it has on the receiving tissues.

Good treatment is never static, but progresses, no matter how slowly, towards better function of mind and body. It is a sound principle (and a wise precaution) to treat the person as though he were suffering from a more serious ailment than is actually present. This minimises the possibility of aberrant reactions (see p. 112), which alarm and distress the patient and worry the therapist. It also prevents the therapist from aggravating the condition of the patient on those occasions when there is a serious underlying illness of which he is unaware and which is as yet undiagnosed.

Choosing whether to stimulate and tonify tissues or whether to sedate and disperse within the tissues

Stimulating and tonifying

Tonifying or stimulating treatment is given to reflex zones which are depleted. These may be in abdominal musculature following surgery there, after childbearing or a stroke, or in organs such as the spleen or kidneys whose function has deteriorated. It is quicker and often more penetrating than the basic palpation movement described in Chapter 4 on page 64, which is used for all assessment. The lymphatic, urinary, gastrointestinal, respiratory and endocrine systems often need to be stimulated.

Reflex zones which are cold, and where the tissues are flaccid and empty, are most in need of stimulating treatment, particularly where their sensation is diminished.

They are treated from all directions (e.g. see Fig. 6.11), and treatment continues until they become warmer, pinker, more resilient and elastic; and either the discomfort is reduced *or* sensation increases. If they are too painful to treat for more than a few seconds, or if there are ANS reactions (see p. 112), the treatment should be continued but in another less painful area of the feet, but returning frequently to these depleted zones for as long as the underlying tissues are unchanged. For as long as the zone remains cold, the skin blanched and pale, with diminished tone of the underlying tissues, the related organ part

and system are not functioning well. It may take several sessions before the tissues begin to respond normally again, but the treatment given at each visit builds upon the systemic improvement gained at previous visits. As normality in the temperature, tone and skin become restored, the need of the underlying tissues for tonifying treatment is reduced. They must be palpated at each visit, and tonified as necessary until the improvement in the reflex zones is sustained. Treatment in these areas creates warmth, moves blood (arterial and venous) and lymphatic fluid and stimulates the GRS and all nervous tissue.

All depleted areas need frequent, rhythmic, gentle but stimulating movements which are repeated regularly, and grow in depth and strength as the tissues become more receptive and responsive to this stimulus. They do not respond to any strong or penetrating movement, being too depleted already. Too much stimulation also imposes too great a strain on the already weakened reflex zones. The patient responds with ANS reactions, feels cold, withdraws inwards and does not feel that he is being helped.

The therapist must at all times be aware of whether and where she is stimulating. All stimulating movements must be delivered by one hand only; the other hand supports the foot and monitors temperature and any exudation on the skin. If she is holding the foot in such a way that she is inadvertently treating more than one area at a time, she will not know which stimulus produced a given reaction.

Sedation and dispersing

When tissues are full, dense and resist the entry of the palpating finger, this fullness needs to be dispersed. Movements which disperse the fullness into surrounding tissues begin slowly, increasing in pace as the tissues begin to respond by feeling lighter and more elastic. Sedating movements either have a slower rhythm and tempo, or involve the still holding of the feet with even sustained pressure applied to an area of, for example, muscle spasm in the lumbar region. The adrenal glands, solar plexus, diaphragm, vocal chords, infected teeth, ears and sinuses, sphincters and specific areas of muscular tension are those which most often need sedating on the feet.

If a reflex zone is too hard, dense and painful to allow rhythmical intrusions into the tissues, they must be sedated. A firm, even sustained hold, directing the stimulus to the very centre of the patient's pain and the 'knot' within the tissues is maintained until there is a release. Usually a small pulse becomes perceptible within the tissues under the tip of the palpating thumb or fingers. This grows stronger and more regular, and usually the resistance is suddenly released, with the reflex zone becoming warm and sometimes flooding with heat. This heat is often noticed by the patient in the corresponding body zone, particularly in the musculature of the spine. The therapist maintains the pressure until the whole of the affected segment of the back feels warm.

This sustained hold, at a depth which is tolerable for the patient but which addresses the pain, is used for all first aid. If ANS reactions are provoked, harmonising strokes are used, and the patient is stabilised with light, sedating touch to the solar plexus, diaphragm and adrenal glands. The therapist should probe and hold more lightly for up to 4 minutes, and always harmonise afterwards.

The balance between stimulation and sedation must be found in each individual patient on each pair of feet.

Using different holds and movements

Support holds

The limb should always be supported whilst the treatment is being given. A number of different holds may be appropriate, depending on the area being worked and on whether the therapist is treating with one or both hands. Some holds for the foot are shown in Figure 6.2.

Treatment movements

The basic treatment movement is the palpation movement using one thumb, as detailed in Chapter 4 (p. 64). However, when working on particular areas it may be more appropriate to use the index finger, the middle and ring fingers, or all three together (the little finger never plays as full a part as do the others).

As her skill develops the therapist can choose to work on both feet at the same time, using both thumbs simultaneously whilst supporting with the fingers (see also Ch. 8, p. 167), allowing for fine alterations in skin, tissue tone and response over a wide area to be gauged and treated accordingly. Or she may work with both hands on one foot, either supporting it with the fingers while treating with both thumbs as above, or supporting with the thumbs and using four to six fingers simultaneously.

In addition to palpation a number of other movements can be used, including circumduction or circling movements, the 'cello grip', milking, sawing and kneading. Examples of the variety of treatment movements available are shown in Figure 6.3.

Incorrect holds and movements

Some holds and movements should be avoided as they put undue stress either on the therapist's joints or on the patient's hand or foot. Figure 6.4 shows some incorrect treatment techniques.

Stroking and holding movements

Any combination of the following harmonising and relaxing strokes and holds may be used.

Effleurage

Deep strokes which are performed in a centripetal direction are called 'effleurage'. In order for effleurage to be fully effective the muscular system of the whole body should be relaxed. This can be achieved if necessary by light stroking of the limbs before beginning effleurage, or the strokes can be used in the later stages of a session when the patient has relaxed sufficiently. It should never be performed over muscles which are contracted. Effleurage has a mechanical effect upon the venous and lymphatic return, which it improves, and may at any time have a reflex response.

Yin-Yang strokes

Yin-Yang and harmonising strokes are used at the beginning and end of every session, whenever

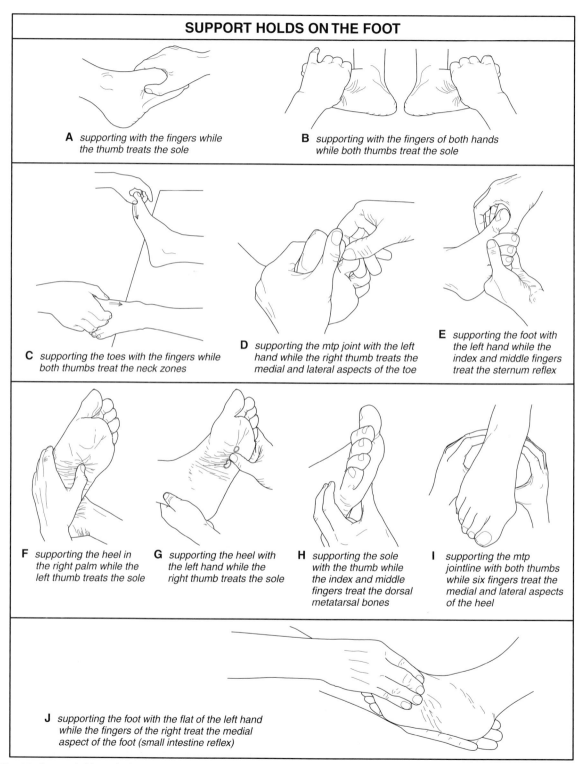

SUPPORT HOLDS ON THE FOOT

A *supporting with the fingers while the thumb treats the sole*

B *supporting with the fingers of both hands while both thumbs treat the sole*

C *supporting the toes with the fingers while both thumbs treat the neck zones*

D *supporting the mtp joint with the left hand while the right thumb treats the medial and lateral aspects of the toe*

E *supporting the foot with the left hand while the index and middle fingers treat the sternum reflex*

F *supporting the heel in the right palm while the left thumb treats the sole*

G *supporting the heel with the left hand while the right thumb treats the sole*

H *supporting the sole with the thumb while the index and middle fingers treat the dorsal metatarsal bones*

I *supporting the mtp jointline with both thumbs while six fingers treat the medial and lateral aspects of the heel*

J *supporting the foot with the flat of the left hand while the fingers of the right treat the medial aspect of the foot (small intestine reflex)*

Fig. 6.2 *Support holds on the foot*

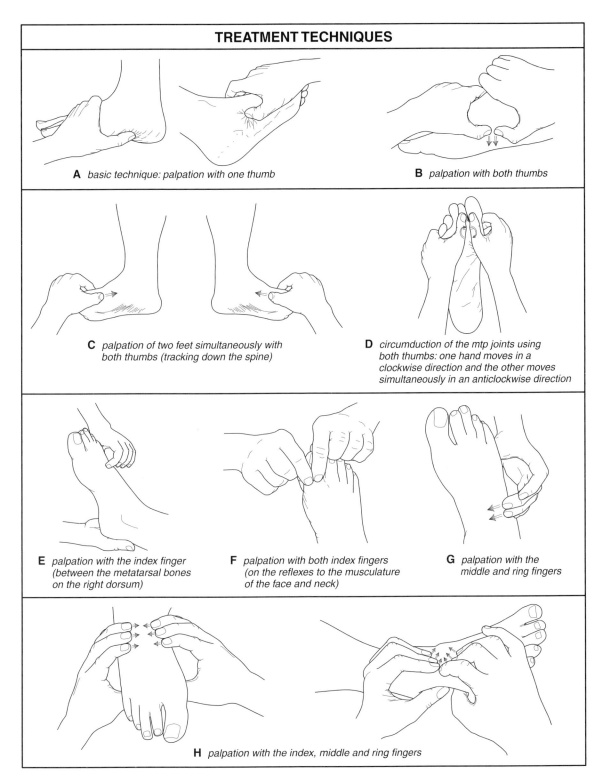

TREATMENT TECHNIQUES

A *basic technique: palpation with one thumb*

B *palpation with both thumbs*

C *palpation of two feet simultaneously with both thumbs (tracking down the spine)*

D *circumduction of the mtp joints using both thumbs: one hand moves in a clockwise direction and the other moves simultaneously in an anticlockwise direction*

E *palpation with the index finger (between the metatarsal bones on the right dorsum)*

F *palpation with both index fingers (on the reflexes to the musculature of the face and neck)*

G *palpation with the middle and ring fingers*

H *palpation with the index, middle and ring fingers*

Fig. 6.3A–H *Treatment techniques (continued on following page)*

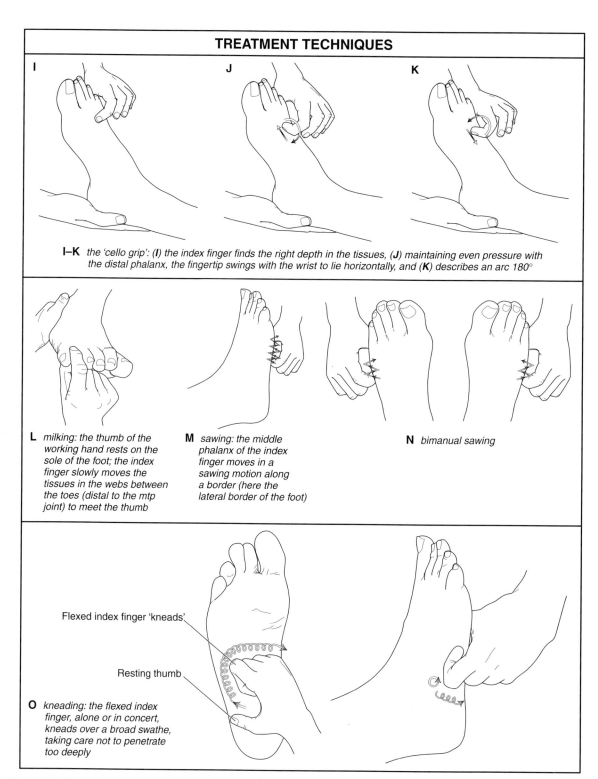

TREATMENT TECHNIQUES

I   **J**   **K**

I–K *the 'cello grip': (**I**) the index finger finds the right depth in the tissues, (**J**) maintaining even pressure with the distal phalanx, the fingertip swings with the wrist to lie horizontally, and (**K**) describes an arc 180°*

L *milking: the thumb of the working hand rests on the sole of the foot; the index finger slowly moves the tissues in the webs between the toes (distal to the mtp joint) to meet the thumb*

M *sawing: the middle phalanx of the index finger moves in a sawing motion along a border (here the lateral border of the foot)*

N *bimanual sawing*

Flexed index finger 'kneads'

Resting thumb

O *kneading: the flexed index finger, alone or in concert, kneads over a broad swathe, taking care not to penetrate too deeply*

Fig. 6.3I–O *Treatment techniques (continued)*

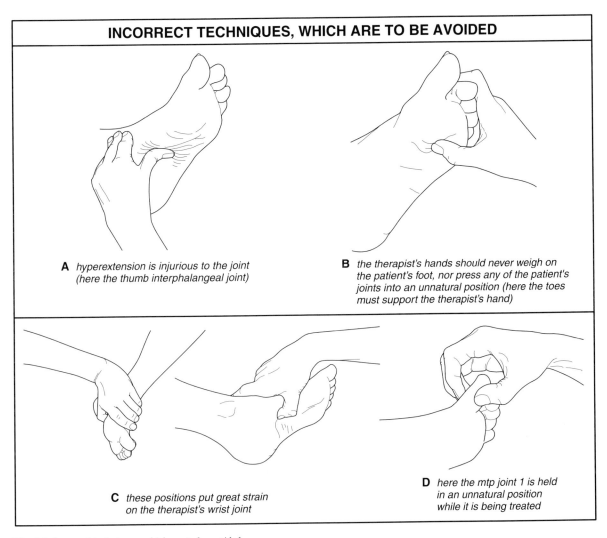

INCORRECT TECHNIQUES, WHICH ARE TO BE AVOIDED

A *hyperextension is injurious to the joint (here the thumb interphalangeal joint)*

B *the therapist's hands should never weigh on the patient's foot, nor press any of the patient's joints into an unnatural position (here the toes must support the therapist's hand)*

C *these positions put great strain on the therapist's wrist joint*

D *here the mtp joint 1 is held in an unnatural position while it is being treated*

Fig. 6.4 *Incorrect techniques, which are to be avoided*

treatment is painful and whenever a respite is needed or wanted.

Without exerting any pressure the whole palm of the right hand of the therapist makes as close contact as possible with the sole of the right foot of the patient. The other hand of the therapist is laid on the patient's lateral right calf. Moving both hands simultaneously, the therapist's right hand stays in contact with the patient's skin and sweeps toward the knee whilst the left hand moves toward the foot,

sweeps down over the dorsum of the feet and toes and both hands are lifted off the skin surface at the same time (Fig. 6.5). This stroke is then repeated on the left foot, with the therapist's left hand placed on the sole and her right hand on the lateral calf. This calming movement can be repeated two or three times on each foot, or as often as is necessary.

Alternatively, the therapist places both of her hands on the soles of the patient's feet (see Fig. 6.5), sweeps up the medial surfaces of the leg, crosses by

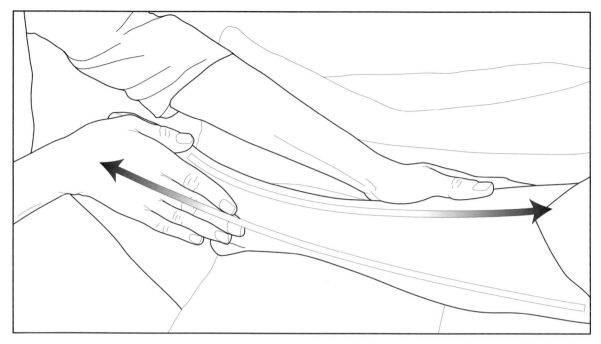

Fig. 6.5 *Yin-Yang strokes on the left leg: up the medial surface and down the lateral surface (then vice versa)*

keeping fingertip contact from medial to lateral aspect of the legs at the upper calf level, and resumes full contact as her hands sweep down the lateral aspect of both legs. This stroking is most effective when even contact is maintained, without either too much or too little pressure being applied, and the movements flow in even strokes both up and down the feet and legs.

The therapist should ask each patient to tell her at assessment which rhythm and level of touch is most comfortable or relaxing. In time the therapist becomes attuned to what best relaxes and comforts each person.

Palm/sole contact

The therapist places both palms of her hands on the soles of the patient's feet, keeping an even contact, and without dorsiflexing the foot or applying any pressure, stays in quiet contact with the feet to relax or calm the patient (Fig. 6.6). If the hands of the therapist are smaller than the feet of the patient, most people prefer to have the therapist's hands in contact with their toes rather than with their heels.

To encourage diaphragmatic breathing

A group of 16 muscles which are small, strong, and rarely attached to bone though often moving bones, are called 'mimetic'. They are the muscles of the face, responding to every human feeling and giving expression to the face. They have also, for the past century and a half, been linked by scientists (notably Sir Charles Bell 1822) to breathing. Respiratory distress in infants is characterised by circumoral pallor, as these muscles are recruited to assist the labouring diaphragm and intercostal muscles. Breathing which is fast, shallow or irregular causes delicate changes to the mimetic musculature and thereby gives the therapist important cues about the physiological and emotional state of the patient. Abdominal or diaphragmatic breathing is at all times beneficial, and any change in expression indicating discomfort or distress during treatment is counterbalanced by encouraging deeper breathing through the treatment.

Taking both heels into her hands and, without lifting the heels from the bed and keeping her fingers and thumbs flat against the surface of the skin (so that the tips do not grip into the tissues), the therapist

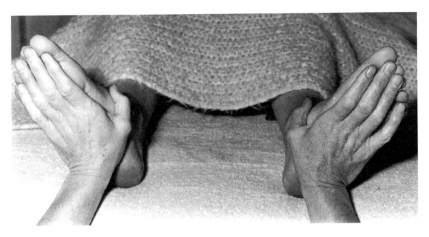

Fig. 6.6 *Palm/sole contact*

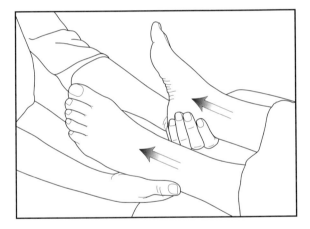

Fig. 6.7 *Without lifting the feet from the bed, traction is applied to both heels*

applies gentle traction on both heels to extend the legs and spine of the patient (Fig. 6.7). This stretching is even more effective if traction is applied while the patient is breathing in and released while he is breathing out.

The therapist does not breathe in and out at the same time as the patient, but should maintain her own breathing pattern and rhythm. This stretching manoeuvre can be repeated as often as necessary until diaphragmatic breathing is established in the patient.

For those people who habitually hyperventilate, and in whom all the feedback mechanisms in the body have become accustomed to an abnormal input,

learning how to breathe effectively again can take weeks or months. Normal breathing, by gradually lowering blood carbon dioxide levels during treatment and allowing the patient to do this for himself, greatly improves any other underlying condition, as long as the associated mental factors which caused him to hyperventilate in the first place are also taken into account.

If the patient is large and his legs heavy (perhaps oedematous) the therapist can take one foot at a time, one hand over the heel and the other over the dorsum, with fingers meeting or almost meeting at the internal and external malleoli, and apply traction to each leg individually.

If at the end of a treatment session the patient is not breathing deeply, this manoeuvre should conclude the session before he is left to rest. To secure the most benefit from this technique, the patient needs to be lying down with spine and neck reasonably straight. If propped up, the incline of the pillows should be as even as possible.

To relax the muscles of the pelvis and hips

The therapist places the palm of her right hand over the external malleolus and surrounding area of the patient's left foot, and her left palm around the internal malleolus and surrounding area. One hand is slowly rotated against the other, so the patient's foot is rotated first clockwise and then anticlockwise, and the pace is increased as the foot relaxes.

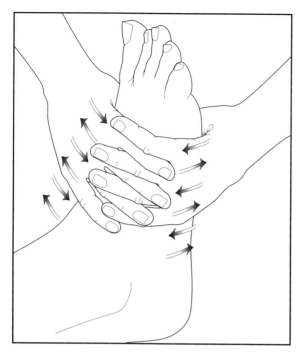

Fig. 6.8 *Wringing the foot: both hands encircle the foot and move simultaneously in opposite directions*

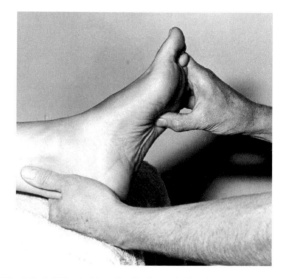

Fig. 6.9 *Sedation hold on the diaphragm/solar plexus*

Alternatively, the left heel is taken into the therapist's left palm (keeping fingers and thumb flat against the skin surface) and, using her right hand, the ankle is slowly and gently rotated to its fullest extent in both clockwise and anticlockwise directions. The procedure is repeated on the right foot.

Toning the muscles of the spine and abdominal wall and relaxation

One hand is placed on top of the other over the dorsum of the foot, with one thumb over the medial border and the other over the lateral aspect. The foot is wrung by moving the hands in opposite directions (Fig. 6.8). This procedure should be omitted, however, in anyone whose feet have delicate or broken skin, or where there are varicose veins.

The reflex zones to the diaphragm and solar plexus

These zones on both left and right feet (see Ch. 8, p. 152) can be touched either individually (Fig. 6.9) or simultaneously (see Ch. 8, p. 174) in a sedating hold,

which is maintained for 30–60 seconds, or until the patient is breathing regularly.

The resting holds used to promote relaxation are summarised in Figure 6.10.

Passive movements

In the patient who is bedfast, is only partially mobile, or who has only limited movement in any of the joints of the feet, passive movements to toes, mtp joint line and ankle should be included as part of any RZT treatment. The whole range of movements — flexion, extension, rotation and circumduction — should be executed (see Fig. 8.2, p. 139). Passive movements are made slowly and gently, they exercise muscles, ligaments and all joint structures without exceeding the range of movement which is possible for the patient in each joint.

Summary of treatment procedure

RZT treatment is most commonly given to the reflex zones of the feet. The reflex zones on the feet and their order of treatment, system by system, are given in Chapter 8. In other cases, treatment may be better

RESTING HOLDS TO PROMOTE RELAXATION

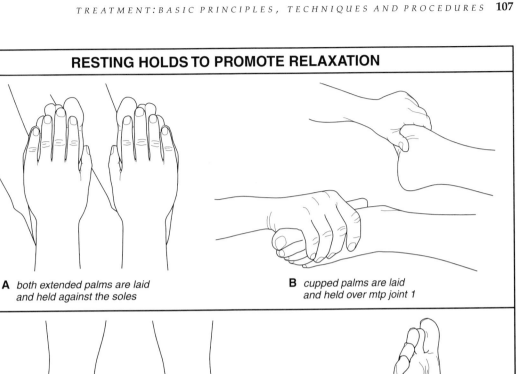

A *both extended palms are laid and held against the soles*

B *cupped palms are laid and held over mtp joint 1*

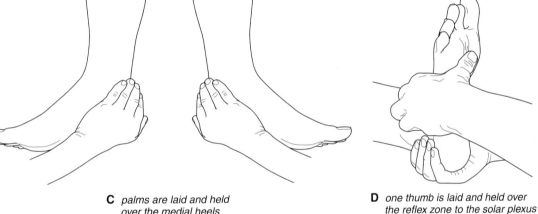

C *palms are laid and held over the medial heels*

D *one thumb is laid and held over the reflex zone to the solar plexus*

Fig. 6.10 *Resting holds to promote relaxation*

given to the hands (Ch. 9), or back (Ch. 10). The teeth also form a complementary reflex zone field (Ch. 11).

The following procedure is recommended for treatment:

1. From the record card the therapist checks which areas of the feet, back or hands need treatment. During the time given over to treatment, she palpates all the reflex zones which at the previous visit have been observed to be disordered, plus the reflex zones of each system in which reactions have been noted. Each reflex zone must also be assessed for alterations in the texture of the skin, tone of the tissues (see Fig. 4.12, p. 69) and also its individual temperature, which can change quickly during treatment.

It should also be observed from which direction the disordered reflex zone is most effectively treated. For example, when treating the lower spine for backache, faster and more effective relief may be obtained if treatment is directed at the sacroiliac joint from the sole of the

A

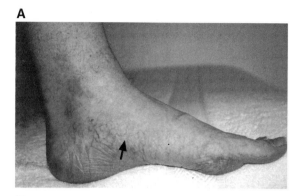

B

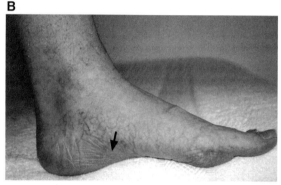

C

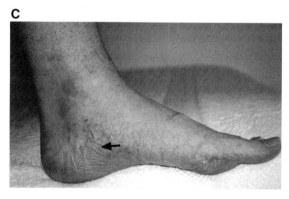

Fig. 6.11 *Treatment of the sacroiliac joint directed: A toward the dorsal aspect; B toward the sole; C toward the heel*

foot in one person, from the dorsum of the foot in another, and from the medial aspect in yet another (Fig. 6.11A–C). The inspecting thumbs or fingers assess the temperature, texture, elasticity and resilience of the tissues, without provoking any unnecessary pain in the reflex zones.

Any system which has reacted to the previous treatment is palpated in its entirety for as long as

there continue to be reactions in that system. Reflex zones to reacting systems always have a heightened sensitivity during the reactive phase.

All of the reactive systems are treated. If the patient reports increased gastrointestinal activity and the resurfacing of an old right shoulder pain which had not bothered him for several years, the gastrointestinal tract and right shoulder are treated as well as all other disordered reflex zones.

2. Each disordered reflex zone is treated for *either*:
   (a) up to 30 seconds — if this length of treatment time is tolerable for the patient; at the end of 20–30 seconds of treatment the reflex zones should be less painful, the skin warm and pink, the underlying tissues more even in texture, and more elastic and resilient when palpated
   (b) or until the discomfort or pain within the reflex zone has eased, which may take between 2 and 30 seconds. Recent or mild disorder responds within a few seconds, and any discomfort disappears. If there is still discomfort or pain after 30 seconds, or if there is still diminished sensation, the therapist should note whether the underlying tissues are still full or flaccid, whether the zone is warm or cool, and whether there are any colour changes in the skin.

If, however, ANS reactions (pallor, cooling, sweating, changes in the rate, rhythm or depth of breathing) take place before the recommended treatment time is over, the therapist should stop treatment and straight away stabilise the patient. This is done by holding and harmonising the feet (see Fig. 6.10) before moving to treat zones which are less acutely disordered, so that the patient, the GRS and the reflex zones are given a respite.

Although it is rare for a person to respond adversely to RZT, there are always exceptions, and the therapist must know how to restore the patient whenever it becomes necessary. The reflex zones to the diaphragm, solar plexus, adrenal gland and sternum are sedated for just as long as it takes to reduce the overactivity of the sympathetic nervous system, and no longer. Harmonising strokes and still holding of the feet have a reflex action on the whole of the nervous system. The still awareness of the therapist who is receptive to small shifts of energy in the feet is reassuring for the patient.

3. During the treatment, the therapist should check regularly with the patient whether the zones which she has found to be disordered cause him discomfort during normal palpation. This develops skill in palpating and the ability to sense changes in tension in those tissues lying immediately below the probing finger. In time, provided always that the therapist refines her sense of touch, and does not rush palpation during treatment, her hands become reliable detectors of almost imperceptible changes within the tissues.

   In order to give good treatment the therapist must exercise her discrimination. A patient will benefit from a well-considered treatment given to three or four of the most disordered reflex zones over 7 minutes and gain little from a treatment to 10 or 15 indiscriminate areas of the foot over half an hour or more.

   As the purpose of RZT is to restore vitality and to ameliorate as far as is possible the disease process, with each treatment the patient should advance towards this goal, however small the steps taken. Although he may not mark great progress in the early stages, the therapist should be reviewing his response at each session.

   Normal treatment palpation is adapted to meet the needs of the patient and his condition. A lighter touch is desired by some, while others prefer a firmer hold on the feet and a deeper and more vigorous probing. The assessment should, however, always be completed using only a delicate, investigative touch.

4. Each of the reflex zones is treated *at least three* and preferably *four times* at each session. Where a zone is too painful to palpate for more than a few seconds, this zone is treated briefly several times during the session, whilst in between treating those areas which are less disordered and using frequent harmonising strokes, or quietly holding the feet until the breathing returns to normal.

5. Optimum treatment time is 20–30 minutes per session, if this can be tolerated.

   If there are many disorders, the therapist should treat first the system or systems showing the most disorder. This is often one of the excretory systems, but any combination of disordered reflex zones can be found.

   It is rarely beneficial to exceed the above time limit. The very sick and those whose nervous and physical resources are overstretched tire quickly and cannot benefit from a longer treatment. They respond better to smaller dosages of RZT at frequent and regular sessions. If there are more disordered reflex zones than can be treated in each 30 minute session, the therapist should treat those she considers to be most disordered.

   When a stipulated time is set aside for therapy, the mind of the therapist concentrates on the disorders most in need of treatment, and treatment time is less likely to be dissipated.

6. As in the assessment session, a rest period of at least 15 and preferably 20 minutes follows each session, during which the patient remains lying down and undisturbed.

7. The feet should be checked for colour and warmth before the patient gets up after the rest period.

8. At the end of the visit the therapist should record any reactions which have occurred (see p. 111), any change in the pattern of disordered reflex zones, the treatment given and any visual changes which have been observed. As treatment is always given to each of the disordered reflex zones and whichever are the reacting systems, it is only necessary to make a note of any departure from this rule.

9. If a reflex zone was painful at assessment and ceases to be painful after one or more visits, it no longer needs to be treated. Reflex zones which were initially sensitive to touch but which normalise with treatment mirror an improvement in function of the internal organs which they reflect. (A healthy reflex zone is not painful to normal touch.) It is not necessary to treat healthy reflex zones unless the person is strained and overtired, when a general treatment to promote relaxation and relieve stress is required.

   Reflex zones which are diminished in sensation at assessment may become acutely painful as treatment progresses. Organs and systems whose function has been depressed are gradually stimulated into more competent activity. Their reflex zones, previously toneless and unresilient, become more springy, warm, and also painful, before they stabilise, when they become again normal to touch, visual inspection and tone.

10. If the feet become tender, so that walking is painful, previous treatments and more specifically the last treatment have been either too penetrating, too stimulating or the time given to treatment has exceeded the limit of what was tolerable for the patient at that time.

    If one or more points on the feet remain or become painful once the treatment session is over, the treatment has been either too penetrating, too long, the pressure too great, or a combination of these factors. However, this may also be an indication of general exhaustion reflected in the reflex zones. In many patients the adrenal gland needs to be sedated, but 'resents' getting more treatment than is necessary. The complaint is registered by tenderness after the session. At the end of a session the patient should walk away 'as though on air'.

11. Once there is no longer any discomfort in the reflex zones, the health of the skin has improved, the temperature of the feet is uniformly warm, and the tissues are resilient, elastic and uniform in tone, treatment is concluded.

12. Sometimes a plateau is reached, in which there are no further reactions, but disorders are still apparent on the feet, and the symptoms have not completely resolved. When this happens — usually because the patient is debilitated, the illness is of long standing, or chronic disease has set in — a break in treatment is indicated. This may be for 8–14 weeks. After this time a new assessment is made, and the most recent findings provide the pattern for this series of treatments.

13. Alternatively, the therapist can treat the hands or the back, whichever is most suitable (see Chs 9 and 10).

14. In principle, treatment is given for as long as it is appropriate, i.e.:

    - as long as there is continuing improvement
    - for as long as reactions persist
    - and for as long as there are disordered reflex zones

- sleep, energy and mood improve
- until a plateau is reached.

Treatment ends when:

- there are no further improvements in function, sleep, energy and mood
- there are no further reactions
- all discomfort in the reflex zones has subsided.

This general pattern of treatment is adhered to, no matter whether the patient presents with headache, tennis elbow, gastric upset, cystitis, menstrual disorders, backache or any other complaint. Each person is first assessed and, according to the findings in the reflex zones, a treatment pattern which is individual to each particular person is decided on. The disordered reflex zones and reacting systems are treated over a period of half an hour, followed by a 20 minute rest period. When the reflex zones are no longer painful, the symptoms alleviated, and any reactions have subsided, the series is concluded.

When treatment needs to be modified

In certain circumstances treatment may need to be modified.

Physical, mental or emotional weakness

In patients who are physically, mentally or emotionally weakened through prolonged or severe illness or stress, palpation, sedation and stimulation are more effective if they are performed slowly. Acutely sensitive and painful reflex zones can be treated if they are palpated slowly and rhythmically, or a sustained gentle pressure applied to the painful area.

Reflex zones to the sciatic nerve, the adrenals, the ears, the kidneys, the sinuses and the lymphatic tissue reflected in the webs of the toes can be exquisitely painful at times, and this degree of pain is a measure of their impairment. Their functions are already depressed, and any rapid, painful or stimulating movements only increase their burden and the patient becomes more shocked. By finding and giving a measured stimulus (i.e. one which is neither too strong nor too provocative) the pain in the reflex zones frequently diminishes.

It should be remembered that effective therapy does not depend on the number of zones treated at each visit, or the length of time spent on the feet. It does depend on the correct choice of debilitated systems and the most disordered reflex zones to be treated at each session

The undulating flow in which are combined the experience of pain, stillness and holding, active treatment, respite, treatment, harmonising and the rest period refresh and revitalise the patient.

In chronic degenerative disease

Chronic illness is the medical challenge of the late 20th century in the West.

The diseases of multiple sclerosis, Parkinson's disease, ankylosing spondylosis, cystic fibrosis and muscular dystrophy cannot be reversed by RZT. Treatment may, however, be useful:

- to maintain function
- to counteract the side-effects (such as constipation) of some medications
- to treat intercurrent infections, e.g. cystitis, bronchitis
- to assist some functional disorders, such as backache, muscle weakness, muscle spasm, etc.
- to relieve symptoms and maintain as much function as possible
- to meet needs of touch and communication.

An assessment is made at the first visit, but the information yielded on palpation is qualitatively different. It is more likely to show a foot insensitive to touch over large areas, and abnormality of many or all reflex zones.

Consensus regarding treatment should be sought between the patient, his family (or carers), medical team and the therapist. Reactions may be minimal, but should be noted. Both physical and psychological responses need to be assessed. Treatment can bring symptomatic relief, and is useful in:

- constipation
- muscle weakness
- urgency or incontinence
- intercostal muscles, diaphragm and shoulder girdle to improve breathing or expectoration.

Treatment is given for as long as it achieves the above purposes. If a plateau is reached, and no further improvement or reaction takes place, RZT should be suspended for a while, and continued after a break of at least 6 weeks, but treatment must always be conditional on the relief it gives.

If there are reactions, however slight, the reacting systems are treated for as long as they persist.

If feeling (sensation) returns to reflex zones which have previously exhibited little or no feeling, they are treated at each session, and mark a positive response to RZT, indicating that further treatment is merited.

RZT may be given twice or three times a week to begin with. When the reactive phase has become established, sessions can be more widely spaced — once weekly or every 10 days.

In terminal illness

The therapist seeks to relieve pain and symptoms, without any expenditure of any energy by the patient. No assessment is made other than a visual examination.

Emphasis is given to calming and harmonising strokes, and to quiet holding of the feet. Just the right amount of touch to reduce pain or other symptoms is used.

Note should also be made of the contraindications and precautions indicated in some conditions (see Ch. 5, p. 77).

Reactions to treatment

The definition of reaction is: '*reciprocal or responsive effects because of activity or interaction with another: response to stimulus, to undergo changes or show behaviour due to some influence*'.

Any effect produced by a stimulus can be called a reaction, such as the experience of relaxation, pain and symptom relief which is felt by most people after treatment. During and after treatment however, other reactions or responses may be noted. The nature, frequency and type of reactions govern all stages of treatment in RZT, whichever body surface is being treated.

All reactions are always a positive response to RZT, whether of relief or whether they cause temporary discomfort. Whatever their form, they are always a reflection of existing pathology in the patient, and are a systemic response on the part of tissues or organs which have been vitiated by infection, chemicals or other noxious influences.

Innate regenerative capacities are mobilised or strengthened by stimuli transmitted to all parts of the body by the GRS. While healthy tissues function at their optimum, tissues which function poorly or inefficiently slough off diseased parts under the impetus of appropriate treatment, in whichever form it is given.

Common features of reactions

These include the following:

- they usually peak within 24 hours of treatment, and generally subside within 48 hours of a session
- they may appear in one system, such as the urinary tract, and remain confined in that system for as long as a course of treatment is needed
- they may appear in more than one system at the same time, for example the gastrointestinal tract and endocrine system; they persist for longest in whichever system has been most prejudiced by the illness
- they may appear first in one system (e.g. respiratory) and appear later in another (e.g. locomotor)
- they may appear after the assessment, but more often become apparent after three to six sessions
- they may last for a few hours or days
- they may be stronger in one person than another, which does not affect the outcome of therapy; their strength, frequency and duration are good indicators of the constitutional strength or weakness, past or present illness, and injury or disorder of the person.

Autonomic nervous system reactions

The essentially motor ANS responds immediately, sensitively and globally to all stimuli. The SNS and PNS are different in structure and function one from another, but are complementary to each other, and their balanced and coordinated function is necessary for health.

When the SNS is stimulated, adrenaline (or acetylcholine in the sweat glands) prepares the body for fright, fight or flight. The pupils dilate immediately: the heart rate increases; the smooth muscle walls in bronchioles and bronchi relax, the spleen puts blood with a high concentration of red blood corpuscles into the circulation, the blood supply to the skin and digestive organs is reduced while that to voluntary muscles is increased, peristalsis stops, sphincters close, sweating increases (notably on the palms of the hands, soles of the feet and forehead) and the hairs on the skin 'stand on end'. The individual is pervaded by a sense of anxiety.

A person who is debilitated, very sick, very young or very old reacts to any stimulus with greater sensitivity than does a healthy person, and reactions are more pronounced. During RZT treatment, ANS responses are triggered: (a) by palpating reflex zones reflecting exhausted function, (b) if the depth and rhythm of treatment is not judiciously measured in relation to the immediate capacity of the patient, or (c) if too much time or pressure is applied to weakened reflex zones.

The therapist needs to observe the patient throughout the treatment session, becoming aware of the first intimation of sympathetic overstimulation, and identifying the weakness from which it arises. The emphasis of treatment is then shifted to harmonising, sedating, or both, and if necessary bringing the session to an end.

ANS reactions are most often noticed during treatment. If they appear some hours afterwards, they suggest that too strong a stimulus has been given.

The following signs in a patient indicate SNS overstimulation:

- pallor
- rapid, shallow breathing
- restlessness
- sweating, which begins as a fine film of perspiration on first the soles of the feet and very soon afterwards the palms of the hands, then spreads to the rest of the body if the stimulus is not moderated

- cooling, of one or both feet (usually the foot on which the reflex zones are most disordered cools first); this gives clues as to which quadrant or quadrants are affected; the person quickly feels cold if his condition is not first stabilised
- a sense of pressure over the sternum, usually associated with difficulty in breathing
- a dry mouth, noticed if the patient starts to lick his lips.

Throughout the session the therapist remains aware of the depth, rate and rhythm of the patient's breathing. Breathing and expression are reliable indicators of ANS and emotional balance, and the therapist must learn to read their cues.

Slow, deep breathing characterizes relaxation, itself an ANS reaction, and is in part responsible for the feelings of well-being after RZT.

If the SNS becomes overstimulated the therapist should take the following steps.

1. Note how long has been spent on treatment so far.
2. Note which reflex zone was being treated at the time, and whether it is full and tense, empty and flaccid, and whether sensation is heightened or diminished, whether it was provoked by sedation or stimulation, and the nature of its disorder.
3. If the zone which was being treated is not apparently disordered, note which system was being palpated, and consider whether it is reflecting developing illness, past trauma, unresolved illness, and in what way function is impaired. Try to discover the relationship of the reflex zones to the patient's complaint.
4. If neither the zone nor the system being palpated were noticeably disordered, the cumulative effect of treatment given at this session is probably responsible. The extent to which the patient is tired, borne down by long or severe illness, and to what extent the capacity and reserves of the GRS have been consumed is demonstrated by the resilience or otherwise of the ANS.

    Placing the palms of the hands against the soles of the patient's feet, or applying gentle traction to the heels, in combination with any of the harmonising strokes or holds previously described, should restore the patient.

No further treatment is given at this visit unless and until the patient recovers normal colour, temperature, breathing pattern, and is at ease. Give a warm footbath, covering both feet to above the ankles in comfortably warm water, and repeat as necessary.

5. Record all reactions, including those perceived by the patient. Weakened zones need cautious treatment at future sessions, responding best to frequently repeated, small stimuli until they become less disordered. They need to be palpated, however briefly, at each session, until normal touch no longer provokes reactions. A measure of the patient's recovery is remarked when zones which were previously labile become tolerant of normal palpation.

    Reassure the patient that reactions are beneficial, short lived and have no lasting effects. Learning how to incorporate the information they provide into therapy demonstrates the experience and skill of the therapist. It is neither possible nor desirable to prevent this reflection of impaired function, but a competent therapist does not overstimulate the SNS unnecessarily.

Uncommonly strong reactions may occasionally occur, and are frightening for the patient, who must be stabilised and reassured.

If patients are frequently overstimulated or become anxious after the session, the therapist's technique is in question. Reflex zones which become painful after the session (which is most likely to happen over the adrenals) suggest that too much treatment has been given to this area.

Commonly occurring reactions

Physical

The urinary system. A diuresis is the most commonly reported reaction. Urinary output is increased, and the urine is usually darker and more concentrated. Changes may be noticed in the frequency, amount, colour, concentration or odour of the urine. Diuresis occurs when the kidneys have been functioning inadequately because of infection, disease within the organ, or deficient liver chemistry.

The respiratory system. Mucous secretions from sinuses or lungs, with increased production of phlegm, sputum or catarrh, may take place. There may also be changes in consistency, odour and colour for a short while. They occur when respiratory illness has been a feature of past illness, and when there is too high a dairy content in the diet in susceptible persons.

The gastrointestinal tract. Bowel function becomes more active. Change in colour, odour, consistency and mucous content of stools is regularly reported. Erosion of defence functions in the lining of the gut, infection, unsuitable nutrition or faulty eating habits are usually responsible for reactions in this tract.

The musculoskeletal system. Joint pains or flitting muscular pains may affect the patient for a short time after a treatment. Pain in the symptom area (such as the back or shoulder) may become more pronounced for a short while after the first few sessions. They are a reflection of unconscious muscular tension, of old illness, or the fact that muscle has been used as a depository for metabolic waste when excretory pathways are clogged or defective.

The genitourinary system. Vaginal or urethral discharges may occur or become more profuse, with changes in consistency, colour or odour. An example of this is given in Case study 6.1. Menstruation may be earlier and heavier for one or two cycles. This is a prelude to a normal cycle being restored.

The skin. Temporary rashes, blotchiness, areas of dry skin or eczema may appear. The reflexes over which they occur is more significant than their

---

CASE STUDY 6.1

A 33-year-old man complained of acute pain in the stomach, which was waking him at least once a night, and he was slightly nauseated at the thought of food. His history revealed that he had suffered from a non-specific urethritis for some years, with a urethral discharge and painful micturition. He had had a 2 year course of antibiotic treatment, but a residual discharge persisted.

On assessment there were mildly painful reflex zones to the stomach, but the overlying skin was pale and cold, and several small blisters were noted. Reflex zones to the upper central incisors were painful; there was some callus over the left shoulder zone, reflecting an old skiing injury. Reflex zones to L4 and L5 were painful, and those of the testes very painful, gauged at level 5. Both feet became cold and clammy. The patient withdrew his feet.

At the second visit he reported that passing urine was painful, and that the discharge was thicker and darker. Treatment was concentrated on the endocrine and urinary systems, all other disordered zones being palpated as well. The feet immediately became chilled and clammy whenever reflex zones in the pelvic area were palpated.

At the third visit the patient reported a heavy, dark urethral discharge and a diuresis.

At the fourth visit the skin over the stomach zone appeared more normal in colour, was less dry and blistered, and was warmer. The patient reported that he was sleeping through the night, and was less troubled by pain in the stomach. However, he was troubled by persistent urethral discharge, and passing urine was still painful. The reflex zones in the pelvic areas continued to provoke ANS reactions. Treatment and harmonising were again interspersed.

At the fifth visit both feet were cold, the patient reported frequent bowel actions and had no appetite. The gastrointestinal tract and all other disordered reflex zones were treated, the stomach zone was now normal on appearance and touch. Reflex zones to the teeth and spine were less painful, and ANS reactions were milder. The feet grew warmer, and towards the end of treatment the whole area over the heels was hot and dry. There was uniformity to the tissue tone — the previously dense knot over the testes had dispersed, the stomach zone was fuller, and the lower part of the spine could be palpated without discomfort.

By the sixth visit the discharge had ceased, appetite had returned, and the patient was untroubled by pain. It was thought that prolonged antibiotic use had disturbed the stomach lining and function. Less disturbance was reflected in this zone than in the testes, and the unresolved pelvic infection was the primary disorder.

Neither the discharge nor the gastric pain had returned 5 years later.

location, particularly on the face, as these are always related to the patient's pathology. The skin is one of the earliest systems in which internal change becomes evident.

Reactions here may also be indicative of previous skin disorders. The skin becomes an accessory organ of excretion when renal function is impaired, in addition to performing its normal excretory activities.

The eyes. There may be an increase in the normal secretion of tears.

The ears. A discharge may be produced, or an existing discharge may become more profuse. Changes in the consistency, colour and odour of an existing discharge may be noticed. More wax may be produced.

The mouth. The appearance of small blisters or gumboils, usually painless, may be noted, and are usually situated round an interference field in the mouth. (See Ch. 11.)

There is sometimes a temporary and unpleasant taste in the mouth, resulting from liver and gastrointestinal dysfunction. A dry or burning sensation on the tongue is felt when the endocrine system is depleted.

Temperature. This sometimes rises, usually in children, who may spike a temperature for a few hours after treatment.

Scars. These may itch or feel puckered. Any of the discomforts associated with scarring may be exaggerated. (See Ch. 7 scars.)

Rarely, a mucous exudate is produced over the scar tissue.

Exacerbation of symptoms. The symptom for which the person came for treatment may be exacerbated for a short while after treatment. Headaches, backache, sinusitis and eczema can worsen before an improvement is noticed.

Temporary reappearance of symptoms of past, unresolved illness. It is not uncommon for people coming for treatment with one complaint to experience reactions in another system, but this only occurs when the system showing reactions has been previously weakened by illness. For example, a person requests treatment for chronic tiredness. The most disordered reflex zones found at assessment are to the lungs. Questioning elicits that he has regularly suffered from bronchitis. He soon begins to have a productive cough, which persists for seven sessions. As treatment progresses the sputum diminishes and at the same time reflex zones to the lungs revert to normal colour and tone on the feet. When resolution takes place, relieving the acidosis in tissues of the GRS, normal energy levels are restored.

Illnesses are sometimes suppressed by medications or become chronic because there is not time or opportunity for convalescence. When internal or external stresses weaken the defence systems, the illness reappears. An example of this situation is detailed in Case study 6.2.

CASE STUDY 6.2

A 32-year-old woman who was having headaches came for RZT. She was 5 months pregnant with her second child. After five sessions she complained that a patch of eczema had reappeared on her back. As a child, and intermittently since, she had suffered from this skin condition, always treating it with proprietary remedies. The eczematous area on her back lay over reflex zones to the lungs, and she confirmed that she had had many chest infections as a child. She was shown some breathing exercises, and advised to do The Lift exercise twice a day (see Appendix II). This eczematous reaction persisted for a further five sessions, the skin being dry and itchy. By the twelfth visit, and without any topical applications, it had disappeared. She was headache free, and remained so for the rest of her pregnancy.

Other reactions

Relaxation. A sense of relaxation is experienced by most people, beginning usually with the assessment, becoming deeper and lasting for longer with each successive session.

Lassitude. This is commonly experienced after the early sessions, and may be profound. Where possible patients should take advantage of this feeling and rest, preferably in bed (rather than in a chair) and be allowed to sleep undisturbed.

It seems that rest is the hardest prescription to take in the late 20th century. Nature has nevertheless dictated that recuperation and healing are helped primarily by rest, and hindered when without it.

Sleep. The quality of sleep is the first improvement noticed by the patient as treatment progresses, and it is a valuable indicator of improvement.

Dreams. These are often reported and described as being vivid.

Diminution of symptoms and pain relief. These may be gradual or sudden, usually becoming apparent to the patient once the reactive phase has peaked and begins to subside.

Mood. Patients may experience labile mood swings, usually in the early stages of treatment. As sleep, energy and relief of symptoms improve, mood becomes more equable. It is, none the less, important for the therapist to spend time listening to the patient, as mood and symptoms have a bearing on one another.

Energy. This improves, markedly for some; as symptoms reduce, sleep, appetite and function improve. This improved energy level is often described by patients as an enhanced coping ability.

Management of reactions

It is an important responsibility of the therapist to distinguish between a reaction, a complication of the illness and concurrent developing illness. If in doubt, medical help should be sought.

Since a diuresis is so common a response to treatment, the therapist should check that the patient who tells her that he is passing more urine is not developing a urinary infection.

Without arousing undue anxiety, the person coming for RZT for the first time should be informed that treatment may be accompanied by a reaction. Their temporary discomforts do not last for long, and are a small inconvenience while 'spring cleaning' is going on. People should be encouraged to note their

reactions, and to bear with them, related as they always are to their present trouble.

However, if the patient is debilitated, the treatment is too long, or the pressure is too strong, the reactions may make the patient feel uneasy, exhausted, or both. If, furthermore, any reactions are marked, persistent or too strong, modify the treatment accordingly. For instance, the therapist could:

- shorten the treatment time
- miss out one or more sessions
- treat the hands rather than the feet or back for one or more sessions
- increase the number of days between each visit, so that instead of treatment two or three times a week, the patient attends every 5 days
- give a warm footbath after the session; the patient should repeat this every 4 hours and before going to bed, and until the reactions subside
- question her technique.

The therapist treats the patient, and waits for the response, which is then dovetailed into the next treatment. A dialogue between the therapy and illness is set up, whose text cannot be anticipated at the first visit.

People in good health do not have strong or prolonged reactions, while those whose complaint is of long duration are more prone to suffer them. People coming for treatment for minor ailments are often surprised by their reactions. For as long as the GRS is able to contain weakness within an area, they feel well.

Reactions only appear when some inner weakness is brought to the surface by treatment.

Treatment is modified at each visit according to whichever reactions the patient is presently experiencing, for example:

- the whole of the urinary system is treated if the patient is having a diuresis
- the lungs are treated if there is productive sputum
- the liver is treated if there has been a persistent bad taste in the mouth
- the endocrine system and pelvic organs are treated when the menstrual cycle is irregular
- kidneys, ureters and bladder are treated if there has been a diuresis.

CASE STUDY 6.3

An 80-year-old woman with osteoporosis suffered from severe backache. An assessment was made and twice weekly treatments begun. After four sessions bowel function became more active, and the reflex zones to the gastrointestinal tract more painful to touch.

Unusually, reactions in this system continued for 6 months, during which time RZT was given at weekly intervals. After this time she no longer needed daily aperients, was able to climb the flight of steps to her flat, and estimated that the pain was some 30–40% less than before starting treatment. Most of the improvement had occurred over the last month. Treatment was concluded once the urgency of her daily bowel movements ceased.

CASE STUDY 6.4

A physiotherapist was treating a 16-year-old girl for a shoulder injury. At assessment she found painful reflex zones to the neck, shoulder girdle and right shoulder, which was judged to be at pain level 2. The appendix was found to be acutely painful, assessed as pain level 5, and the surrounding area was tender to level 3 or 4. The skin over this area had a pink blush, and was warmer than the rest of the foot. The physiotherapist advised the mother to take her daughter to the general practitioner. The girl was found to have a subacute appendicitis, and was immediately admitted for surgery.

Two weeks later she returned for physiotherapy. On RZT palpation the physiotherapist found that reflex zones to the neck and right shoulder remained disordered, but the reflex zone to the appendix and surrounding abdominal area was virtually pain free. The temperature, colour and contour had returned to normal.

During the reactive phase, reflex zones are more painful than they are before reactions begin. Small changes of colour and texture appear on the skin over the reflex zones, and the temperature may alter.

RZT should be given at regular intervals for as long as reactions persist. When normal function returns to previously reacting systems, treatment is no longer needed. This invariably coincides with a sense of well-being. When reactions cease and there has been only partial relief of the symptoms (usually in people who have long-standing chronic illnesses) a break in treatment of at least 2 months is advised. A new assessment is made when resuming therapy, and at each visit treatment is given to all reflex zones which are disordered, as well as to those reacting to the previous treatment session.

Case study 6.3 documents an example of reactions over the course of a treatment.

The therapist should tailor her treatment so that the patient is not overwhelmed by the reactive phase. And if, at some stage, the recuperative processes impel the patient to rest or sleep, no harm is done.

At the end of each session the therapist should record all reactions which have either occurred during the treatment, or been reported by the patient, as well as any changes noted in the reflex zones.

Follow-up

A follow-up some 8–12 weeks after a course of treatment clarifies to what extent improvement has been maintained.

The patient is asked to complete and return a questionnaire 8–12 weeks after treatment ends, in which an appraisal of the treatment and improvement is made. Alternatively, he is asked to return for a follow-up visit. It is usual for improvements to continue to be noticed after a series of treatments is ended. A follow-up shows whether any symptoms have not been relieved, or have recurred. The therapist and patient can evaluate the effects of RZT, and, if necessary, an appropriate referral can be made.

If at any stage during treatment symptoms worsen, unexplained or strong reactions appear or persist, or there is a deterioration in the patient's condition then the necessary medical referral must be made. Case study 6.4 is an example of such a circumstance.

Although there may be a short period of discomfort or inconvenience during the reactive phase, the reliable signs of temperature, skin condition, tissue tone and reflex zones are noted at each visit. If a steady improvement is observed in these indicators, the underlying resilience of the patient is improving.

Summary

- Economy of effort is important for both participants, and enhances the patient's recovery.
- The therapist should not spend longer on the feet, back or hands than is necessary.
- The therapist needs to choose carefully which areas/zones/systems will be treated at this session, and accept that there may be changes to this pattern as treatment progresses.
- There are times when more communication is needed and demanded, usually for the very young, the very old and the very ill. There are times when the patient wishes to share some important information, which always has a bearing on his illness, and it then becomes necessary to leave off treatment and listen to what he has to say. When this happens, the therapist should not lose contact with the feet but continue to hold them supportively and keep them covered, but not divide her attention between giving treatment and listening to an important expression of feeling. Once the patient is calm again the treatment can be resumed, but may need to be modified in the remaining time.
- The therapist should not overtire the patient. RZT delivers a stimulus to the GRS, and is met by a response. A GRS which is weakened is less resilient and has a more limited recuperative capacity than has a healthy GRS. Any increased demands which are laid upon this system impair its function still further. 'The least amount of treatment to do the most good' is a wise maxim for any sick person.
- The therapist should not allow the treatment to become a repetitive routine. Since repetition and rigidity rapidly lose their savour for both patient and therapist, the latter should try not to repeat continuously the same movements from one foot to another or one treatment to another. She should rather follow the clues presented by the visual and palpable changes in the feet as they occur, so that she is treating what needs care today and not what needed care a week ago.
- Illness always provokes an emotional response in the sick person, of which the therapist should take cognisance.
- Most therapists feel relaxed and alert after giving treatment. If the therapist feels tired, heavy or dull, she should question her posture and technique, ask whether she is overtired, ask whether she is relaxed while giving treatment, and whether it is only in this particular situation that she becomes exhausted and, if so, question whether this is a straightforward exchange between the patient and herself. It is possible that the therapist and the patient can have different goals in view and, if so, they should be discussed.
- The therapist should not allow herself to be hurried or pressured. Rather give a short session, concentrating on the areas most in need of treatment, in an unhurried and calm atmosphere. Loss of sensitivity and perception tend to be the first casualties of haste, and it is well nigh impossible for the patient to feel relaxed in such a milieu.
- Eliminate as many distractions as possible during the session.
- At no time should the legs of the patient be supported on the knees of the therapist. The resulting lack of support for the patient's legs inevitably leads to overextension of the joints of his knees. This position is uncomfortable and stretches all the muscles at the back of his legs. For the therapist the weight of the legs in one position on her thighs is distracting, as well as impeding the venous and lymphatic return. If she is treating several people consecutively this may become prejudicial to her own well-being. Furthermore, there is insufficient space between her body and the patient's feet to allow her movements to be flowing and unhindered. The space over her lap needs to be free and, depending on which areas she is treating, she needs to be able to move one or both feet into whichever is the most comfortable working position for the patient and for herself.
- It cannot be sufficiently emphasised that to achieve its maximum effect, treatment must be

given to the primary disorder as reflected in the reflex zones. The symptoms which bring the patient for treatment are, except in the case of injury, referred to dermatome and myotome because the functioning of one or more internal organs has become impaired. Treatment given to a symptomatic area may be pleasant, comforting and give some relief. It does not, however, address the disorders of biochemistry deep within, whose disturbance has given rise to either the pain, skin rash, sinus discharge, headache or low back pain. RZT offers most to the patient whose discomfort or pain are causing him to suffer when the therapist learns to trust her own findings of disorder in the reflex zones, and learns to treat them appositely.

- While assessment follows the same pattern for all patients at the first visit, it will soon be remarked that the effect is not the same on everyone, that not all people like, want or respond to the same treatment, and that, although reactions appear in similar systems, their pattern and intensity is different in every person who comes for treatment.

Thereafter treatment is bound to vary because of their different make-up and past histories. Each individual treatment is adapted and tailored to the immediate need of each patient. This may (and often does) vary from session to session. One or both thumbs, one or more fingers, one or both hands, diverse rhythms and tempos in alternating depths or tempi are used according to the location and severity of the disorder and the immediate disposition of the patient. If the feet become cool or clammy, active treatment is replaced by harmonising and stroking movements which allow the patient to assimilate and respond to the stimulus he has just received. Any reflex zone whose treatment provokes SNS reactions should be treated individually and slowly, alternating touch between these and less disordered reflex zones.

- By being aware of the responsiveness or otherwise of the patient, either as he comments on his progress, or by the slight changes occurring on the feet from one visit to another, as well as the reactions, no two treatments are ever the same.

Reference

Bell Sir C 1822 Of the nerves which associate the muscles of the chest, in the actions of breathing, speaking and expression. Philosophical Transactions 2:284–312

7

Treatment: further techniques

Introduction

In addition to the basic treatment techniques outlined in Chapter 6, in certain circumstances other techniques may be required. For instance, sometimes it is impossible to treat the main reflex area because of injury or disability. In these cases the use of a reciprocal (or cross-) reflex on another part of the body provides a solution. Reflex zones to teeth also provide a method of treating areas of the body for which there are no reflex zones, and to supplement other treatment (see Ch. 11, p. 206). At other times the therapist may become aware of the need to treat an interference field, often arising from a scar. Finally, specific treatment of reflexes to the nerve pathways and muscles may be a valuable addition. Each of these special techniques is discussed in the following sections.

Reciprocal or cross-reflexes

Reciprocal reflexes (also called cross-reflexes) are those areas on or below the skin which mirror injury to other parts of the body (mainly joints and muscles), which are their functional equivalents in other limbs, and to which they are related, probably via the nervous system. They can be used by therapist and patient to reduce pain and strengthen the effects of treatment.

Pain resulting from injury (or surgery) in any joint or major muscle group causes a reciprocal pain in the same locus

- in the equivalent joint on the contralateral (opposite) side of the body

CASE STUDY 7.1

An elderly woman had sustained a Colles fracture of her right wrist. She had fallen 2 weeks previously, the arm was in a plaster cast, and the pain (most acute at the fracture site) was keeping her awake at night.

The reciprocal reflex was found on the left wrist, and responded painfully to palpation, as did the reciprocal reflex in her right ankle. Fairly deep and stimulating touch to these areas relieved the pain considerably within 2 minutes in the reciprocal reflexes. The right wrist was more comfortable in about 20 minutes' time.

She was shown which sites her family should treat, and within a few days the pain was much reduced, and she was sleeping through the night.

- in the reciprocal joint on the same side of the body.

Frictions, vigorous palpation or sedation of all the reciprocal reflexes helps to reduce pain at the site of injury.

The technique can be used as first aid immediately after injury, several times a day thereafter, or both. Case study 7.1 contains an example of this.

Technique

Deep, vigorous, circular movements are made over the sites of reciprocal pain. Frictions will also serve the purpose, if they are not too painful for the patient to bear. Continue to treat the area vigorously for about 2 minutes, until there is a good vascular response, the area is pink and warm, and the pain has lessened. Treatment must be directed toward the tissues of the centrally painful area, and should not create a friction burn on the skin.

Each joint is related to its reciprocal joint on similar surfaces (i.e. medial relates to medial, lateral to lateral, anterior to anterior and posterior to posterior) whether on the knee, elbow, or any other joint.

In practice:

- an injury to the left shoulder is treated on the same aspect of the right shoulder and the left hip

- a pain on the right posterior aspect of the elbow is treated in the same location on the contralateral (left) elbow posteriorly and the posterior aspect of the right knee
- a pain on the anterior aspect of the left elbow is treated on the anterior aspect of the right elbow and the anterior aspect of the left knee
- a bruise on the anterior aspect of the left upper arm is treated on the anterior aspect of the right upper arm and the anterior aspect of the left thigh.

The following are reciprocal areas of the body (Fig. 7.1):

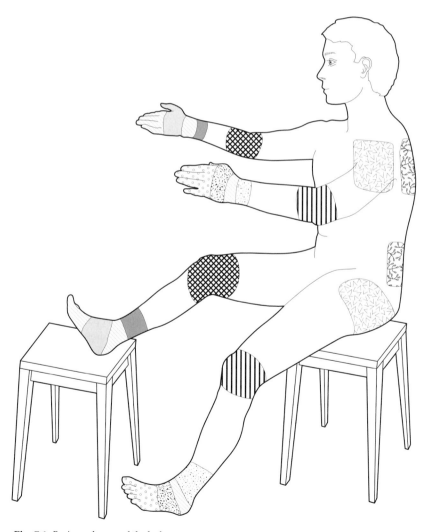

Fig. 7.1 *Reciprocal areas of the body*

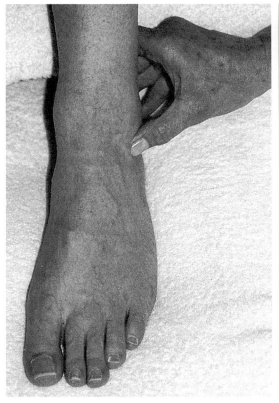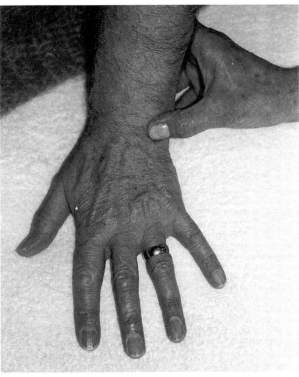

Fig. 7.2 *The ankle and wrist as reciprocal reflexes*

- fingers relate to toes
- feet relate to hands
- ankles relate to wrists (Fig. 7.2)
- lower legs relate to lower arms
- knees relate to elbows (Fig. 7.3)
- thighs relate to upper arms
- hips relate to shoulders
- the left side of the back relates to the right side of the back.

Practical applications

After surgery to the knee, the elbow on the same side and the contralateral knee are treated, on the same surface as the surgical incision.

After surgery to the base joint of the big toe, the base joint on the opposite foot and the base joint of the thumb on the same side are treated (Fig. 7.4).

It is necessary to locate the painful point precisely; if the injury is to the medial aspect of the knee the reciprocal reflex lies on the opposite knee, on the medial aspect and at exactly the same level. The elbow (on the same side of the body as the injury) is bent to a right angle, resembling the knee. The second reciprocal reflex lies on the medial aspect and at the same level on the elbow as does the injury on the knee.

Following an amputation the opposite limb is treated right around the circumference of the limb at the level of the amputation. This stimulates healing and relieves pain.

It has regularly been observed by therapists that reflex zones in the feet can also have reciprocal reflexes. While the mechanism for this is not yet understood, and possibly arises from CNS connections, the cardinal rule of reflex zone therapy is that all painful and disordered reflex zones are treated until the pain is relieved.

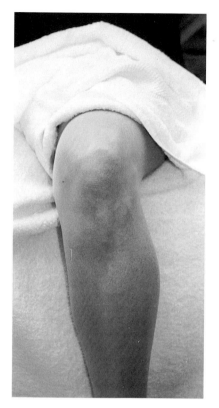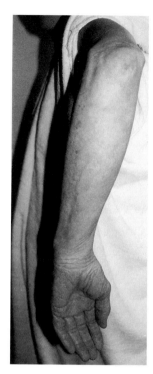

Fig. 7.3 *The knee and elbow as reciprocal reflexes*

Treating scars

The treatment of scars is of special importance in reflex zone therapy because scars may act as an interference field or may at some time become an interference field (see Ch. 2, p. 34).

Many therapies are aware of the problem which scars may present and have evolved a number of treatments to minimise their effects. Neural therapy, acupuncture, herbalism and connective tissue massage are some which have well-described methods of treatment.

A scar is the result of a protective mechanism by which the body heals itself after injury. When blood escapes from vessels, clotting agents cause coagulum to form into which fibroblasts migrate. They are followed by newly formed capillaries sealed with granulation tissue. Collagen fibres are laid down and rigid scar tissue closes the wound. After about 8 days

a thin, intact new skin covers the surface of the wound. When healing is competent the reparative processes work so well that within a matter of weeks it may be difficult to see where there has been a break in the skin. In a deep incision, healing and repair of the underlying muscle and tendon continue for weeks, but the outer epithelial covering which is at the risk of infection entering from outside closes quickly. This type of repair, with all layers accurately approximated, is called 'healing by first intention'.

When a wound has been infected, when a drain is left in the wound to aid outflow of pus, when it is known that stress will result in an area if the edges are sewn together, a wound is left open to heal from the base upwards, the cavity filling with granulation tissue. This is termed 'healing by second intention'.

The scars formed by first or second intention healing are firm and integrated if the GRS is healthy, if there is no infection, and if hydration, nutrition and

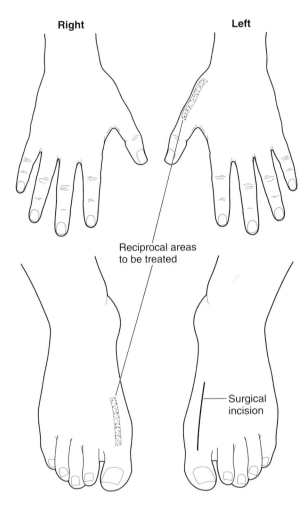

Right **Left**

Reciprocal areas
to be treated

Surgical
incision

Fig. 7.4 *Reciprocal reflexes to be treated after Keller's operation to the left foot*

rest are ample and adequate. In clinical practice there are frequent complaints of:

- constant tightness in the scar
- changes in sensation in the scar when the weather and/or barometric pressure changes
- feelings of tingling or itching in the scar
- complaints that even light clothing feels heavy over the scar or a part of it
- superficial and deep pain in the scar
- sensitivity to the lightest of touches on the scar.

One or more of the above suggests the likelihood of an interference field beneath the scar.

Any scar, however small or large, however old or recent, however changed in sensation or untroubled, may give rise to a disturbance field. This is more likely to happen if:

- the wound was infected and healed by second intention
- inclusions, e.g. gravel, thorns, glass splinters, cloth fibres, talcum granules, etc. remain in the wound. Some insect bites contain toxins which remain sealed up in the wound and create an interference field.

For this reason *all* scars are treated in RZT.

The scars which are most amenable to treatment on the feet are those of the body surface, including the oronasopharynx. The scar of, for example, a healed gastric ulcer is treated with the basic technique previously described. If there is an interference field in the scar it always shows on the feet (Fig. 7.5) and gives rise to reactions during or shortly after treatment. If there is no interference field the corresponding reflex zone is neither painful nor disordered.

A disturbed scar in the body mirrors itself in precisely the same location in the feet. That is, a scar on the left upper arm is reflected on the left foot over the fifth metatarsal bone. This may be accompanied by a less intense pain in the same location on the right foot. It is interesting to find that if there is one area of a fibrous scar which is more painful than areas adjacent to it this is mirrored in the reflex zones to the scar on the feet. As in the body, only a part of a scar may become a disturbance field (often where there has been a drain, an infected stitch or an inclusion).

Reflected scars in the feet may be recognised as follows:

- the skin may be changed in colour or texture
- a ridge or one or more fissures may be visible
- the contour of the tissue may be changed
- a depression, a raised area with puffiness or an abnormal density of the subcutis is seen or
- the area is painful to normal palpation.

In general, reflex zones which reflect scars on the body surfaces are more easily identified over the midline, over the medial and lateral aspects of the heel, and over the dorsum of the feet, where the

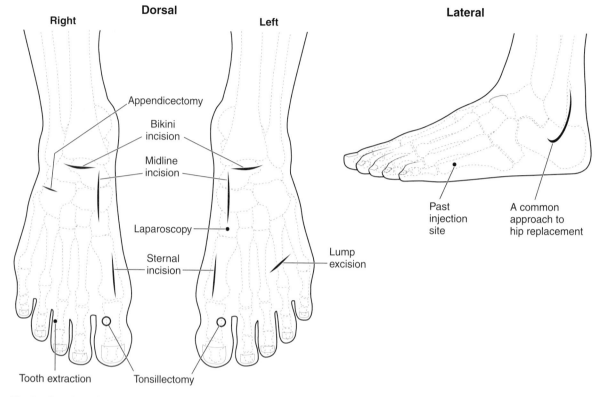

Fig. 7.5 *Locations of some scars reflected on the feet*

reflex zones to muscles abound. If they are disordered, they are treated. Treatment is given to relieve the load on the GRS. A secondary benefit may be a cosmetic improvement in the look of the scar. If the reflex zone is painful because it reflects an interference field, and is appropriately treated, the patient should notice:

- normal sensation returning to the fibrous tissue (usually within 48 hours)
- a diminution in symptoms (over the period of a month)
- that her energy level has improved — owing to a reduction of load on the GRS (over the next few weeks)
- functional improvement
- the scar tissue becoming softer and approximate more in appearance to normal skin within a few weeks.

Treatment procedure

Scars can be treated through their reflex zones on the feet, by the application of scar cream to the scar itself and by intradermal injection underneath the scar tissue.

Treating scars on the feet

Once a scar has been identified as such, it is treated as a disordered reflex zone, within the session.

1. The therapist needs first to identify exactly on the feet the length and extent of the painful/disordered reflex zones relating to the scars. They might be the size of a pinprick, a few millimetres in length, or a rounded area.
2. The index finger or thumb is used to palpate the area in very small steps.

A

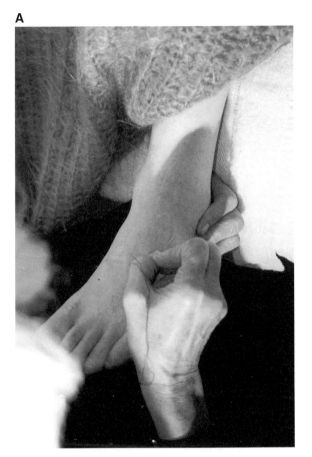

B

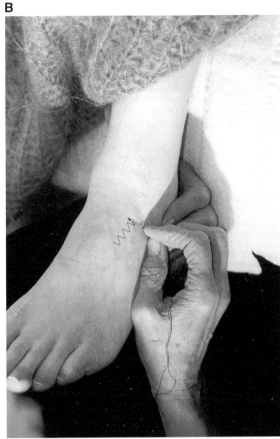

Fig. 7.6 *Treatment of a scar: **A** lightly scarify the skin in a weaving (zigzag) pattern; **B** work along the length of the disordered reflex zones*

3. If a reflex zone is painful, a note is made of where it is and firm, even, sustained pressure is applied over the area until the pain in the reflex zones subsides.

4. Very careful observation of the patient is necessary during the procedure. Signs of SNS stimulation, of the resurfacing of painful recollections, require a short break in treatment. A note is made of the area being treated at the time, while the therapist continues to hold the feet supportively, and allows the patient to talk if she wishes to do so. Harmonising measures can

be used if necessary and the therapist should proceed further only when it is acceptable to the patient.

5. Using his nail or a sterile needle, and without scratching or breaking the surface, the therapist then lightly scarifies the surface of the skin (Fig. 7.6A) and then, as though weaving, criss-crosses over the painful area in order to promote a hyperaemic response in the underlying tissue (Fig. 7.6B).

6. Firm, even, sustained thumb or finger pressure is repeated over those reflex zones which were

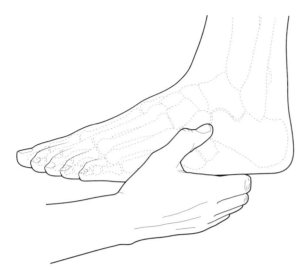

Fig. 7.7 *Sedation of the scarified zones*

painful (Fig. 7.7). The pressure is maintained until the pain disappears. If it does not completely disappear, the thumb is released, the therapist waits for a few seconds, and then the sedation is repeated. More often than not the pain will be less acute than at the first palpation.

7. The session is ended with those of the harmonising measures which most restore the patient, she is covered warmly and, as with all treatment, she is allowed to rest for 20 minutes. She should not be allowed to leave until the energy (whether emotional or autonomic) which is so often released when a scar is treated has been integrated and balanced, and she is composed. A record is made of the treatment that has been given, and any reactions.

8. At the next visit the therapist discusses any changes which the patient has noticed since her treatment, and once more the reflex zones to the scar are checked.

The subsequent course of action depends on whether the pain in the reflex zones has lessened or remained the same (it is extremely rare for them to have become more painful). Depending on the effects of the last treatment and how the patient is feeling, the therapist may:

(a) decide that there is no need for any further treatment to scar tissue; one treatment

may have provided the stimulus that was required to restore the GRS around the scar tissue

(b) repeat the treatment within the session or

(c) should the patient prefer it, give a normal treatment and defer further treatment for a few sessions

(d) decide to use one of the 'energetic' creams, either alone or in conjunction with treatment of the reflex zones, or

(e) refer the patient for neural therapy if there is no change in the painful/disordered reflex zones or the symptoms after five or six treatments on the feet.

Postoperative scar treatment on the feet to aid pain relief. First aid, in the form of a firm, even, sustained hold over the area corresponding to an incision or tissues which have been handled, can be given as often as necessary to help relieve pain. Case study 7.2 is an example of this.

Reflex zones can become painful with lightning-like speed after an accident or surgery, sometimes as quickly as 30 seconds. Sometimes other factors mask the pain, but changes in the tissues are usually evident within a few hours. When giving first aid to relieve pain, a firm and unwavering hold to the depth which is tolerable for the patient is applied to the most painful area until the pain recedes. If there is no relief after 4 minutes, and touch has been directed

---

CASE STUDY 7.2

A 30-year-old woman was in hospital having had a lump removed from her breast at about 2 p.m. At 5 p.m. she was nauseated and in considerable pain, despite a pain-relieving injection an hour beforehand.

The reflex zones to the solar plexus on both feet were sedated for 60 seconds, and then the area on the dorsum of the right foot which corresponded to the recent incision was sedated for some 2 minutes until the pain receded in the foot. She vomited suddenly and without effort, after which both nausea and the pain in her breast receded and she slept comfortably for a few hours.

correctly, it is unlikely that there is going to be any further effect.

Energetic cream

Plant- and herb-based creams designed to have a beneficial influence on scars are as old as herbal medicine in all medical cultures, and have recently been prepared in some European countries. They act on the scar and its underlying tissue by affecting the bioelectric potential of cells surrounding the scar tissue.

The usual mode of application is to cream the length of the scar tissue lightly twice a day. It generally takes about 4 weeks for the full effects to be noted, and repeated applications may be necessary over a period of months. The cream can be used continuously without ill effect, and is preferred by some patients to an injection. If the area of scarring is extensive, such as a burn over the abdomen or the face, one of the 'energetic' creams is the preferred treatment with which to begin. If painful areas or insensitive areas remain in the scar tissue, neural therapy can be given to these smaller areas at a later date.

Cream can also be applied to any surgical scar on mucous membranes, such as haemoroidectomy or episiotomy and dental extractions, but should not be applied until the skin has closed and the wound healed.

Residual disturbed scar tissue is sometimes seen after open heart surgery, patients complaining that even the lightest touch of clothing irritates the sternal scar tissue. The irritation becomes less intense if one of the energetic creams are used. Case study 7.3 gives an example of this treatment.

CASE STUDY 7.3

A 41-year-old woman gave birth to her first baby by caesarian section, and all had gone well except that 3 months later she was still troubled by a 'stitch', which pulled constantly at one point in the scar. As she was unable to travel anywhere from her remote location, an energetic cream was applied to the scar tissue twice daily, and she reported that she had ceased to be longer troubled by the stitch or any tight feeling in the scar at the end of 6 weeks.

Treatment by injection — neural therapy

Local anaesthetics such as procaine or lidocaine, when injected, repolarize depolarized cells, allowing cell membranes which have become permeable to become resealed. This technique is used in nerve block and the treatment of interference fields. The homeopathic preparation of Sensiotin (Atropine sulfuricum Dil D5 0.5 ml and hypericum perforatum Dil D5 0.5 ml) is also used to infiltrate scar tissues and relieve an interference field. Usually one single injection is sufficient, and the results are marked within a few hours or days. The treatment needs to be prescribed, and all the usual procedures associated with injections have to be heeded. Case study 7.4 gives some examples of this treatment.

Any scar, no matter how old, how small and seemingly insignificant, should be treated if its corresponding reflex zone on the feet is disordered. Reciprocal reflexes over any scar tissue can be palpated to see if they are painful, and treated accordingly.

It should be remembered that emotional events have physical consequences (e.g. an outpouring of adrenaline, a rise in blood pressure, a fall in blood sugar). These physiological mechanisms, especially if often repeated owing to stress, will affect the proper functioning of the GRS. The capacity of the GRS depends on many factors, including:

- genetic endowment
- endocrine capacity
- nutritional state
- sense of purpose in life and the way in which one relates to others.

If there is an overlay of distress, depression or isolation, all physical functioning is undermined. This includes responses to scar tissue treatment. The GRS tries to work optimally for the survival of the organism even in episodes of great deprivation such as war or starvation. A strong sense of purpose seems to supply energy when most needed. But accident, injury and disease can overwhelm the GRS, just as can thoughts and feelings. In RZT the whole person should constantly be borne in mind, not just the physical manifestation. The cardinal rule of RZT is that all painful and disordered reflex zones reflect the internal situation, and they should be treated.

CASE STUDY 7.4

1

A middle-aged woman teacher attended a physiotherapist complaining of pain in her back and left knee which she had had for some months. Her history revealed that she had suffered from gastric problems for many years.

Examination of her feet revealed a large scar, 4 mm in diameter, on the left plantar heel. At the age of 18 a verucca had been deeply excised, and since then she had not been able to bear her full weight on that foot. Assessment revealed painful reflex zones to the small intestine, to the back and to the endocrine system. After six sessions, during which her gastric upset was beginning to improve, she was referred for neural therapy.

The scar tissue was infiltrated with 2 ml of Sensiotin (a homeopathic preparation of Atropine sulfuricum Dil D 5 0.5 ml and hypericum perforatum Dil D5 0.5 ml). Although the injection was painful there was an immediate sensation of release in the scar tissue, and she was able to put more weight on the heel immediately after the treatment. There was a rapid improvement over the next few days in the scar, back and knee pain, but full weight bearing was still not possible.

The injection was repeated a few months later, being much less painful on this occasion. Within a few hours the scar was pain free, she was fully weight bearing, walked evenly, and the back and knee were pain free within a fortnight. Her gastrointestinal disturbances improved over the next 3 months. Since the second injection, 2 years ago, she has not had to take any sick leave. Neural therapy was the preferred form of treatment in this patient, over and above RZT.

2

A woman in late middle age was suffering from large, damson-sized, raised, pallid and itchy patches on her skin. She also complained that she had recently been much troubled by constipation, despite trouble-free bowel movements for decades. The first patch had appeared on her left upper arm 2 years previously, slowly followed by others, but over the past 6 months she had never been without a dozen. Added to the itchiness was an increasing pain, which was beginning to keep her awake at night. Its distribution had spread from her left upper arm to the left chest, first the front and then the back, and then to the right upper arm. There were no patches below the elbows and none below the waist, either front or back.

At the first visit the reflex zones were assessed; those to the stomach, left adrenal, left kidney and large intestine were moderately painful, but there was an exquisite pain over the reflex zone to the deltoid muscle on the left upper arm, causing her to blench. On further questioning she said that she had become run down 2 years ago whilst caring for a close relative who was dying, and had taken a holiday to recuperate. Before leaving England she had been inoculated by injection into the left upper arm. Shortly afterwards the first patch had appeared. The injection puncture had created an interference field in a debilitated subject. The almost invisible scar was treated with frequent application of scar cream.

After the initial assessment there was an exacerbation of the patches, a diuresis and an improvement in bowel function.

After six treatments at twice-weekly intervals her skin and bowel function had returned to normal.

3

A young professional woman was participating in a course and offered herself as a patient for neural therapy. She had been involved in a serious car accident some 4 years beforehand and had several long and ragged scars on her arm, one on her face and a raised fibrous scar on her knee. Whilst the scars were being infiltrated with Sensiotin she became pale and shaky and closed her eyes. A supportive group held her hands and comforted her.

After a cup of tea and a rest she disclosed that at the first needle prick she had vividly relived her reception into hospital, and saw again the doctor examining her knee — which was excruciatingly painful — and the panic she felt believing that she would never walk again.

She was sufficiently recovered to go home at the end of the day, and was cheerful the following morning. Some weeks later she wrote to say that since having the injections she was no longer waking up with nightmares during which she relived the accident. The nightmares had started after she left hospital and occurred at least once a week, and the lethargy from which she had suffered since the accident had disappeared.

At a meeting 4 years later she confirmed that the benefits had been lasting, and said that at the moment of the injection into her knee she had felt herself becoming emotionally freed from the memory of that night.

After a scar has been treated, either on the feet, with one of the scar cream preparations or by injection, the therapist should look for the following:

- lightening of distress — this feeds into and strengthens the GRS
- any improvement in the whole symptom picture of the person
- the scar itself; the desired effect is achieved when:
  - the dense fibrous tissue becomes more elastic and less 'tight'
  - the colour becomes less livid or blanched
  - when appearance, movement and function of that segment of the body improves, and pain, hypersensitivity, or both, in the scar and the reflex zones diminishes.

Whilst a cosmetic improvement is pleasing, it is secondary to relieving the strain on the GRS.

Scars may also be cross-reflexed (see p. 123). That is, an operation on the right hip may result in a painful reflex zone over the area of the left hip, or over reflex zones to both hips. All the painful zones are treated.

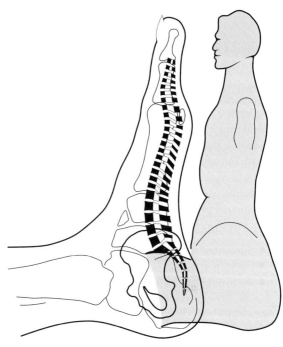

Fig. 7.8 *Walter Froneberg's conception of the seated human form, and the levels of the spine, mirrored in the reflex zones of the feet (compare with Hanne Marquardt's depiction, Fig. 1.11 on p. 18) (Developed by Walter Froneberg, copyright Norbert Gosch and A. Froneberg, reproduced with kind permission)*

Manual neurotherapy (MNT)

MNT has evolved from a combination of several manual therapy techniques. The method was developed in Germany in the 1950s by Walter Froneberg after a comparative study of many specific forms of nerve and muscle massage and of chiropractic. This gave him an insight into certain aspects of motor innervation in postural and kinetic dysfunction. After studing RZT with Hanne Marquardt, he has developed her ideas (Fig. 7.8), and refined a method of localising and treating reflex zones to the nerve pathways on the feet, which then became incorporated as an important component of MNT (Froneberg & Fabian 1992).

Manual neurotherapy combines three elements:

- reflex therapy of the nervous system on the feet
- specific muscle and nerve massage
- modified joint mobilisation.

In MNT the spine is of central importance, providing a scaffolding for the whole body and protection for the spinal cord. Segmental disturbances of the spine can be evaluated in the light of its known anatomical and physiological functions. Nerves conducting afferent and efferent impulses form an interconnecting pathway between the spine, joints, soft tissues and the intestines. The three elements of MNT allow the extent of disturbance in peripheral and central innervation to be assessed, and segmental, anatomical, mechanical, visceral and psychological relationships to the clinical picture to be taken into consideration.

Assessment

MNT procedures require a holistic assessment, which is informed by:

- taking a history of the motor and autonomic dysfunctions
- general examination of the entire musculoskeletal system

- palpation
- careful observation of the reaction of reflex points in the feet and their continuing assessment.

Treatment technique

The purpose of MNT is to relieve dysfunction in the skeletal motor and autonomic nervous systems. Combining the three basic techniques of reflex therapy, nerve and muscle massage and joint mobilisation allows any concealed interactions of disorder between spine and periphery to be revealed. Reflex points of the nervous system are distinguished on the feet as belonging to either:

- the central/autonomic nervous systems
- the cranial nerves
- the arteries, veins and lymphatic channels;

or:

- the motor nervous system
- the musculature (Fig. 7.9)
- the pelvic ligaments and supports.

Reflex therapy to the nervous system

The technique of reflex therapy to the nervous system on the feet involves the exact localisation of each point, and an appropriate pressure stimulus, while simultaneously assessing the intensity and duration of each individual response.

By interpreting each reaction and response as it occurs, treatment can be directed and controlled at the moment it is applied. Treatment of the nervous system enhances the capacity of organs and structures whose function has become depressed through conditions such as inflammation, spasticity and other neuropathies to respond to therapeutic stimuli. It also balances the ANS, restoring synergy to its sympathetic and parasympathetic arms.

Nerve and muscle massage

The nerve and muscle massage, which is specific to MNR, involves performing relief promoting frictions in particular directions along cutaneous and deep peripheral nerve pathways. This massage is accompanied by investigative palpation:

- in the paravertebral area
- in the tissues to detect the smallest variations in texture
- in the painful and affected areas.

The advantage of this preparatory massage of nerves and muscles is evident in the improvement which takes place within the affected tissues, and parallel beneficial changes in the corresponding reflex zones in the feet.

Modified joint mobilisation

The modified joint mobilisation is a method of normalising the mechanical and neural function of disturbed joints in the spine (due to segmental disorder) or in the extremities. This form of mobilisation is characterised by its multisegmental effect, and is gently carried out with and without impulsion in the physiological area of joint play. Important protective mechanisms are built into the way such movements are made in order to prevent any overstimulation. Nerve reflex therapy is given before mobilisation and the specific nerve and muscle massage appropriate to the disorder which is being treated is given after the mobilisation.

The task of the therapist is to analyse and reflect on segmental relationships in combination with the elements making up MNT. This helps him to get to know the many details of the clinical picture in relation to the coordinated function of the nervous system, and allows him to integrate them into therapy.

A comprehensive and detailed knowledge of the CNS and ANS as well as that of the musculoskeletal system is necessary for the practice of MNT. Therapists are expected to have become competent in their practice of RZT before proceeding to learn this advanced technique.

Nervous structure reflexes are in the main found and treated on the dorsal and medial aspects of the feet. Pinpoint precision in the treatment of these minute reflexes, which are located at varying angles to the skin surface, lead to safe and effective treatment with this specialised technique. As nervous system responses are so rapid and their effects on vital organs so profound, the technique is best learned under an experienced mentor, and hence only the principles of MNT have been outlined.

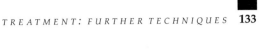

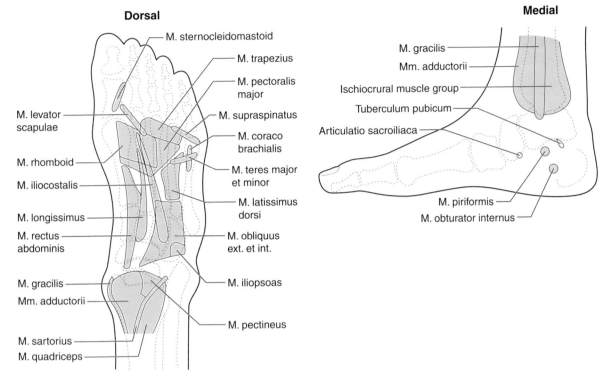

Dorsal

- M. sternocleidomastoid
- M. trapezius
- M. pectoralis major
- M. supraspinatus
- M. coraco brachialis
- M. teres major et minor
- M. latissimus dorsi
- M. obliquus ext. et int.
- M. iliopsoas
- M. pectineus

- M. levator scapulae
- M. rhomboid
- M. iliocostalis
- M. longissimus
- M. rectus abdominis
- M. gracilis
- Mm. adductorii
- M. sartorius
- M. quadriceps

Medial

- M. gracilis
- Mm. adductorii
- Ischiocrural muscle group
- Tuberculum pubicum
- Articulatio sacroiliaca
- M. piriformis
- M. obturator internus

Lateral

- Ischiocrural muscle group
- Tractus iliotibialis
- M. obturatorius ext. et int.
- M. iliopsoas
- Mm. glutaei
- M. quadratus lumborum
- M. psoas major
- Articulatio cubiti

- M. vastus lateralis
- M. rectus femoris
- M. tensor fasciae latae
- M. obliquus ext. et int.
- Regio brachialis anterior
- Articulatio humeri
- M. triceps brachii

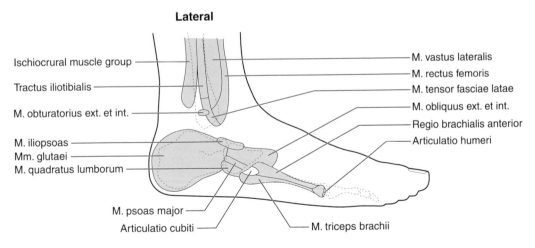

Fig. 7.9 *Musculature on the feet (Developed by Walter Froneberg, copyright Norbert Gosch and Axel Froneberg)*

Reference

Froneberg A, Fabian W 1992 Manuelle
  Neurotherapie/Nervenreflextherapie am Fuss, 1st edn.
  Haug Verlag, Heidelberg

The reflex zones of the body

8

The feet

Reflex zones of the head

The big toe

The structures of the head are mirrored as reflex zones over all 10 toes (see Fig. 8.3). The big toes are an exception in that, as well as corresponding to all the structures found in zone 1, they also mirror in miniature all the reflex zones of the head.

Consider both big toes as representing the head. The dorsum of both big toes is the reflex zone mirror to the face, the right half of the face and neck being reflected in the right big toe, and the left half of the face and neck reflected on the dorsum of the left toe (Fig. 8.1). The lateral aspects of both big toes represent the sides of the head and neck (left on the left toe and right on the right toe) (Fig. 8.7), and the plantar aspect of both big toes represents the back of the head and neck (Fig. 8.4).

Each of the big toes can be divided into 5 zones, zone 1 lying in the midline and zone 5 being the most lateral (Fig. 8.1).

The assessment is begun by rotating the big toe at its articulation with the first metatarsal head in as wide an arc as possible. Any limitation of movement in the patient's neck is revealed by this manoeuvre. The toe is commonly seen to be dorsiflexed when the head is habitually flexed over the cervical spine. Limited plantar flexion of one or both toes reflects an equal limitation in extension of the cervical spine. One palm surrounds mtp joint 1 and counter-rotates while the other hand applies light traction to the big toe by holding it at the level of the interphalangeal joint space between the index and middle fingers.

This hand slowly and gently rotates the toe first in a clockwise and then in a counter-clockwise direction for two or three rotations in order to explore how freely the head and neck rotate (Fig. 8.2).

Dorsal aspect

The full surface of the distally rounded top of the toe represents the vault of the skull, and the articulation of the proximal phalanx with the head of the metatarsal, represents the head of the sternum. The toenail represents the forehead and the base of the toenail the orbital ridge. Between the two landmarks of the base of the toenail and mtp joint 1 lie the reflex zones of the face and neck, including the upper and lower incisor teeth on that side (Fig. 8.1).

The *body and spinous process* of cervical vertebra 1 (C1) lie in zone 1 at the base of the distal phalanx (Fig. 8.1), and reflex zones to the rest of the cervical vertebrae lie on the medial aspect of the big toe, with the reflex zone to the 7th cervical vertebra lying at the base of the proximal phalanx of the big toe.

Reflex zones to the *transverse processes* of the vertebrae lie on the lateral border of the big toe in zone 5 (Fig. 8.1), and extend from a level just distal to the interphalangeal joint space to mtp joint 1.

The transverse processes of cervical vertebrae 3, 4 and 5 on the left foot relate to the heart. (The phrenic nerve comes mainly from the fourth cervical nerve and runs down the neck and side of the mediastinum to supply the diaphragm with motor fibres. Sympathetic fibres from the superior cervical ganglion are also derived from here. Painful reflex zones here should be treated in tandem with any other disordered reflex zones to the heart.)

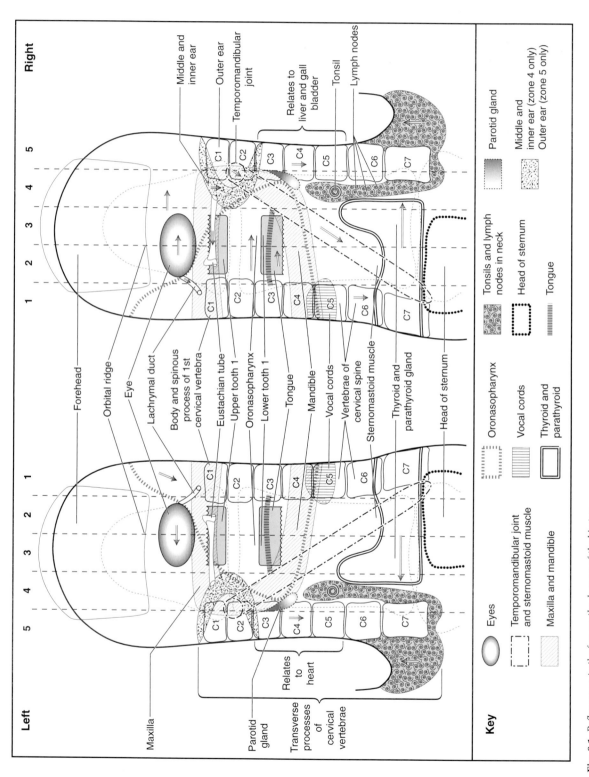

Fig. 8.1 *Reflex zones to the face on the dorsum of the big toe*

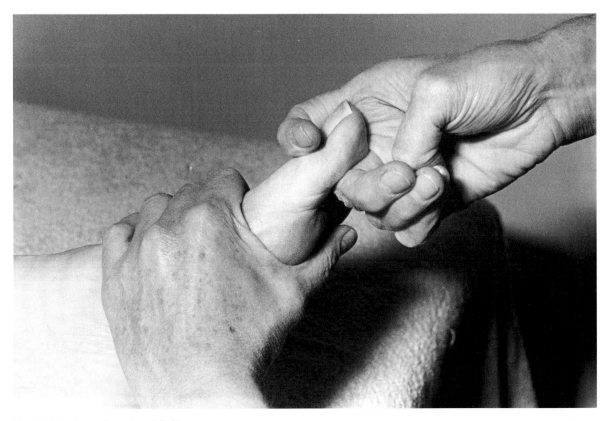

Fig. 8.2 *Traction and rotation of the big toe*

Case study 8.1 gives an example of this treatment.

The transverse processes of cervical vertebrae 3, 4 and 5 on the right foot relate to the liver and gall bladder, and should be treated in combination with these organs whenever they are found to be disordered. They are usually found to be disordered when there is established liver disease, and are frequently painful when there are reactions involving the liver.

Reflex zones to the *forehead* are covered by the toenails, but can still be palpated on the nail, which is at times surprisingly painful to normal touch. The *orbital ridge* (along the line of the eyebrow) lies along the base of the toenail. The *maxilla* lies along the proximal third of the distal phalanx, articulating with the head of the *mandible* at the lateral base of the distal phalanx. The *ramus* lies along the distal third of the proximal phalanx of zone 5, and the body across the middle phalanx of the proximal

phalanx at approximately the level of C4, forming the lower jaw.

The highest point of the *oronasopharynx* lies just distal to the base of the toenail in zone 1 and extends across zones 1–4 at its lowest border at the level of cervical vertebrae 3–4. Like all mucous membranes in the body, the mucous membranes of the oronasopharynx are made of secretory epithelium, and show in daily practice a curious connection with the mucous membranes of the pelvic outlet. It has been observed that persistent infections of the nose and throat which become chronic are often succeeded by infections of the linings of the urethra, bladder, vulva and vagina. The reverse is also seen, and babies or children who have recurrent attacks of cystitis or vulval thrush which become chronic are prone to develop infections of the nose and throat as they grow older. Careful palpation at assessment shows which areas need treatment.

CASE STUDY 8.1

A middle-aged woman with high blood pressure (180/140) was referred to the physiotherapist for treatment for a stiff and painful left knee which she had had for 6 months.

At assessment both feet were hot and dry. Tissue tone around the small area of the reflex zone to the seventh cervical vertebra on both feet reflected heart disorder. Reflex zones to the third, fourth and fifth cervical vertebrae were painful at level 4, the reflex zone to the heart at level 2, to both kidneys at level 3, to the left adrenal at level 4, to the right adrenal at level 2, and to the spleen at level 2. The tissue tone over the spleen had superficial resistance but beneath this was reduced in tone, and over the spleen the skin was pale and transparent. Reflex zones to both knees were painful at level 2. Teeth 28 and 38 were painful at level 2. The tissue tone of the small intestine was uneven, there being several knots and areas of flaccid, toneless tissue. SNS reactions were provoked by palpation of the adrenals and the transverse processes of C3, C4 and C5 on the left foot.

At the next visit the adrenals were sedated. The heart, cervical spine, spleen, kidneys, small intestine, teeth and knees were treated. The feet became cold after about 20 minutes and treatment was concluded.

At the third visit the patient stated that she felt pleasantly relaxed, and that she was having periods of tiredness, increased bowel action and diuresis, which were interpreted to be reactions. Similar treatment was given to that of previous visit, but only 20 minutes was tolerated.

At the fourth visit the feet were less hot, she was still very tired but relaxed, diuresis persisted, and early, heavy menstruation was reported. Tissue tone over the small intestine was less abnormal, the sympathetic

reactions less marked, and 25 minutes of treatment to the same disordered zones and those of the endocrine system was tolerated.

At the fifth visit the feet were less hot and dry. Tissue tone around the seventh cervical vertebrae was more resilient. The skin over the spleen and adrenals was faintly flushed, and flaking away over the small intestine. The patient had little appetite, and reported that she had lost her taste for meat and tea. Diuresis and tiredness persisted, she had had flitting joint pains in the left shoulder girdle, but she felt better than for many months. Reflex zones to the kidneys, adrenals and small intestine were more painful than they had been at assessment. There was more resilience over the reflex zone to the spleen and 30 minutes of treatment was tolerated.

At the sixth visit her appetite was still depressed, she had an unpleasant taste in her mouth and a continuing diuresis. She was at the same time beginning to sleep well, the left knee was less painful and she was free of her usual dull, heavy headache. The reflex zones to the adrenals were painful at level 3, and there were no longer any sympathetic reactions. The adrenals were sedated, the liver (because of the unpleasant taste in her mouth) and all disordered zones treated.

Her progress after this was steady and unremarkable. Twelve treatments were given in all, at the end of which the feet were still hot over the toes but otherwise warm, tissue tone had improved everywhere, and only the spleen and adrenals were still painful. Her blood pressure had fallen to 140/105 and the GP had reduced her hypotensive medicines. She was without pain and stiffness in her knee and free of headaches, and had become proficient at relaxed abdominal breathing.

The *temporomandibular joint* (TMJ) lies at the lateral articulation of proximal and distal phalanges on the border of zone 4–5. The masseter and the temporalis are two important muscles acting on this joint. They are the principal muscles of mastication and, working together, are strong enough to support the weight of the whole body. Treatment of these muscles is achieved by treating the TMJ. The joint is quickly affected by tension, which, if sufficiently severe or continuous, leads to pain and stiffness in almost any area of the neck and face. The TMJ is an important

first aid point for relieving tension, and should always be sedated, never stimulated. It is often found to be painful in people suffering from headaches, face, neck and shoulder pain, in those with ear and dental problems and in those who grind their teeth.

From a mechanical point of view, the TMJ is also that joint furthest away from the feet, and the last at which any accommodation to different leg lengths or disabilities of the hips or spine can be made. Any shortening, however minimal, of the leg and any spinal deviation must be accommodated here by the skeletal framework. A stiffening hip or knee joint reflects discomfort in this reflex zone on one or both sides from its earliest stages.

The *sternomastoid muscle* runs from the TMJ in zone 4–5 to the medial head of metatarsal 1. This large, strong, superficial muscle protects all the vital structures of the neck, bending it forwards and to each side, and tilting the head backwards. Any limitation of movement of the head and neck in any of these directions is reflected in an equal limitation of rotation at the same angle in the big toe.

Unrelieved tension on one side of the neck causes the toe on that side of the body to become dorsiflexed. This is frequently observed in children with torticollis. When the torticollis is severe, the reflex zone is thickened and cord like. All grades of dorsiflexion are seen on one or both big toes. Each accurately reflects the degree of flexor contraction of the neck musculature. It is a rewarding area to treat in the elderly whose respiratory vital capacity has become diminished through postural disorder. It should be sedated when there is any acute muscular spasm in the neck muscles.

Traction of the big toe followed by clockwise and anticlockwise rotation (see Fig. 8.2), maintaining gentle traction during the manoeuvre, combined with sedation of this reflex zone, helps to relieve muscle spasm, stiffness and pain in the neck, whether caused by tension, from holding the head for too long in one position (e.g. when working at a VDU) or from postural defects.

The *external ear* is also found lying on lateral zone 5 at this level, and extending over the lateral aspect at the interphalangeal joint line. Disorders of the hip and/or TMJ can be reflected in the reflex zones of the outer ear.

The *internal ear* lies medial to this in zone 4, over the interphalangeal joint line. Discomfort in the reflex zones to the middle ear may arise from:

- infection, either local or generalised, when the reflex zone is hot and sharply painful
- mechanical causes, such as tension in the TMJ, too noisy an ambience
- reflection, e.g. from neurological disorders or from disorders of the small intestine.

The *eustachian tube* runs from the middle ear in zone 4 to the nasopharynx in zone 2, and is found just distal to the interphalangeal joint line. Discomfort in the eustachian tube may be due to:

- infection — local or general
- mechanical causes — as in flying, fast elevators and mountain climbing
- reflection, e.g. when the primary disorder lies in the fallopian tube or inguinal canal.

Reflex zones to the *eyes* lie across zones 2 and 3, just proximal to the base of the toenail. Discomfort in the reflex zones to the eyes may be due to:

- disease or degradation of the eye itself, e.g. glaucoma, cataract
- infection, local or generalised
- mechanical, such as the need for new glasses or working at a computer or VDU whose screen is too high, low or nearby
- secondary complication of other disease such as jaundice, thyrotoxicosis, diabetes, hypertension, renal impairment, drug addiction, etc.

The reflex zone to the *lachrymal duct* runs from the inner canthus of the eye in zone 2 to the nasopharynx in zone 1. Discomfort in the lachrymal duct may be due to:

- infection of the duct or of the eye
- mechanical causes (narrowed or blocked) or excessive dust or other irritants in the atmosphere
- secondary effect of illness (such as rheumatoid arthritis) when the secretion of tear fluid is diminished or absent
- a side-effect of drugs, particularly the hypotensive agents, a common side-effect of which is to reduce the secretions of this duct, resulting in 'dry eyes'.

The reflex zones of the *superficial cervical lymph nodes* (which drain lymphatic fluid from the face and the scalp) and *deep cervical lymph nodes* (which drain lymphatic channels from the whole of the head and neck) lie on the lateral border of the proximal phalanx of the big toe, over zones 4 and 5. The unencapsulated lymphoid tissue of the tonsils is a particularly important defence at the entrance to the respiratory and alimentary tracts. Their reflex zones lie at the midpoint on the lateral border of the proximal phalanx. The skin shows changes over the area after repeated tonsillar infections or tonsillectomy.

Discomfort in the reflex zones to the lymph nodes in the neck may be due to:

- infection, either local to the head, neck and throat, or generalised
- acute or chronic respiratory disease
- acute or chronic gastrointestinal disorder
- allergic reaction
- immune system compromise; infections, drugs, radiotherapy, prolonged illness or exhaustion, unrelieved stress, exposure to toxic materials and inadequate nutrition are common causes of immune system depletion
- secondary effects of other illness, such as cystitis, hepatic or renal insufficiency
- reflection, e.g. when the primary cause lies in the small intestine or pelvic region and all lymphatic tissues have become secondarily involved in the resulting disease process.

The reflex zones to the *vocal cords* extend across zones 1 and 2 in the region of C4 and C5. The vocal chords are sensitive to dust, chemicals, using the voice in noisy conditions and having to frequently speak loudly or to shout, and are strained by poor postural habits. Tension causes a tightening of the vocal chords, and the greater the tension, the higher the pitch of the voice becomes. (Sedation (see p. 98) of the vocal chords is used as a first aid measure to relieve tension in the neck and throat from physical and emotional causes.)

Reflex zones to the *thyroid* and *parathyroid glands* lie across zones 1, 2 and 3, and occupy the proximal quarter of the proximal phalanx. Disorder in the reflex zones of the thyroid and parathyroid glands may be due to:

- primary endocrine disorders — one or more of the glands may be over- or underactive
- secondary effects of endocrine imbalance elsewhere, as in pregnancy, and for a few months after delivery of the baby
- dietary deficiencies
- reflection, e.g. the primary disorder lies in the ovaries and uterus in women or the testes in men; this zone is commonly uncomfortable in

young men at puberty, and in women who are subfertile or who frequently miscarry their pregnancies

- exposure to radiation.

Reflex zones to the *tongue* are found over the interphalangeal joint line on zones 1 and 2. Glossitis is associated with malnutrition, acute diarrhoea and vomiting, and the late stages of most illnesses.

Reflex zones to the *parotid glands* are found in zones 4 and 5 on both toes. They are painful when their secretions are diminished as a side-effect of some medicines, if they are infected, when there is dental infection and, rarely, when internal stones are forming.

Reflex zones to the *incisor teeth* in zone 1 lie at the articulation of the distal and proximal phalanges — the upper tooth on the distal and the lower tooth on the proximal phalanx.

Reflex zones to all *bones*, *muscles* and *nerves* are found across the surface of both big toes in small scale, and across the dorsum of all ten toes.

All the reflex zones to the face are found in larger scale over all 10 toes (Fig. 8.3), and are treated as part of the wider picture in tandem with all other disordered zones, those which are most abnormal being most in need of treatment. For instance, the pain of trigeminal neuralgia can sometimes be ameliorated if the painful reflex zones are sedated for up to 4 minutes at the point of maximal discomfort. If neuralgia occurs over the right maxilla and under the eye, a careful palpation of the reflex zones over the second and third toes of the right foot usually reveals acutely painful reflex zones, or, if the condition is of long standing, diminished sensation. They are held in the firm, sustained sedation hold for up to 4 minutes. The second and third toes on the left foot should also be palpated in case pain is also reflected here.

All reflex zones have to be palpated once in the assessment.

Plantar aspect

The following reflex zones are found on the plantar aspect (Fig. 8.4).

Across the top of the toe is the *skull vault*, across the interphalangeal joint line is the *skull base* (Fig. 8.5).

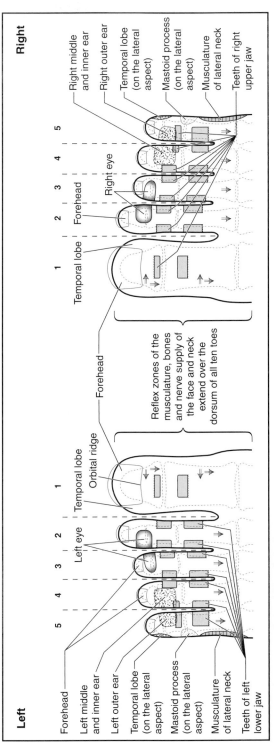

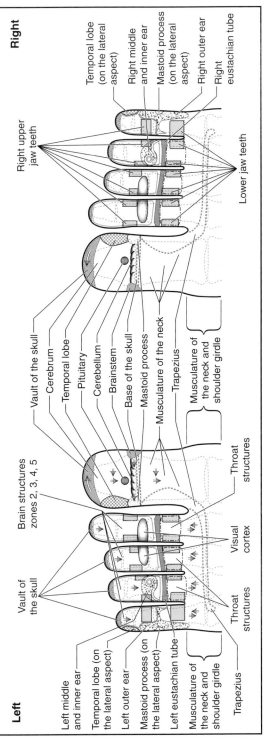

Left

Forehead

Left middle
and inner ear

Left outer ear

Temporal lobe
(on the lateral
aspect)

Mastoid process
(on the lateral
aspect)

Musculature
of lateral neck

Teeth of left
lower jaw

Temporal lobe

Orbital ridge

Left eye

Forehead

Reflex zones of the
musculature, bones
and nerve supply of
the face and neck
extend over the
dorsum of all ten toes

5   4   3   2   1

Right

Right middle
and inner ear

Right outer ear

Temporal lobe
(on the lateral
aspect)

Mastoid process
(on the lateral
aspect)

Musculature
of lateral neck

Teeth of right
upper jaw

Right eye

Forehead

Temporal lobe

5   4   3   2   1

Fig. 8.3 *Reflex zones to the head (dorsal view)*

Left

Vault of
the skull

Left middle
and inner ear

Temporal lobe (on
the lateral aspect)

Left outer ear

Mastoid process (on
the lateral aspect)

Left eustachian tube

Musculature of
the neck and
shoulder girdle

Trapezius

Brain structures
zones 2, 3, 4, 5

Visual
cortex

Throat
structures

Throat
structures

Vault of the skull

Cerebrum

Temporal lobe

Pituitary

Cerebellum

Brainstem

Base of the skull

Mastoid process

Musculature of the neck

Trapezius

Musculature of
the neck and
shoulder girdle

Right

Right upper
jaw teeth

Temporal lobe
(on the lateral
aspect)

Right middle
and inner ear

Mastoid process
(on the lateral
aspect)

Right outer ear

Right
eustachian tube

Lower jaw teeth

Throat
structures

Fig. 8.4 *Reflex zones to the head (plantar view)*

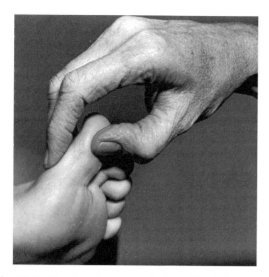

Fig. 8.5 *Treating the reflex zones to the base of the skull*

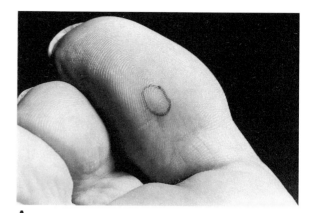

A

Just above the interphalangeal joint line is the cerebellum. *Brainstem* structures are found in zone 1 of the big toe, overlying and just distal to the interphalangeal joint line. Between skull vault and cerebellum is the *cerebrum*. Just above the cerebellum is the *pituitary*, which is usually the most prominent point on the pad of the big toe (Fig. 8.6).

Between the interphalangeal joint line and mtp joint 1 are the *muscles supporting the neck* and the *upper shoulder girdle*, while at the lateral edge are the upper fibres of the *trapezius muscle*.

Lying at the lateral edge of the plantar aspect of the big toe is the *temporal lobe*, found between the skull vault and the mastoid process, which lies adjacent to and just above the skull base.

Lateral aspect

On the lateral aspect of the big toe lie the following:

- the structures found on the lateral neck
- the muscles supporting the neck
- the ear
- the mastoid
- the temporal lobe (see Figs 8.1, 8.3, 8.4).

Medial aspect

On the medial aspect are reflex zones to the cervical spine (see Figs 8.1, 8.3).

B

Fig. 8.6 *A The reflex zones to the pituitary; B enlarged reflex zones to the pituitary on both feet in a patient with left hemiplegia*

The second toes

Dorsal aspect

The dorsal aspect (see Fig. 8.3) mainly corresponds to reflex zones to the *bones, muscles and nerve supply* of the face in zone 2, whilst the toenail represents the *forehead* in zone 2, and beneath this the *eye* on that side of the body.

Reflex zones to the *teeth* in zones 2, 3 and 4 are found on the medial and lateral aspects of the second, third and fourth toes, with a small overlap occurring onto the dorsum and plantar aspects. The teeth in zone 1 lie on the dorsum only, and the wisdom teeth in zone 5 are found on the dorsum, with an overlap onto the medial aspect. The teeth of the upper jaw lie just distal to the interphalangeal joint space, and those of the lower jaw just proximal to it (see Fig. 8.3).

Plantar aspect

The plantar aspect (see Fig. 8.4) bears reflex zones to:

- the *skull vault* zone 2 distally
- the *visual cortex*
- structures of the *brain* in zone 2
- the *eustachian tube*
- structures at the *back of the throat*
- the medial and lateral borders of *the teeth*, overlapping from the medial and lateral aspects of the toe.

Medial aspect

The medial aspect (see Figs 8.3 and 8.4) bears reflex zones to:

- the structures of the *brain* in zone 2
- the upper and lower second *teeth*, whose reflex zones extend across the whole aspect of the medial aspect and have a small overlap on the dorsal and plantar aspects
- the *sinuses* and *lymphatic tissue*
- *lymph nodes* and channels.

Lateral aspect

The lateral aspect (see Figs 8.3 and 8.4) bears reflex zones to:

- the structures of the *brain* in zone 2
- the upper and lower third *teeth*, whose reflex zones extend across the whole lateral aspect of the toe, with a small overlap on the dorsal and plantar aspects
- the *sinuses* and *lymphatic tissue*
- *lymph nodes* and channels.

The third toes

Dorsal aspect

The dorsal aspect (see Fig. 8.3) bears reflex zones to:

- the lateral half of the *eye* on that side of the body
- *bones, nerves and muscles of the face* in zone 3
- *teeth* of the upper and lower jaw at the medial and lateral margins.

Plantar aspect

The plantar aspect (see Fig. 8.4) bears reflex zones to:

- the *skull vault* zone 3 distally
- the *visual cortex*
- structures of the *brain* in zone 3
- the *eustachian tube*
- structures at the *back of the throat*
- *teeth* of the upper and lower jaw at the medial and lateral margins.

Medial aspect

The medial aspect (see Fig. 8.7A) bears reflex zones to:

- the *brain* structures in zone 3
- the upper and lower fourth *teeth*
- the *sinuses* and *lymphatic tissue*
- *lymph nodes* and channels.

Lateral aspect

The lateral aspect (see Fig. 8.7B) bears reflex zones to:

- the *brain* structures in zone 3
- the upper and lower fifth *teeth* on that side
- the *sinuses* and *lymphatic tissue*
- *lymph nodes* and channels.

The fourth toes

Dorsal aspect

The dorsal aspect bears reflex zones to:

- *bones, nerves and muscles* in zone 4

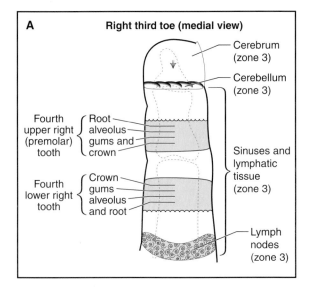

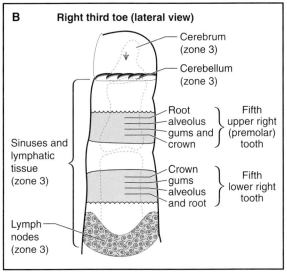

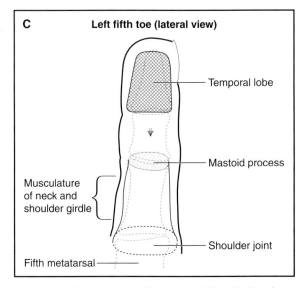

Fig. 8.7 *Diagram to show the arrangement of reflex zones on:* **A** *the medial and* **B, C** *the lateral aspects of the third and fifth toes*

- the *inner* and *middle ear*
- *teeth* of the upper and lower jaw at the medial and lateral margins.

Plantar aspect

The plantar aspect bears reflex zones to:

- the *skull vault* zone 4 distally
- structures of the *brain* in zone 4

- the *inner* and *middle ear*
- the *eustachian tube*
- structures at the *back of the throat*
- *teeth* of the upper and lower jaw at the medial and lateral margins.

Medial aspect

The medial aspect bears reflex zones to:

- structures of the *brain* in zone 4
- the upper and lower sixth *teeth* on that side
- the *sinuses* in that zone
- *lymph nodes* and channels.

Lateral aspect

The lateral aspect bears reflex zones to:

- *brain* structure of zone 4
- the upper and lower seventh *teeth* on that side
- the *sinuses* and *lymphatic tissues*
- *lymph nodes* and channels.

The fifth toes

Dorsal aspect

The dorsal aspect bears reflex zones to:

- *bones, nerves and muscles* in zone 5
- the *external ear* (the auricle and auditory meatus)
- the upper and lower eighth (wisdom) *teeth*.

Plantar aspect

The plantar aspect bears reflex zones to:

- the *skull vault* zone 5 distally
- structures of the *brain* in zone 5
- the *external ear*
- the upper and lower eighth *teeth*.

Medial aspect

The medial aspect bears reflex zones to:

- *brain* structures of zone 5
- the upper and lower eighth *teeth*
- the *sinuses*
- *lymphatic nodes* and channels.

Lateral aspect

The lateral aspect (see Fig. 8.7C) bears reflex zones to:

- the *temporal lobe* of the brain
- the *mastoid* area
- *musculature of the neck* and *shoulder girdle*.

Toe webs and bases

In the webs of the toes, distal to the mtp joint line, are found reflex zones to all the *lymphatic structures* within the neck and the throat (see Figs 8.24 and 8.25).

In the remaining area between the bases of the toes and mtp joints 2–5 on both plantar and dorsal aspects lie reflex zones to *musculature of the neck* and of the *shoulder girdle*.

A record should be made of all those reflex zones in which pain, disordered sensation, skin or tissue tone has been found. If there are many disorders in the head zones, it is suggested that a separate record card showing reflex zones to the face be used when there is a concentration of disordered reflex zones over this area. As the therapist becomes more experienced she usually finds that she is able to complete her records at the end of the session. During the early stages of her practice, however, she may want to record her findings at assessment after each system has been palpated in its entirety.

The musculoskeletal system

These reflex zones are found on all four aspects of both feet (Figs 8.8 and 8.9). The spine, being a central structure, is reflected equally in zone 1 of both the left and right feet.

Medial aspect

On the medial aspect are found the reflex zones to the bones, muscles and neural pathways of the spine. These include the:

- *cervical spine*, lying medial to the proximal phalanx of the big toe
- *thoracic spine*, medial to the first metatarsal bone
- *lumbar spine*, medial to the first cuneiform and the navicular bones
- *sacrum*, which begins at the articulation between the navicular, talus and calcaneum bones and extends along the medial calcaneum (Fig. 8.10); the reflex zone to the *sacroiliac joints* are also found over this articulation

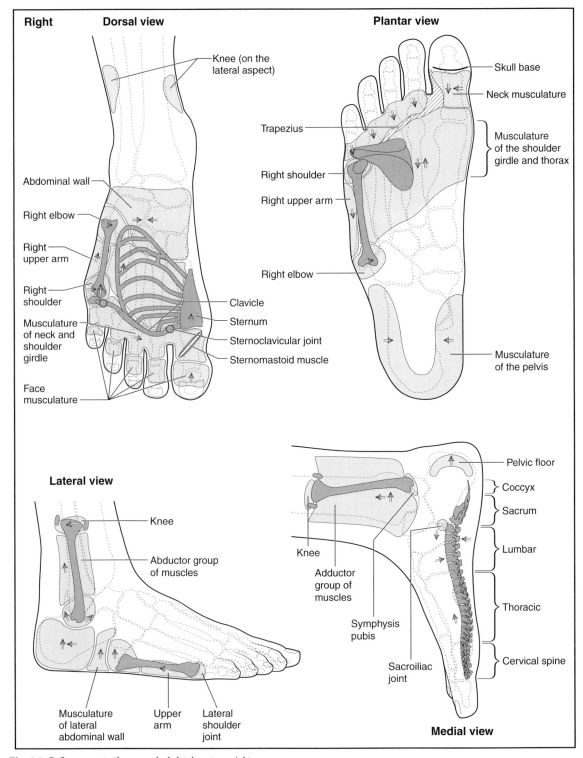

Fig. 8.8 *Reflex zones to the musculoskeletal system: right*

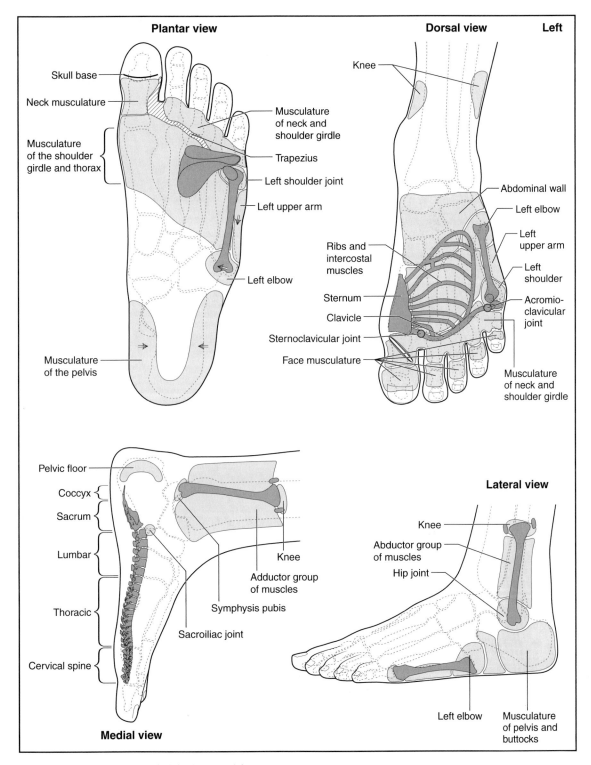

Fig. 8.9 *Reflex zones to the musculoskeletal system: left*

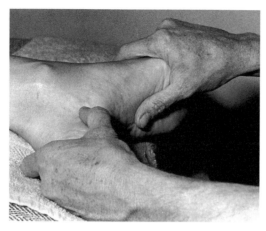

Fig. 8.10 *Treating the reflex zones to the coccyx and sacrum. Without allowing any weight to be transmitted to the foot, the right hand holds the foot, the fingers of the left hand support the foot while the thumb palpates the zones.*

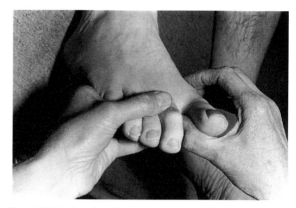

Fig. 8.11 *Treating the reflex zones to the sternum*

- *coccyx*, medial to the middle third of the calcaneum (Fig. 8.10)
- *symphysis pubis*, within a crescent just inferior and posterior to the internal malleolus
- *musculature of the pelvic floor*, lying over the large area of the medial calcaneum
- *medial musculature of the thigh* (the *adductor* group), medial to the tibia and extending about a handsbreadth proximally from the internal malleolus
- *knee*, which lies the patient's handsbreadth above the internal malleolus.

Dorsal aspect

On the dorsal aspect lie reflex zones to the:

- *face*, over the toes
- *neck*, between the mtp joint line and the proximal interphalangeal joints on all toes
- *sternum*, occupying approximately the distal two-thirds of the first metatarsal, towards the midline (Fig. 8.11)
- *clavicle*, extending from mtp joint 1 to mtp joint 5, the *sternoclavicular joint* at the head of the first and second metatarsals, and the *acromioclavicular joint* at the head of the fourth and fifth metatarsals
- *ribs*, extending across all five metatarsal bones

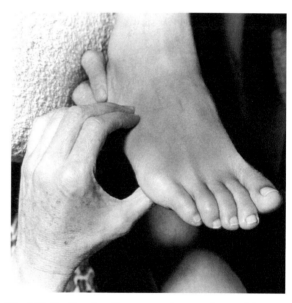

Fig. 8.12 *Treating the reflex zones to the musculature of the abdominal wall*

- *shoulder joint*, which occupies the whole of mtp joint 5
- *upper arm*, which lies over the fifth metatarsal
- *elbow*, surrounding the base of the fifth metatarsal
- *musculature of the shoulder girdle*, which covers the distal third of all five metatarsal bones
- *intercostal muscles*, which overlie all five metatarsal bones
- *musculature of the abdominal wall*, which covers all the tarsal bones (Fig. 8.12).

Lateral aspect

On the lateral aspect are found reflex zones to the:

- *shoulder joint* (its lateral aspect), surrounding mtp joint 5
- *upper arm* (its lateral aspect), lateral to the fifth metatarsal
- *elbow* (its lateral aspect), lateral to the base of the fifth metatarsal
- *hip joint*, lying in a crescent immediately inferior to the external malleolus:
- *musculature of the pelvic girdle*, lying over the lateral aspect of the calcaneum
- *musculature of the lateral thigh* (the *abductor* group), overlying the fibula, extending approximately a handsbreadth above the external malleolus
- *knee*, overlying the fibula, distal to the external malleolus by the patient's handsbreadth; this mainly reflects structures of the lateral knee.

Plantar aspect

On the plantar aspect are found the:

- *musculature of the neck and shoulder girdle,* overlying the proximal phalanx of the big toe, the proximal phalanges of the second, third, fourth and fifth toes and the mtp joint line
- *trapezius muscle,* from the head of the fourth and fifth metatarsals across the mtp joint line to the lateral articulation of the proximal and distal phalanges of the big toe
- *musculature of the shoulder girdle and thorax,* extending from the length of the fifth metatarsal to the midline of the foot, and from the mtp joint line to the bases of the metatarsals
- *shoulder joint,* over the articulation of the head of the fifth metatarsal and the proximal third of the proximal phalanx of the fifth toe
- *upper arm,* lateral to the fifth metatarsal bone
- *elbow joint,* over the base of the fifth metatarsal bone
- *musculature of the buttocks and pelvis,* in a wide border around the medial, lateral and posterior calcaneum.

The cardiovascular system

Since the heart is virtually a midline structure, its reflex zones are distributed over the dorsal, plantar and medial aspects of both feet, although they lie over a larger area on the left foot than on the right (Figs 8.13 and 8.14).

Plantar aspect

On the plantar aspect are found the reflex zones to the cardiovascular system:

- overlying the distal half of the first metatarsal bone on the right foot
- overlying the distal half of the first and medial half of the second metatarsal bones on the left foot.

Dorsal aspect

On the dorsum the zones are found:

- overlying the distal half of the first metatarsal bone on the right foot
- overlying the distal half of the first and medial half of the second metatarsal bones on the left foot. The *aortic arch* in the midline lies distal to the heart zones, and is larger over the medial head of the first metatarsal on the left
- the *aorta* and *vena cava* can be treated over the midpoint of the first metatarsal up to their bifurcation over the navicular bone.

Medial aspect

On the medial aspect these zones are found overlying the distal half of the first metatarsal bone on both feet. (When treating the reflex zones to the heart on either dorsal or plantar aspects of the foot, include the midline zones in both assessment and treatment (Fig. 8.15).)

The respiratory system

The reflex zones to the respiratory system are distributed over the dorsal and plantar metatarsal bones on both feet (Figs 8.16 and 8.17).

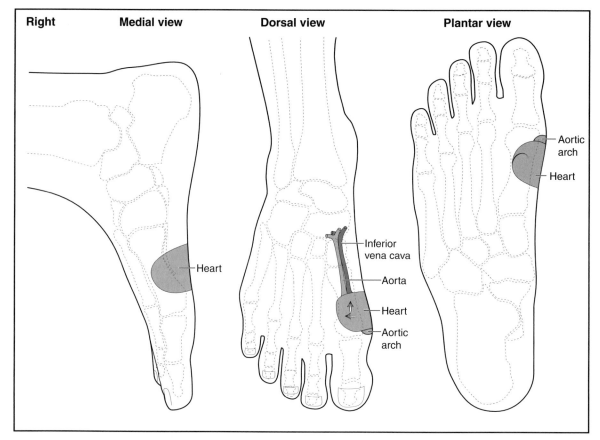

Fig. 8.13 *Reflex zones to the heart: right*

Plantar aspect

The plantar aspect bears the reflex zones to the:

- *trachea*, overlying the first metatarsal bone on both feet
- *lungs*, overlying the second to fifth metatarsal bones on both feet
- *diaphragm*, the anterior attachment arching from the midpoint of the first metatarsal bone to the base of the fourth/fifth metatarsal, and the posterior aspect arching from the base of the first metatarsal (equivalent to the base of the 12th thoracic rib) to the base of the fourth/fifth metatarsal bones
- *solar plexus*, the midpoint of the second metatarsal bone extending to overlap both first and third metatarsal bones (treating the whole area of the diaphragm also affects the solar

plexus, improving respiratory function and filling the bases of the lungs).

Dorsal aspect

The dorsal aspect bears the reflex zones to the:

- *oronasopharynx*, on the dorsum of both big toes
- *vocal cords* in zone 1, at the midpoint of the proximal phalanx on the dorsum of each big toe
- *trachea* in the midline, overlying the first metatarsal bone on both feet;
- *lungs*, overlying the second to fifth metatarsal bones on both feet
- *diaphragm*, arched from midpoint of the first metatarsal bone to the base of the fifth metatarsal bone.

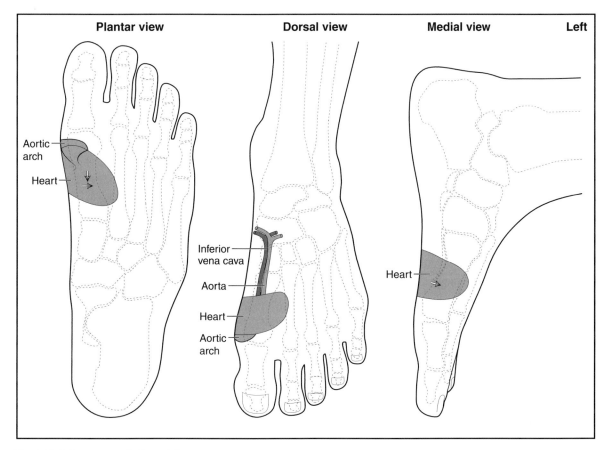

Fig. 8.14 *Reflex zones to the heart: left*

The urinary system

The reflex zones of the urinary system are found on the plantar, medial and dorsal surfaces of both feet (Figs 8.18 and 8.19).

Plantar aspect

The plantar aspect bears reflex zones to:

- the *kidneys*, at the bases of the second and third metatarsal bones on both feet
- the *ureters*, which track down from the bases of the second and third metatarsals over the second cuneiform bones, the navicular and the calcaneum; when the toe is dorsiflexed, the flexor tendon hallucis longus becomes

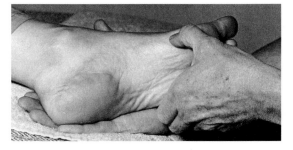

Fig. 8.15 *When treating the reflex zones to the heart on the dorsum the therapist should include zones in the midline in assessment and treatment*

prominent (Fig. 8.20), and the ureters lie medial to this tendon.

Medial aspect

The medial aspect bears reflex zones to:

- the *bladder*, which lies below the internal malleolus (the bladder has long been treated as the small (often puffy) area adjacent to the sacrum; because of the complex innervation of the bladder, with both sympathetic and parasympathetic as well as CNS fibres, some of which emerge from the lumbar and sacral spine, treatment here is also effective
- the *ureters*, which track from the plantar aspect over the distal third of the calcaneum to meet

the reflex zone to the bladder just below the internal malleolus.

Dorsal aspect

The dorsal aspect bears reflex zones to:

- the *kidneys*, at the bases of the second and third metatarsal bones on left and right feet.

The gastrointestinal system

The reflex zones of the gastrointestinal system are found over all four aspects of both feet (Figs 8.21 and 8.22).

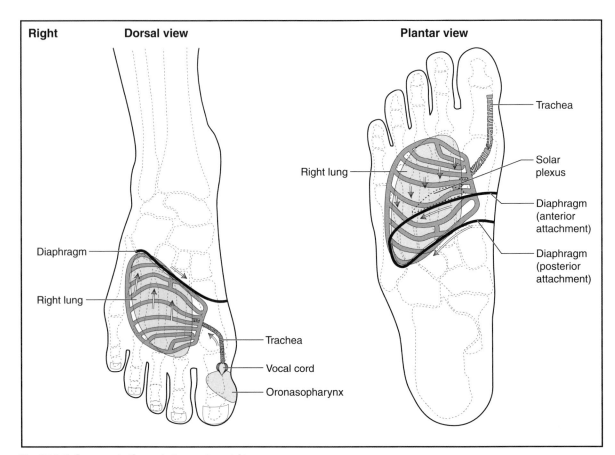

Right   **Dorsal view**   **Plantar view**

Trachea

Solar plexus

Diaphragm (anterior attachment)

Diaphragm (posterior attachment)

Right lung

Diaphragm

Right lung

Trachea

Vocal cord

Oronasopharynx

Fig. 8.16 *Reflex zones to the respiratory system: right*

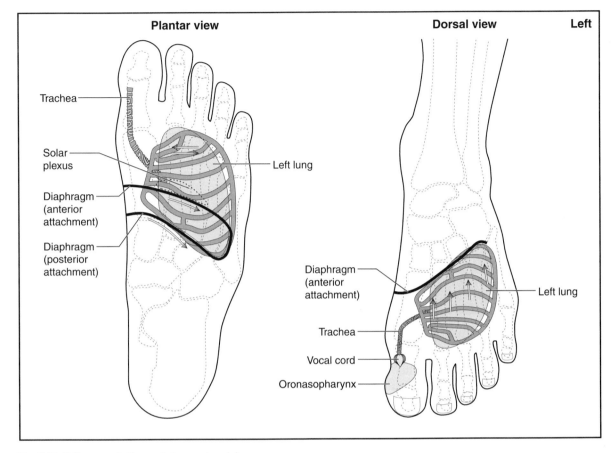

Fig. 8.17 *Reflex zones to the respiratory system: left*

Plantar aspect

The plantar aspect bears reflex zones to the:

- *oesophagus*, beneath the first metatarsal bone on both feet
- *cardia* (entrance to the stomach, where the oesophagus passes through the diaphragm), on the left foot only, at a point approximately one-third distal to the base of the first and second metatarsal bones
- *stomach*, overlying the bases of both first metatarsal bones
- *pyloric sphincter* (whose thickened circular fibres prevent food from passing too rapidly into the duodenum), on the right foot only, at the base of the first and second metatarsal bones
- *duodenum*, which lies on the right foot

- *liver*, overlying the proximal third of the fourth, third, second and first metatarsal bones on the right foot, with a small tongue extending over the base of the first metatarsal bone on the left foot
- *gall bladder*, lateral to the pyloric sphincter, towards the base of the third metatarsal bone
- *pancreas*, spanning the articulation of the first cuneiform and metatarsal bones on the right foot, and the articulation of first, second and third cuneiform and metatarsal bones on the left foot; the pancreas has many digestive as well as endocrine functions, and is treated with whichever is the most disordered system — the therapist, being mindful of the fact that the picture of painful and disordered reflex zones can and often does change at each successive visit, adapts and tailors her treatment accordingly

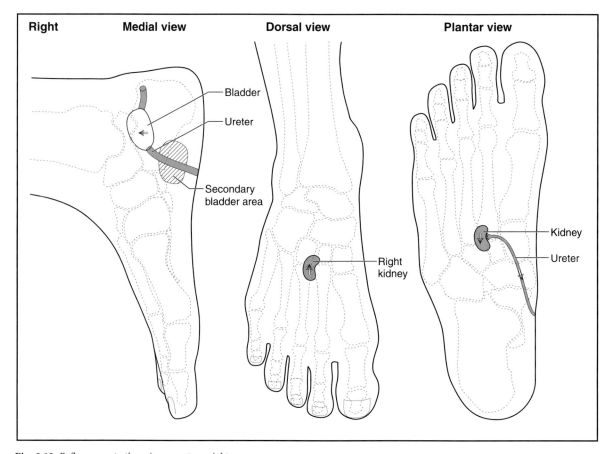

Fig. 8.18 *Reflex zones to the urinary system: right*

- *jejunum* and *ileum*, overlying the arched tarsal bones on both feet (Fig. 8.23)
- *ileocaecal valve* and *appendix* (separating the small from the large intestine), sharing the same reflex zone on the lateral articulating surface of calcaneum and cuboid bones in zone 4 on the right foot only (the reflex zone to the ileocaecal valve is most easily found by resting the fingers of the left hand over the dorsum so that the joint of the thumb wraps round the lateral border of the foot below the level of the base of the fifth metatarsal, where it fits well into the cuboid indentation; the tip of the thumb is directed towards the midline of the foot, but palpates zone 4)
- *ascending colon*, the first part of the large intestine, overlying the calcaneal, cuboid and base of the fifth metatarsal bone on the right foot, where it bends sharply at the *hepatic flexure* before it becomes the
- *transverse colon*, which stretches across the abdominal cavity and also spans all the cuneiform bones of both feet, bending sharply at the *splenic flexure* at the base of the fifth metatarsal on the left foot, then becoming the
- *descending colon*, overlying the base of fifth metatarsal, the cuboid and calcaneal bones on the left foot, and itself bending sharply to become the
- *sigmoid colon*, overlying the articulation of the calcaneal and talus bones, on the left foot only.

Dorsal aspect

The dorsal aspect bears reflex zones to the:

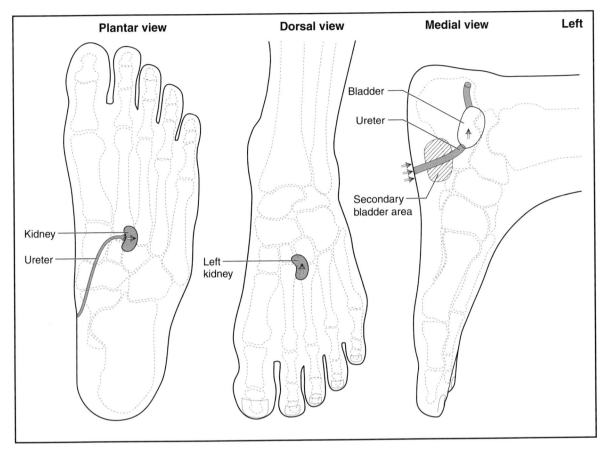

Fig. 8.19 *Reflex zones to the urinary system: left*

- *mouth*, overlying the distal, medial half of the proximal phalanx on both feet
- *oesophagus*, over the first metatarsal bone on both feet
- *gall bladder*, between the bases of the third and fourth metatarsal bones, on the right foot only
- *ascending colon*, overlying the cuboid bone in zone 5 on the right foot
- *appendix*, where the calcaneum and the cuboid bones meet, in zone 4 on the right foot only
- *descending colon*, overlying the cuboid bone in zone 5 on the left foot.

Lateral aspect

On the lateral aspect are found reflex zones to the:

- *ascending colon*, alongside the cuboid bone on the right foot

- *descending colon*, alongside the cuboid bone on the left foot.

Medial aspect

On the medial aspect are found reflex zones to the:

- midline structures of *rectum* and *anus*, found on the medial aspect of both heels alongside and proximal to the reflex zone to the coccyx
- *stomach, liver, pancreas, small intestine* and *transverse colon*, which are all influenced by treatment of the spine at the levels from which their nerve supplies are derived (reflex zones which are painful or disordered over, for example, the lumbar spine, should be treated in conjunction with painful reflex zones to those organs and structures to which they are related).

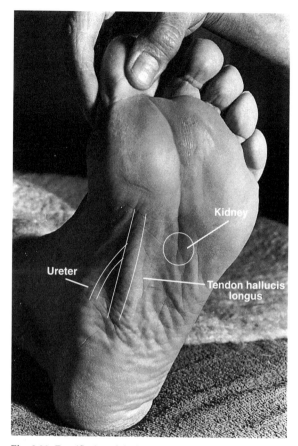

Fig. 8.20 *Dorsiflexion of the big toe to show the tendon of flexor hallucis longus*

The lymphatic system

The reflex zones to the lymphatic system are distributed over all four aspects of both feet (Figs 8.24 and 8.25).

Dorsal aspect

On the dorsal aspect are found the reflex zones to the:

- lymph nodes draining the *oronasopharynx*, lying on the big toe and overlying the interphalangeal joint on both feet
- *tonsils*, on the dorsum of each big toe, at approximately the midpoint on the lateral border of the proximal phalanx;
- lymph nodes of the *neck*, on the lateral aspect of the proximal phalanx of the big toe in zone 4–5,

and distal to the mtp joint line in the webs between all 10 toes (Fig. 8.26).

Note: The tissues in the webs of the toes are best assessed and treated with the thumb resting on the plantar foot, at or just above the mtp joint space, while the flexed index finger of the same hand steadily rolls the subcutaneous tissues between the toes like a wave before its fingertip, until thumb and finger meet (Fig. 8.27). The thumb stays in its original position on the sole of the foot, and the index finger 'milks' the subcutaneous tissue from the dorsum towards the sole, bringing about a good vascularisation of these tissues. This movement is painful when the reflex zones to these lymph nodes are unhealthy, so it must always be performed quite slowly and gently until the pain diminishes, as it does when the zones improve. Neither the skin nor the tissues should be pinched at any time, and the therapist should avoid any unnecessary friction on the skin.

- *mediastinal lymph nodes*, between the distal halves of the first and second metatarsal bones, and the proximal halves of the proximal phalanges of the first and second toes on both feet; these often form a callused cord over this area when there is long standing respiratory distress
- *apical lymph nodes*, lying just proximal to the heads of the first to fourth metatarsal bones, between the axillary lymphatic tissue and that of the mediastinum
- *thymus*, beneath the head of the first metatarsal bone, behind the sternum on both feet
- lymphatic tissue of the *breasts*, overlying the middle third of the second, third and fourth metatarsal bones on both feet
- lymph nodes of the *axilla*, proximal to the head of the fourth and fifth metatarsal bones on both feet;
- lymphatic tissue of the *spleen*, overlying the base of the fourth and fifth metatarsal bones on the left foot only
- lymphatic tissue of the *appendix*, on the right foot only, where the cuboid and calcaneum articulate laterally
- *inguinal lymph nodes* in the groin lie along the length of the articulation of the talus with the tibia and fibula on both feet, i.e. in the fold of the ankle.

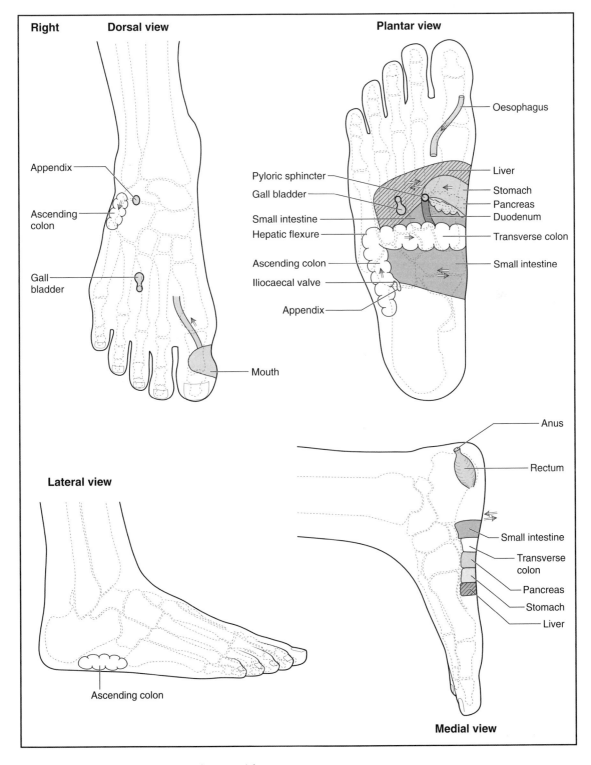

Fig. 8.21 *Reflex zones to the gastrointestinal system: right*

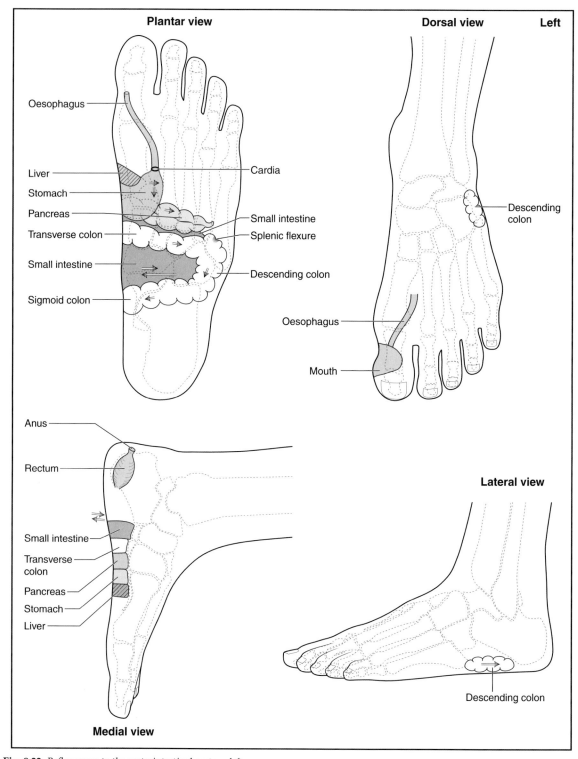

Plantar view

Oesophagus

Liver
Stomach
Pancreas
Transverse colon
Small intestine
Sigmoid colon

Cardia
Small intestine
Splenic flexure
Descending colon

Dorsal view **Left**

Descending colon

Oesophagus

Mouth

Anus
Rectum

Small intestine
Transverse colon
Pancreas
Stomach
Liver

Lateral view

Descending colon

Medial view

Fig. 8.22 *Reflex zones to the gastrointestinal system: left*

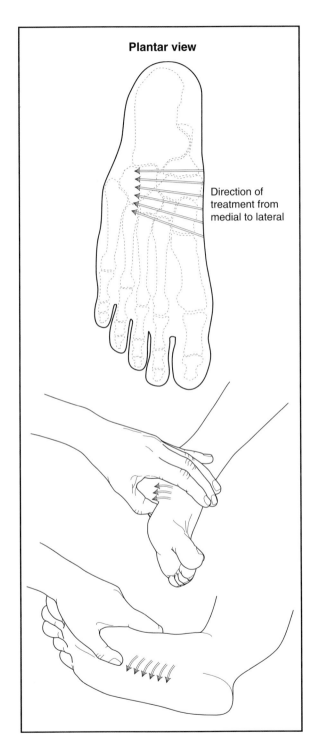

Plantar view

Direction of treatment from medial to lateral

Fig. 8.23 *Tracking across the reflex zones to the small intestine*

Plantar aspect

On the plantar aspect are found the reflex zones to the:

- lymph nodes in the *throat* and *neck*, in the webs of all 10 toes, distal to the mtp joint line
- *mediastinal lymph nodes*, lying between the distal half of the first and second metatarsal bones and the proximal third of the proximal phalanges of the first and second toes
- lymph nodes of the *axilla*, lying below the head of the fourth and fifth metatarsal bones on both feet
- lymphatic tissue of the *spleen*, overlying the bases of the fourth and the medial half of the fifth metatarsal bones on the left foot only
- lymphatic tissue of the *appendix*, on the right foot only, where the cuboid and calcaneal bones meet
- lymphatic tissue investing the *pelvic organs*, beneath the calcaneum (although as this tissue is so densely woven it is often more effective to treat these zones on the medial and lateral aspects of the heels; it is, however, responsive to treatment in young people and those who have been bedfast for long periods).

Medial aspect

On the medial aspect are found reflex zones to the:

- *thymus*, medial to the first metatarsal
- lymph nodes of the *pelvis*, overlying the medial aspect of the calcaneum;
- lymphatic nodes and vessels of the *thighs*, overlying the medial aspect of the Achilles' tendon on both feet, and extending proximally about a handsbreadth from the level of the internal malleolus towards the knees.

Lateral aspect

On the lateral aspect are found the reflex zones to the:

- lymph nodes of the *pelvis*, overlying the lateral aspect of the calcaneum;
- lymphatic nodes and vessels of the *thighs*, overlying the lateral aspect of the Achilles' tendon on both feet, extending proximally for a

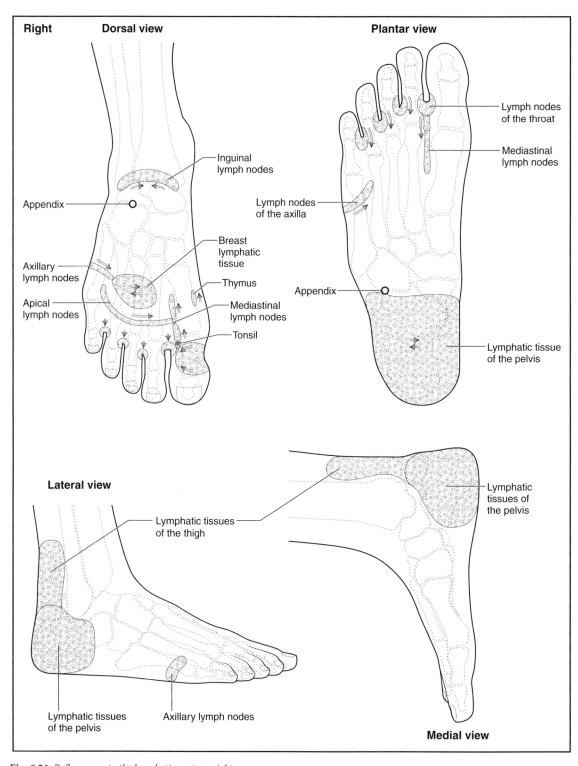

Fig. 8.24 *Reflex zones to the lymphatic system: right*

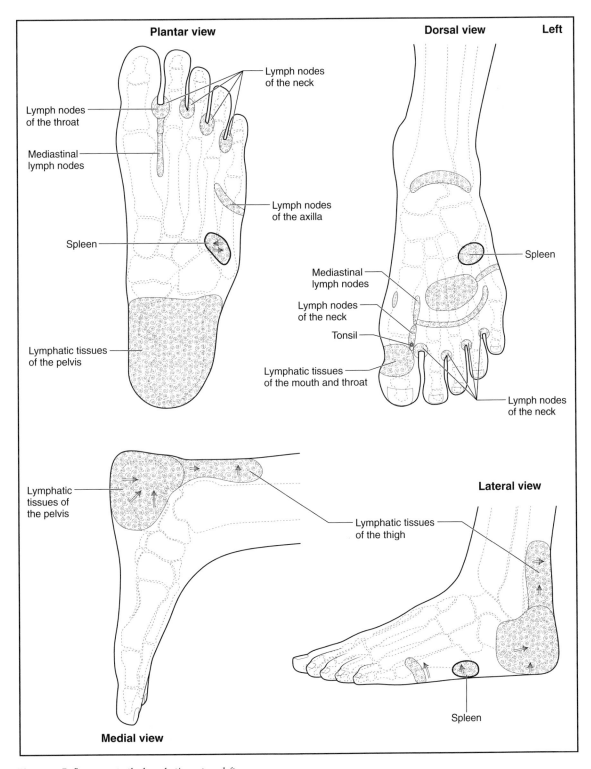

Fig. 8.25 *Reflex zones to the lymphatic system: left*

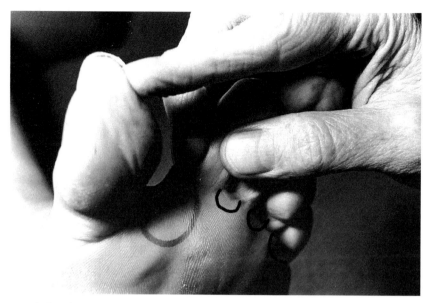

Fig. 8.26 *Reflex zones to the lymph nodes in the neck reflected in the webs of the toes*

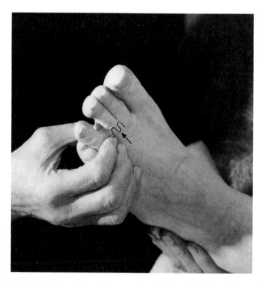

Fig. 8.27 *Treating the reflex zones to the lymph nodes of the neck*

handsbreadth towards the knees from the external malleolus

- *spleen*, over the base of the fourth metatarsal bone
- *axillary lymph nodes*, proximal to the head of the fifth metatarsal bone.

The endocrine system

Hormones (each bearing chemically distinct proteins and their own 'chemical address') are released directly from the endocrine glands into the bloodstream, which carries them to their target organs. The pituitary, lodged within the skull and partially attached to the hypothalamus, connects the endocrine system to the hypothalamic centre of the ANS. Here are directed those life-sustaining functions which take place below the level of conscious awareness.

The reflex zones of the endocrine system are distributed over all four aspects of both feet (Figs 8.28 and 8.29).

Dorsal aspect

On the dorsal aspect are found the reflex zones to the:

- *thyroid* and *parathyroid* glands, over the medial two-thirds of the proximal third of the proximal phalanx of the big toe on both feet
- *fallopian tube* and the *inguinal canal*, along a narrow line across the width of the talus where it articulates with the tibia and fibula, just distal

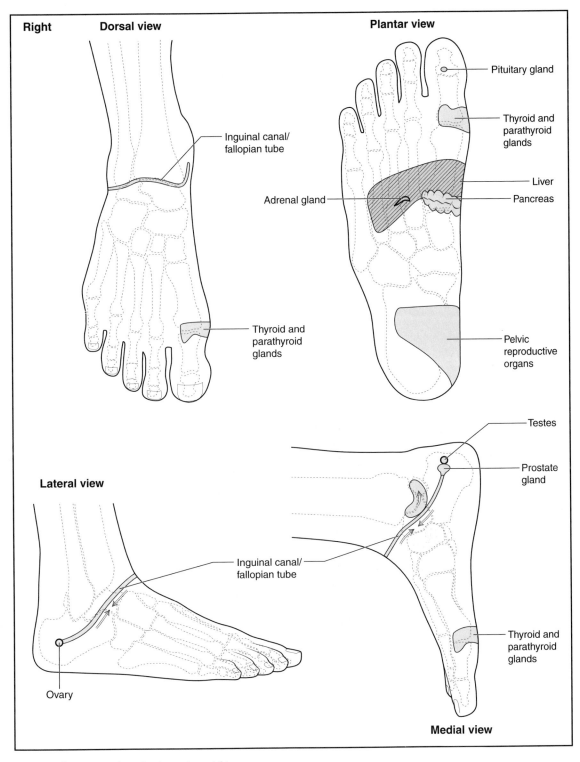

Fig. 8.28 *Reflex zones to the endocrine system: right*

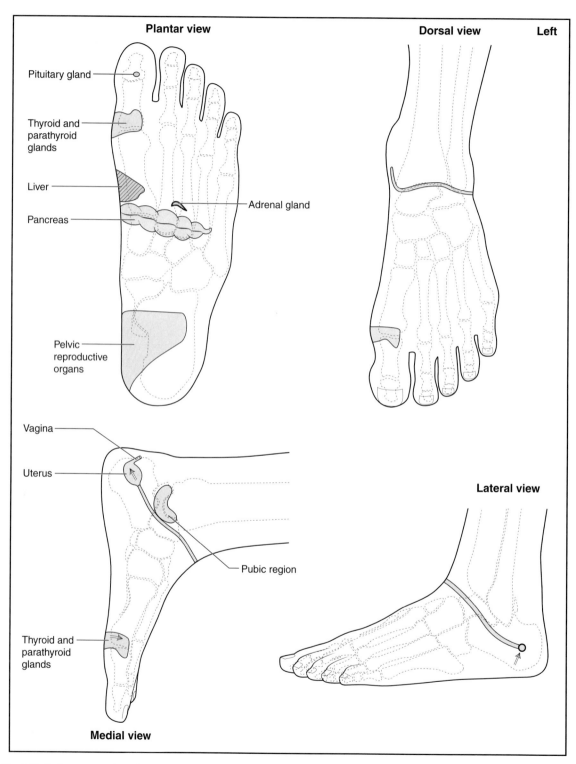

Fig. 8.29 *Reflex zones to the endocrine system: left*

to the ankle fold (although these structures are not endocrine glands, they are included in treatment of this system).

Plantar aspect

On the plantar aspect are found the reflex zones to the:

- *pituitary gland*, on the pad of the big toe on both feet
- *thyroid* and *parathyroid glands*, overlying mtp joint 1 on both feet
- *adrenal glands*, just distal to the expanded bases of the second and third metatarsal bones of both feet
- *pancreas*, the head overlying the proximal base of the first metatarsal and the distal third of the first cuneiform bone on the right foot, with the body and tail lying across the bases of the first, second and third metatarsals and the distal third of the first, second and third cuneiform bones on the left foot
- *liver*, which has both exocrine and endocrine functions, and is the largest endocrine gland of all and may be treated with either system
- *reproductive organs*, over the calcaneum.

Medial aspect

On the medial aspect are found reflex zones to the:

- female *uterus* and *vagina*, the male *prostate* and *testes*, over the posterior half of the calcaneum
- *fallopian tube* and *inguinal canal*, extending from the dorsal aspect of the foot to lie across the medial talus and calcaneum before connecting with the reproductive organs
- structures of the *pubic region*, lying in a semicircle inferiorly to the internal malleolus
- *thyroid* and *parathyroid glands*, which are influenced by treatment over the articulation at mtp joint 1.

Lateral aspect

On the lateral aspect are found reflex zones to the:

- *ovaries*, lying at a point midway on an imaginary line drawn from the external malleolus to the angle of the heel

- *fallopian tube* and *inguinal canal*, extending from the dorsal aspect to lie across the lateral talus and calcaneum, before connecting with the ovaries and abdominal wall.

All the reflex zones of the feet reflecting our present knowledge and understanding of their location are shown together in Figures 8.30 and 8.31.

Using the fingers and both hands for assessment and treatment

With practice the therapist should become sufficiently skilled at using all her fingers and both hands together to be able to complete the assessment in 30–40 minutes. Disordered reflex zones can be competently treated in the 25 to 30 minutes of normal treatment time if the dosage is accurately gauged. By adopting from the beginning a disciplined approach to treatment the therapist is able to focus on those areas most in need of attention. Assessment of all the reflex zones on each big toe is best done individually one at a time and, if time does not permit at the first visit, it can be completed at the second.

It is usual for one thumb, usually that of the dominant hand, to be favoured while learning to locate reflex zones and developing method in assessment and treatment over the first few weeks or months of practice. Once the therapist has become confident of her ability to detect subtle variations of disorder in the tissues by palpation, and to identify all the reflex zones, and has learned to judge the amount of time needed for each individual session, first one or more fingers and then both hands can be used in unison on either one or both feet (see Ch. 6, p. 99).

Advantages

This facilitates distinctions between:

- subtle differences in tissue tone in both feet
- changes in skin texture
- difference in levels of discomfort in affected reflex zones.

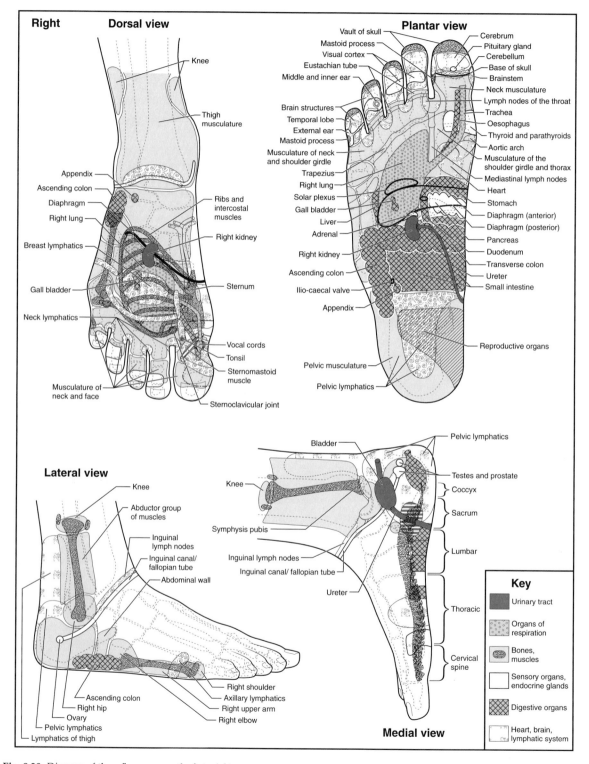

Fig. 8.30 *Diagram of the reflex zones on the feet: right*

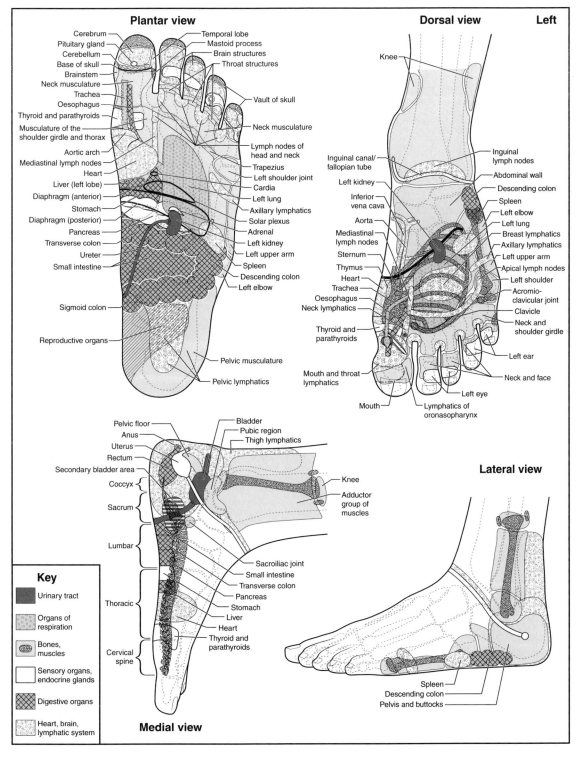

Fig. 8.31 *Diagram of the reflex zones on the feet: left*

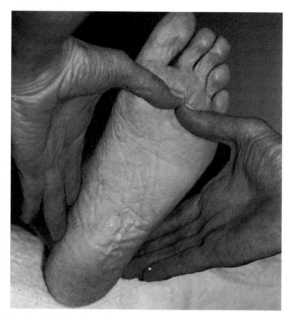

Fig. 8.32 *Supporting the metatarsal heads with both thumbs*

Furthermore, a greater stimulus, more evenly distributed, is delivered to the GRS. Using both hands enables the therapist to treat large areas in a shorter time, her hands returning to treat the disordered zones of the lungs, abdominal wall, intestines and pelvic lymphatics many times. In between, small areas such as the tonsils, appendix or adrenals can be treated individually with one thumb or finger, and the emphasis then shifted to less painful areas of the foot before returning to these frequently vulnerable areas. Because of the enlarged area of skin contact, any change in temperature or perspiration of either foot is likely to be noticed more quickly. As the therapist becomes increasingly ambidextrous, her movements become more rhythmical and balanced. Finally, all patients prefer it.

When using both hands the most convenient place for the thumbs to rest is at the heads of the second and third metatarsal bones (Fig. 8.32). This allows the therapist to support the foot and hold it in the desired position for and during treatment. Also, there are no reflex zones in this vicinity which are likely to be overstimulated by this hold.

Note: At no time should the therapist's thumbs be placed over the reflex zones to the kidneys, the adrenal glands or the solar plexus, as these reflex zones might, however inadvertently, be unduly stimulated by such prolonged pressure. In those who are ill, weak, or those in whom these reflex zones are already painful, even slight pressure soon results in overtreatment.

Very few people feel comfortable when their toes are either plantarflexed or dorsiflexed by the weight of the therapist's hands, which should always be in contact with the skin surface, but the patient should not feel their weight. Once the thumb has become proficient at the basic technique (Fig. 8.33A), the therapist should begin practising with the index fingers (Fig. 8.33B), then introduce the third and fourth fingers, using each one singly to begin with, and then in combinations adapted to whichever part of the foot is being treated (Fig. 8.33C). The little finger rarely plays any active part in palpation, but as it rests on the skin it is used as a sensor for and remains alert to changes in temperature, perspiration or tension.

While it is generally best to carry out the assessment and treatment using both hands synchronously for palpation and holding, it is at times necessary to revert to working with just one thumb or finger while treating one small surface or a particularly painful reflex zone.

Method

The same principles apply to using the fingers as the thumbs.

1. The relaxed wrist lies in a straight line with the forearm.
2. Each finger joint is kept in slight flexion. Overextending any joint is detrimental to its structure in the long term, and often causes pain in the short term.
3. The palpating fingertip or tips are always held level with the wrist.
4. The first contact with the skin is made by the tips of the fingers. Any alteration of temperature in individual reflex zones, of the condition of the skin — whether rough or even, and particularly dryness or moisture — are noted, and then any palpable changes there may be in the immediately underlying tissues.

A

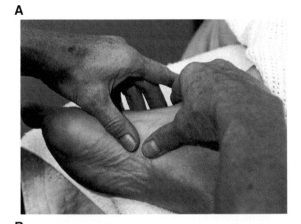

B

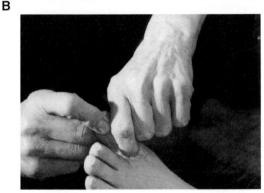

C

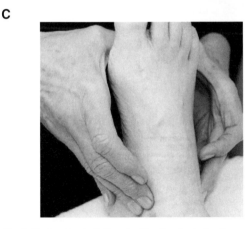

Fig. 8.33 *A using both thumbs; B using the index fingers; C using the fingers of both hands*

At the same time the therapist needs to be aware of the patient's response to what she is doing. Using both hands has the capacity to intensify the treatment, and the frail person reacts

more quickly than another to any stimulus. As is well known, the borderline between a therapeutic stimulus which has its intended effect and one which becomes toxic because it is too strong is a fine one; it is preferable that the patient be undertreated rather than overtreated.

5. This is followed by the same even movement of the fingers as they flow into the subcutaneous tissues in the active phase, and are immediately allowed to be retracted from the tissues in the passive phase, during which time the tissues resume their normal contour before the next movement is made. There is as much to be noticed about the resilience of the tissues during the passive as during the active phase.

6. The muscles of the hand, wrist and forearm should be relaxed before the fingers are advanced by no more than a millimetre or so to probe the next reflex zones.

Using both hands for the assessment

Using both hands and all fingers to perform an assessment in a methodical way allows a clear pattern of observations to be developed. Either both hands are used in palpation or, for those areas where bimanual treatment is awkward, one hand supports the foot and monitors any changes while the other is the treating hand, and is more attentive to what is being palpated.

Since reflex zones to the lungs, breasts, ribs and intercostal muscles lie over the dorsal metatarsal bones, which are generally less protected by muscle and fat, it is advisable to work in the spaces lying between the metatarsal bones and not to work directly over bones and their periosteal covering, which lie so closely underneath the skin. Both hands working together are perfectly adapted to working on the dorsum of either foot, but it is generally less effective to treat the dorsum of left and right feet simultaneously. For this reason, most of the assessment and much treatment on the dorsum is given to one foot at a time.

Also, any one area of the foot may require more intensive treatment than its counterpart. The area of the hip joint is also unwieldy to assess or treat on both feet at the same time, and frequently either just the medial or the lateral aspect of a heel need to be treated. For such zones the basic technique is employed — one hand giving treatment, the other supporting and holding the foot.

The following sequence is recommended for bimanual assessment, followed by some well-adapted holding positions and suggestions for treatment. All assessment and treatment are interspersed with harmonising measures as called for by the patient's responses.

The zones of the head

Each big toe is rotated individually.

With the fingers resting on the dorsum, the thumbs palpate across the vault of the skull on both feet. Resting the straight index fingers on the dorsal aspects, the thumbs palpate both *plantar* surfaces.

Resting the straight index finger on the lateral surface, the thumbs palpate both *medial* surfaces.

Resting the outstretched thumbs on the plantar surface, the index fingers palpate each *dorsum* of the big toe.

Resting the outstretched thumb on the medial surfaces, the index fingers palpate each of the *lateral* aspects.

Resting as much of the straight index finger as possible along the toe gives support and reduces the possibility that the thumb and index finger will be used for palpation on two surfaces at the same time. This is even more necessary when using both hands. Learning to assess and to treat one zone at a time is an essential skill in RZT. It leads to accuracy in the recorded findings and reduces the possibility of overstimulation.

This same procedure is repeated on the plantar, medial, dorsal and lateral surfaces of all other four toes of both feet, the therapist's right hand being used to treat the patient's left foot and vice versa.

The locomotor system

If the patient's hip and knee joints allow it, his feet can be moved about a foot apart. Pain in the lower spine is, however, aggravated by abduction and external rotation of the legs, and they should not be separated wider than any stiffened joints allow. Skilful use of small cushions makes treatment more comfortable for the patient and easier for the

therapist. If the patient is suffering from acute sciatica it may be better to treat one foot at a time, particularly during an acute episode.

Both of the comfortably separated feet should be treated together. The fingers rest on the dorsum while both thumbs track down the length of the medial aspect of the feet to palpate the reflex zones to the spine. Both thumbs simultaneously palpate a semicircle beneath the internal malleolus, the reflex zones to the symphysis pubis and the pubic area.

Working on both feet, the thumbs are used to palpate the plantar surface of the shoulder joint, around mtp joint 5. Using both thumbs to support the feet along the mtp joint line on the plantar surface, the index fingers palpate first the lateral shoulder joint and then the dorsal shoulder joint on both left and right feet at the same time.

The thumbs then palpate the plantar reflex zones to the upper arm and the elbow on both feet. The index fingers palpate the lateral and then the dorsal reflex zones of the upper arm and elbow.

Both thumbs then palpate the musculature of the plantar shoulder girdle on both feet, starting at the metatarsal heads and tracking proximally towards their bases.

As mentioned already, the dorsum of each foot is best assessed individually. With one foot covered, the thumb or fingers palpate the reflex zone to the sternum. With one supporting thumb on the plantar mtp joints, the therapist palpates the dorsal shoulder girdle (and at the same time the reflex zones to the lung and the breast on that side) with one or more of the fingertips, in the spaces between the bones, tracking proximally from the metatarsal heads towards the bases. This is repeated on the other foot.

Covering one foot, and keeping both thumbs at the heads of the metatarsal bones (or alternatively on the base of the first and fifth metatarsal bones), the index, middle and ring fingers of both hands together are used to assess the dorsal arch of the foot, the abdominal wall (Fig. 8.34). The same assessment is made on the other foot.

For the hip joint the following method of holding the foot with one hand and treating with the fingers of the other hand is comfortable for the patient. To work on the right foot, the therapist covers the left foot and places it in a comfortable position some distance away, where it will not be incidentally

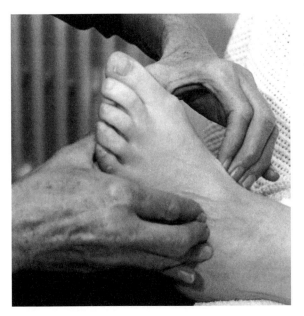

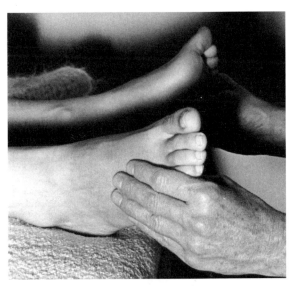

Fig. 8.35 *Assessing and treating the lungs*

Fig. 8.34 *Working on the abdominal wall, tracking across the dorsal arch using the fingers of both hands*

touched while the other foot is being treated. The therapist's right hand supports the right heel of the patient in her palm. The thumb of the left hand is positioned over the mtp joint line or over the base of the fifth metatarsal. The tips of the *left* middle and ring fingers are used, slightly flexed, to palpate a wide semicircle around the external malleolus, the reflex zones to the hip (see Fig. 8.30).

The tips of the middle and ring fingers of both hands track seamlessly up the reflex zones to the abductor and adductor muscles, on the medial and lateral aspects of the lower leg, and to the reflex zone to the knee. Alternatively, both thumbs may be used to track distally from the knee towards the malleoli in broad bands to cover the whole area of these reflex zones. To work on the left foot, the right foot is covered, the left heel supported in the therapist's left palm, and the *right* middle and ring fingertips used to palpate the hip joint, then both hands are used for the musculature of the thigh.

The heart

Resting the fingertips on the dorsum of the foot, both thumbs palpate the reflex zones to the plantar heart

from the midline on the medial aspect of the foot to the lateral borders of its reflex zone, or, tracking proximally from its upper to its lower borders. The legs are so positioned in slight outward rotation that there is enough room for the therapist to treat both feet adequately without her hands coming into contact with each other. The dorsal reflex zones are approached by resting the length of the thumbs along the plantar mtp joint line, and using the tips of the middle and ring fingers to palpate the dorsal reflex zones, starting at the midline and tracking towards the lateral foot.

The respiratory system

To assess the lungs on the plantar aspect, the fingertips of the therapist's left hand are rested on the dorsum of the patient's right foot, and the right hand on the dorsum of the patient's left foot (Fig. 8.35). Both thumbs then track proximally from the metatarsal heads towards their bases as often as is necessary to cover this large surface.

Track from the medial aspect of the feet along the reflex zones to both the upper and lower attachments of the diaphragm. The reflex zone to the solar plexus lying along this line is then palpated (Fig. 8.36).

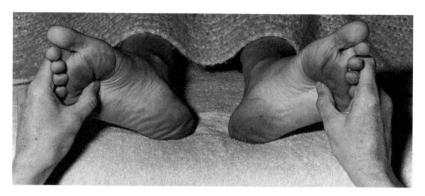

Fig. 8.36 *Using both hands to sedate the solar plexus/diaphragm*

Assessment of the lungs on the dorsum is made on one foot at a time. The area over the dorsal metatarsals includes the thoracic wall, lungs and breast tissue. It is not necessary to palpate three times over different areas; a single careful assessment of the whole surface will indicate which reflex zones need treatment. The therapist does not always know from the symptoms and history which of these systems is ailing (the patient may have come for treatment of a stiff knee), and must wait for reactions to clarify the picture. The heel is supported with either hand while the index finger of the other, starting from the metatarsal heads, tracks proximally between the bones toward their bases.

The urinary system

The dorsal reflex zones to the kidneys are individually assessed with an index finger on first one foot then another. Approaching the plantar aspect, both feet are comfortably separated, slightly outwardly rotated, and both thumbs are used to palpate the reflex zones to left and right kidneys simultaneously. Without lifting the thumbs from their position in the kidney zones, the little fingers are used to dorsiflex the big toes briefly in order to show the flexor tendon hallucis longus and then immediately allow them to return to their normal position. The thumbs, in a smooth and continuous movement, then track proximally (medial to the tendon) along the reflex zones to the ureters, cross the lower spine and then cross the medial aspect of the heels to treat the bladder on both left and right heels.

Gastrointestinal tract

Both feet are uncovered to the ankles and set a comfortable distance apart. Using both thumbs the therapist tracks down the reflex zones to the plantar oesophagus, and then down the reflex zones to the stomach on both right and left feet, starting from the midline. (The dorsal oesophagus will have been assessed already during palpation of other systems overlying the dorsum in zone 1.)

To assess the reflex zones to the small intestine, the therapist tracks from the midline towards the lateral aspect of the foot, one thumb palpating the arch of each foot.

The left index finger is used to palpate the dorsal reflex zone to the gall bladder on the right dorsum, and the thumb on the plantar gall bladder.

The left thumb is used for the plantar reflex zone to the appendix and the left index, middle or ring finger for its dorsal reflex zone.

The large intestine is best assessed following the direction of peristalsis. For this, either thumb tracks distally along the reflex zones to the ascending and then towards the midline over the transverse colon on the right foot; then it tracks laterally along the reflex zones to the rest of transverse colon on the left foot. The left or right thumb, whichever is more comfortable, follows the descending colon proximally, and then tracks toward the midline over the sigmoid colon. Both thumbs, or index, or index and middle or middle and ring fingers are used to palpate the reflex zones to the rectum and anus on the medial heels.

The liver is assessed with both thumbs tracking either from the midline towards its lateral border, or from its upper to its lower border. The pancreas is assessed by both thumbs, starting from the midline, the left tracking in a lateral direction across the articulation of the cuneiform with first metatarsal on the right foot, the right thumb tracking laterally across the articulation of cuneiform with the first to third metatarsals on the left.

The lymphatic system

An index finger is used to palpate the reflex zones to first one and then the other tonsil individually. Resting the thumbs on the plantar foot just distal to the mtp joint 1, and the index fingers just distal to the dorsal mtp joint 1, the reflex zones in the webs of the toes are 'milked' by bringing the fingers towards the stationary thumbs, and gently creating a wave-like motion in the tissues (see Fig. 8.27, p. 164). Both thumbs palpate the reflex zones to the plantar lymph nodes of the axilla on both left and right feet at the same time. With the thumbs resting along the mtp joint line the fingertips assess these zones on the dorsal and lateral aspects.

If the findings are equivocal when palpating between the metatarsal bones, the reflex zones to the breast may need to be assessed individually. In this case a different approach (i.e. tracking from the midline in a lateral direction with the index, middle and ring fingers) is suggested and, if the findings are still ambiguous, tracking from the lateral margin towards the midline, one foot at a time.

The tips of the middle and ring fingers of the right hand palpate the reflex zone to the spleen on the dorsum of the left foot, and then both thumbs, tracking laterally across the fourth and fifth metatarsals, are used on the plantar foot.

The pelvic lymphatics on the medial and lateral aspects of the heels are assessed on one foot at a time. Using both hands, the index, middle and ring fingers commence from the angle at which plantar/medial and plantar/lateral surfaces meet, and are directed towards the posterior margin of the heel as the entire surface of this large area is palpated. The thumbs lie across the mtp joint line or at the bases of the first and fifth metatarsals. Alternatively, both thumbs track across this area from the superior border of the calcaneum towards the plantar foot, the fingers lying over each other across the dorsum of the lower shin, or, with the heel resting on the fingers of one held over another, both thumbs can track from the plantar margin proximally towards the malleoli.

To palpate the dense tissue of the plantar heel below the calcaneum the therapist uses both thumbs tracking toward each other, the fingers resting over the fold of the ankle.

The lymphatics of the thigh are assessed with the middle and ring fingers of both hands tracking proximally towards the knee on either side of the Achilles' tendon. The thumbs rest on the plantar calcaneum. Alternatively, with all fingers resting on the dorsum of the shin, the thumbs track over the lateral and medial aspects of the lower third of the leg and meet on the posterior surface.

There is no reflex zone to the spleen on the right foot, though there may be reciprocal pain over this area if there is impaired function of this organ. The reflex zone to the appendix is often found to be painful, treated individually, and may also give rise to reciprocal pain on the left foot.

The endocrine system

Both thumbs palpate the reflex zones to the pituitary on the plantar aspect of both big toes. The fingers lie across the dorsum of the feet and not over the toes.

Both thumbs, beginning from and including the midline, palpate the reflex zones to the thyroid and parathyroid glands on the plantar aspect. Similarly, both index fingers are used to palpate their reflex zones at the base of the big toe on the dorsum, treating both feet simultaneously.

Both thumbs palpate the reflex zones to the adrenal glands.

Both thumbs palpate the reflex zones to the pancreas in zone 1 on the right foot and across zones 1, 2 and 3 on the left foot, as already described.

With one foot covered, and with both thumbs resting on the metatarsal heads, the middle and ring fingers are used to palpate the reflex zones to the medial uterus and lateral ovaries (or prostate gland and testes). Using the same fingers the therapist then tracks along the dorsal arch of the foot just distal to the ankle fold for the reflex zone to the fallopian tube and inguinal canal, and this assessment is then repeated on the other foot.

As the assessment draws to a close, an increasingly light and effortless touch is used. The stroking movements at the end of the assessment should be barely perceptible for either patient or therapist. The patient is finally left warmly covered to rest.

Using both hands for treatment

On the dorsum

Both index fingers can be used to treat the small areas of the dorsum of the toes, tracking from distal to proximal end. This is particularly appropriate on the big toe for treating the neck and thyroid areas.

Between the metatarsal bones, one finger may rest on another to give added depth to palpation.

Over the tarsal bones, one or more fingers of one or both hands can treat in a lateral, oblique, medial, or distal to proximal direction over disordered reflex zones to maintain a stimulus or if a reflex zone is too painful to bear much direct treatment.

Over the ankle fold, both thumbs may approach each other from the medial and lateral margins of the foot, or the middle and ring fingers of each hand may weave to left and right between the malleoli to treat this area.

On the medial aspect

Both thumbs may be used to treat specific areas of the spine, tracking from the dorsal aspect of the foot to the plantar, or from plantar to dorsal aspect. The thumbs may approach each other from opposite directions, crossing frequently and obliquely over disordered zones.

The index, middle and ring fingers of one hand treat the spine by tracking from dorsal to medial aspects over painful reflex zones at any level, while the heel is supported in the palm of the other hand. Both index fingers are effective in treating the cervical spine, tracking from the interphalangeal joint to mtp joint 1. With one hand lying over the dorsum and the other hand lying over the plantar foot, one thumb tracks obliquely from plantar to dorsal and one from dorsal to plantar, frequently criss-crossing painful zones, as though weaving or plaiting.

If the medial aspect of the heel requires treatment (see Fig. 6.2I, p. 100) the leg is slightly outwardly rotated, the lateral aspect of the heel rests on one of the therapist's hands while the tips of the index, middle and ring fingers of the other hand are used, slightly flexed, for treatment.

Both thumbs may be used to treat the medial aspect of the heel, tracking either from the plantar aspect towards the internal malleolus, or with the thumbs approaching each other from different directions over the heel.

When the tissues of the lymphatics on the medial aspect of the lower leg are very painful they can be treated with gentle stroking movements by the middle and ring fingers of one or both hands interspersed with light palpation until they are able to tolerate stronger treatment.

On the plantar aspect

Both thumbs treating together in the same direction can be used to treat from distal to proximal, medial to lateral or obliquely. Both thumbs may approach each other from opposite directions, and either pass each other to treat an area intensively, or approach a painful reflex zone from many different points of a compass, meeting in the centre until the tissues feel less 'full' or 'empty'.

The index, middle and ring fingers are used to treat the large areas of the gastrointestinal tract. If the left foot is being treated, its lateral aspect rests on the therapist's right palm, her left thumb lying along the dorsal mtp joint line and the left fingers tracking obliquely under the arch of the foot from lateral to medial midline.

On the lateral aspect

From fifth toe to the external malleolus the most satisfactory way of treating these areas is with the index and middle fingers of one hand tracking from distal to proximal while the heel is supported in the palm of the other hand.

On the lateral aspect of the heel, the middle and ring fingers treat either obliquely from the cuboid to the posterior margin of the heel, or from the plantar margin towards the external malleolus, or a combination of these.

The zones are treated from all directions, the therapist passively and gently stretching all the muscles and joints around each area, and beginning all treatment of dorsal and plantar surfaces in the midline.

Each individual treatment is adapted and tailored to the immediate need of each patient. This may (and often does) vary from session to session. One or both thumbs, one or more fingers, or one or both hands are used, according to the location and severity of the disorder. If the feet are cool, active treatment stops and harmonising strokes are given, allowing for the stimulus to be assimilated and a response evoked.

9

The hands

Introduction

As hands are more exposed to the elements and a greater variety of temperature and pressure stimuli than the feet, their reflex zones are often less sensitive to palpation.

Advantages of using the hands

Advantages include:

- in cold climates hands are more accessible than the feet
- they provide an alternative surface if there is injury, infection, a plaster cast, or if part of the lower limb has been amputated
- the very frail and the elderly respond well to RZT of the hands
- they can be used for those who cannot lie prone for back treatment, or for those who cannot lie supine for foot treatment
- they are readily available for first aid
- they are usually easier for the patient to treat herself, either to relieve symptomatic pain or as an adjunct to a treatment.

Disadvantages

The feet, being often confined and less well cared for than the hands and bearing the whole weight of the body, are in general more responsive to RZT, and a course of treatment is best begun on the feet.

Distribution of zones

In the anatomical position the palms face forward and the thumbs outwards. To find the reflex zones on the hands, however, the palms are laid onto any flat surface (the equivalent of placing both soles of the feet on the ground), the palms reflecting the dorsal aspect (or back) of the body. The dorsum of the hands reflects the ventral aspect (or front) of the body (Fig. 9.1).

With some variations, the distribution of reflex zones on the hands is similar to that on the feet (Fig. 9.2). Organs and structures lying in the left half of the body are found in the left hand, and those lying in the right half of the body are found in the right hand.

Treatment to organs is mainly given on the palms (Fig. 9.3), and to bones, nerves and muscles on the dorsum.

Reflex zones can be found 7 to 10 cm (3 to 4 inches) proximal to (or above) the wrist in the adult.

The central structures of spine and bladder, which lie in the midline of the body, are found on the medial aspect of the hands when the palms are facing downwards. Exceptionally, the heart and the stomach are best treated in zone 2 on the palms where they overlie the second metatarsal bone. The thyroid and parathyroid lie on the lateral border of zone 1, against metacarpalphalangeal (mcp) joint 1 in the web between thumb and index finger.

Reflex zones of the head and neck occupy the largest area, lying over all four aspects of the phalanges of the fingers. Structures of the thorax are

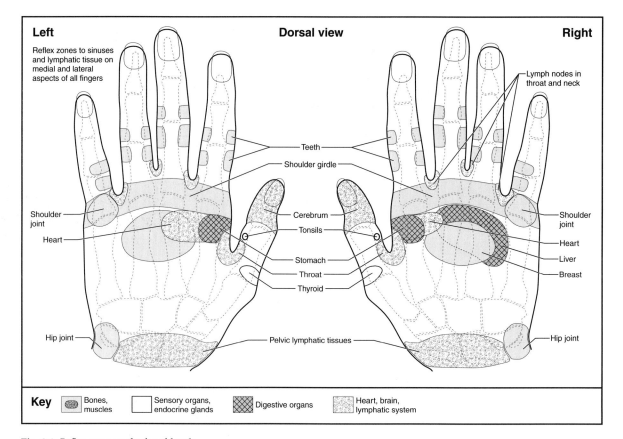

Fig. 9.1 *Reflex zones on the dorsal hands*

found over the metacarpal bones. Structures of the abdomen are found over the carpal bones. Structures of the pelvic region are found over the wrist, where they cover a smaller area of the hands than on the feet.

The fifth body zone extends to the smallest finger on the lateral part of the hands. Here lie reflex zones to the shoulders, elbows and hips.

Harmonising strokes

Yin-Yang strokes on the hands are performed in opposite directions to those used on the feet. This is because they are carried out in the same direction as the meridian flow, and these are in opposite directions for the hand meridians and the foot

meridians. Therefore, Yang strokes flow from the tips of the fingernails over the dorsum of the hand and up the forearm, whilst Yin strokes flow from the midarm towards the palm and fingertips.

Keeping both palms in close but not heavy contact with the skin, the therapist strokes with one hand from the midarm to the palmar fingertips while the other hand simultaneously strokes from the dorsal fingertips to the midarm.

Treatment

This follows the same pattern as that described for the feet. Except when symptomatic relief or first aid are the object, the first session is always devoted to an assessment of all the reflex zones.

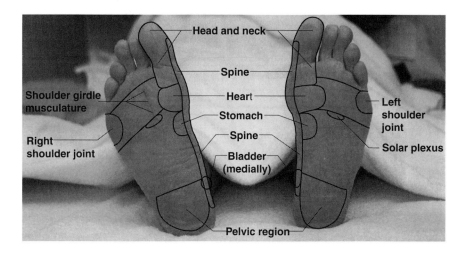

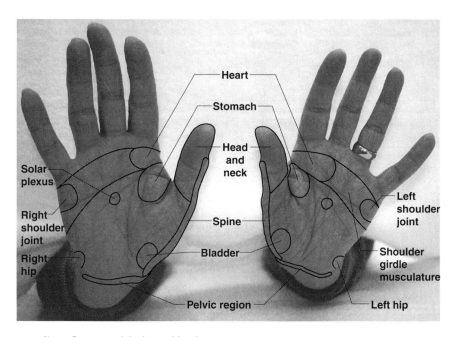

Fig. 9.2 *Some corresponding reflex zones of the feet and hands*

Thereafter all disordered and painful reflex zones are treated two or three times a week. A treatment time of 30 minutes is adhered to unless this proves too long for the very frail. If there are reactions (which tend to be less marked in RZT of the hands) the reacting system is also treated.

A record is kept of all findings on assessment, all treatment given and any reactions which may occur.

Once improvement has reached a plateau, or the reactions have ceased, and the reflex zones are no longer painful, treatment is discontinued. In the frail it can be continued for as long as it is supportive.

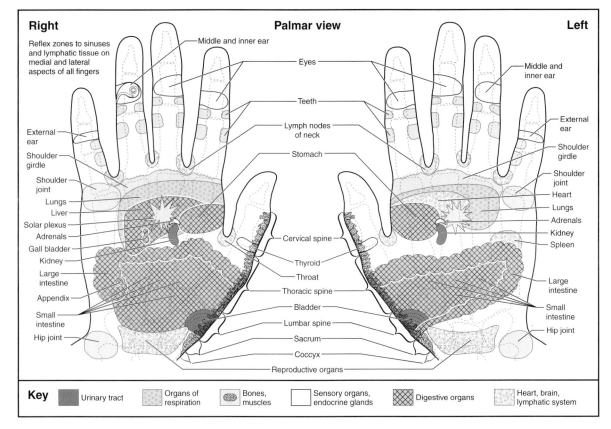

Fig. 9.3 *Reflex zones on the palmar hands*

First aid and self-treatment on the hands to supplement RZT

The patient may, if she wishes for it, be given a small diagram showing which areas to treat. As with feet, it is always better to start with a small stimulus, and treating disordered reflex zones on the hand for 2 minutes three times a day is a good general rule. On those occasions when the need for symptomatic or pain relief is ongoing, the patient can treat the necessary reflex zones more often, and for longer periods.

As on the feet, treatment on the hands can be overdone, and if the reactions of tiredness, nausea, a sense of anxiety or heightened pain in the reflex zones are heightened or severe, the frequency and intensity should be reduced.

Treatment on the hands is usually given to symptomatic or painful areas such as the sinuses,

ears, eyes, teeth, lymphatic tissues of the throat and neck, stomach disorders and injured joints, either as first aid, or at the same time as treatment which is directed towards the primary, underlying cause of the illness is being given on the feet or back.

Symptomatic treatment and first aid

Although any reflex zone in the hand can be treated with benefit, some are more frequently used for first aid than others.

The teeth

These lie distally and proximally to the proximal joint spaces on index, middle and ring fingers. However, on the thumbs only the dorsal and lateral aspects distal and proximal to the single joint line are the site of the central incisors. On the fifth toe the wisdom teeth lie on the medial and dorsal aspects only.

Sedation. When there is infection of a tooth or the surrounding gums, firm pressure and sedating movements are given to relieve pain. The painful reflex zone is held steadily, without increasing or decreasing the depth of the hold. The tissues usually feel taut and tense, and a pulse can be felt below the thumb or the fingertip applying pressure. The pulse usually increases in strength and frequency, then fades as it becomes more regular. This is accompanied by easing of the pain in the affected part.

Tonification. Sedation is followed by tonifying movements of the local lymphatic drainage, which is usually intensely painful, and is a first aid measure until a dentist can be seen. The sedation hold is repeated as often as necessary. At the same time, if the lymphatic tissue in the webs between the fingers is pink or painful, they are vascularised (milked) in the same way as the webs between the toes. Applying light but firm pressure to the subcutaneous tissues, the index finger gradually moves the tissues in a small, wave-like ripple right through to the palmar surface (Fig. 9.4). The thumb stays in the same position between the metacarpal heads on the palmar surface. The reflex zones to the urinary system are treated in any infective episode, and the reflex zone to the stomach if infective material is swallowed.

Treatment of a dental site following dental work or extraction and any disordered lymphatic tissues of the neck and throat promotes the healing process in gums and bony cavities.

The sinuses

These reflex zones are found on the medial and lateral surfaces of the index, middle and ring fingers, the lateral surface of the thumb and the medial surface of the little finger. If the sinus pain is acute, they are best treated with a sedation hold over all their painful reflex zones until the acute pain subsides, and then stimulated for a few minutes every 2–3 hours, when the tissues are treated as vigorously as the pain allows. The therapist should also treat the lymphatic tissues in the finger webs and the urinary system.

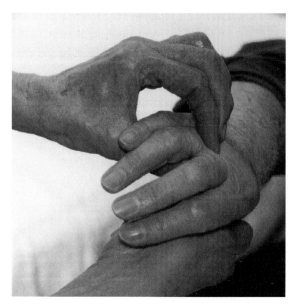

Fig. 9.4 *Milking the webs of the fingers*

The lymphatic tissues of the neck and throat

These reflex zones are concentrated in the webs between the thumb and index finger, and all the other fingers.

They can be sedated as described above for acute pain, such as ear or throat ache, and tonified to stimulate the lymphatic flow. The movements should be repeated as often as possible, at least every 4 hours.

Ear infections

These reflex zones lie over the proximal phalanges toward the bases of the ring and little fingers.

For acute pain in the ear, sedation to these areas can be repeated every half hour. The therapist can stimulate (by milking) the lymphatic drainage of the throat and neck as often as possible, using very slow movements to begin with, as these zones are also acutely painful when the ear is infected.

Painful or stiff neck

The therapist should find the precise reflex zone (or zones) which is most painful on the medial aspect of the proximal phalanx of the thumb on either the left or right hand or both.

Sedation. The area is sedated. The therapist also treats reflex zones at the base of the spine which are usually also painful, similarly with the shoulder girdle. This frequently brings immediate relief, and can be repeated for 2–3 minutes several times a day during the acute stage.

Tonification. When the acute episode is over, and to maintain the improvement, the spinal reflex zones which were disordered should be self-treated regularly by the patient, with fairly vigorous sawing movements along the length of the spine, but particularly over the neck and lower spine (Fig. 9.5).

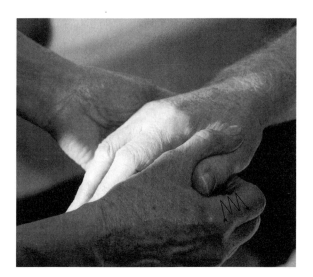

Fig. 9.5 *Tonifying reflex zones to the neck in a sawing motion*

Shoulders

Pain or injury to a shoulder joint is treated by finding the painful reflex zones on either the ventral, lateral or dorsal aspect of the fifth metacarpal joint.

Injury on the ventral aspect of the thorax is reflected onto the dorsum of the hand, that on the lateral aspect onto the lateral aspect of the hand, and if a dorsal (back) injury has been sustained it is reflected onto the palmar aspect of the hand.

Careful palpation around the head of the fifth metacarpal bone should pinpoint the reflex zone, which is sedated for 2 to 3 minutes, at least until the discomfort in the zone is relieved. The painful reflex zones are treated three or four times a day, for not longer than 5 minutes each time. Painful reflex zones in the shoulder girdle and neck are treated at the same time.

Gastritis, indigestion or hyperacidity of the stomach

The therapist should sedate the reflex zone to the stomach at the base of the first metacarpal bone (on both hands) and then gently but consistently milk the web between the base of the thumb and the index finger. The solar plexus is also sedated (see below).

Nausea, fainting, restlessness and anxiety

By cupping the palm of one hand and placing the other thumb over the most concave area, the reflex zone to the solar plexus is found (Fig. 9.6). This is the most useful first aid point on the hands, which can be used either by itself or in conjunction with any

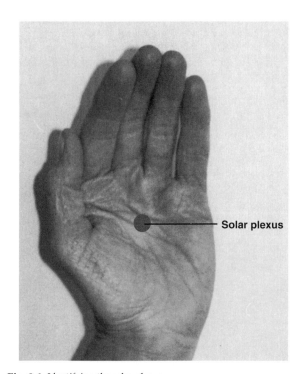

Solar plexus

Fig. 9.6 *Identifying the solar plexus*

other treatment, for physical or psychological distress.

Sedating this point reduces any sympathetic overexcitability and has a soothing effect. One of the effects of treating this is to relax the voluntary striped muscle of the diaphragm, so that breathing becomes more efficient. It can be held for up to 4 minutes at a time, and repeated as often as necessary, with the following caution. Too long or too strong a pressure on this area has the opposite effect to that which is desired. SNS reactions, pain or a feeling of faintness show that the pressure has been too deep, too strong, or been applied for too long.

Pain in the thoracic spine

The reflex zones along the length of this area are sedated. They lie along the medial aspect of the first metacarpal bone. An even pressure is maintained over the painful areas until the pain in the back eases, after which it can be treated with the basic treatment method every few hours or as necessary.

Pain in the lumbar spine

Sedation. The area (which is usually acutely painful) is sedated along the carpal bones for a maximum of 4 minutes or until the pain eases. The reflex zones to the abdominal muscles are sedated on the dorsum. The treatment also treats any painful reflex zones in the cervical spine.

Tonification. As the reflex zones become less painful tonifying treatment may be used. This consists of sawing movements up the pad of the thumb towards the forearm (Fig. 9.7). When an injury is acute a compensatory (and protective) muscular tension appears in the upper spine. The treatment is repeated as necessary. The therapist should also tonify the gastrointestinal tract three or four times a day for no longer than 3 minutes each time. Pain in any part of the spine which is not due to injury reflects either pathological changes elsewhere in the body or degenerative changes within the spine itself, and the cause of the pain should be sought.

An example of treatment to the lower spine is detailed in Case study 9.1.

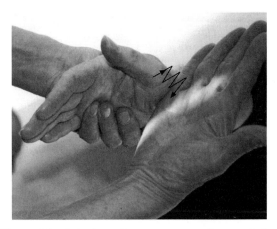

Fig. 9.7 *Stimulating by sawing movements to reflex zones to the lumbar spine and sacrum*

CASE STUDY 9.1

A 28-year-old nurse arrived at work one morning complaining of severe low back pain, constipation and general malaise. She had had several such episodes over the past 5 years, but they were becoming more frequent. As time did not allow either an assessment or treatment on the feet, the most painful reflex zones over the lower spine were identified, sedated until the tension within the tissues began to normalise, and the whole spinal region and small and large intestine were tonified fairly vigorously. The total time spent in treatment was 6 minutes.

At the end of this time the lower back pain was largely relieved, and she was able to work out the remainder of her shift, although she felt tired and lethargic. A further 4 minutes were spent on first aid before she left for home. The following morning she reported that her constipation had been relieved, her back had remained comfortable and warm, and that she had slept well. Although still tired, she was not troubled by malaise or lethargy.

A course of treatment was arranged at her convenience; meanwhile she continued to treat her hands herself two or three times a day, and found that over a period of 3 weeks her backache had ceased to cause her pain and stiffness.

Pain in the sacrum and coccyx

The therapist sedates the proximal, medial aspect of the scaphoid, deep into the joint space, for no longer than 4 minutes at a time. The upper spine is treated if painful reflex zones are found there, and the musculature of the abdominal wall over the dorsum of the hand. This should be repeated as often as necessary.

These measures are used for first aid and to relieve pain, and to complement other treatment whose purpose is to discover the underlying causes of pain or discomfort. Persistent pain which does not respond to treatment calls for further investigation.

Treatment to the reflex zones of of the hands, back and feet should relieve discomfort and strengthen function at all levels. Where an improvement is not possible it is used to sustain present function and because touch is comforting for almost everyone.

Pain in the hip joint

A wide area around the head of the ulna is sedated for up to 4 minutes, by which time the pain should ease. This is repeated as often as necessary. Reciprocal reflexes (the opposite hip joint and the shoulder on the same side of the body) should also be treated. The musculature of the thigh and lower spine also needs treatment.

Pain in the knee joint

Some three fingerswidth proximal to the head of the ulna is one of many reflex zones to the knee. If the injury is on the lateral knee, the therapist should look for the corresponding reflex zone on the lateral arm, if it is on the medial aspect of the knee, he should look for the reflex zone over the radius. The most painful reflex zones are sedated for up to 4 minutes, and the musculature of the thigh distal to the knee zones is tonified. The therapist should treat the reciprocal reflexes.

Retention of urine

Sedation of the solar plexus is given for about 30 seconds before tonification of the reflex zones to the bladder over the proximal carpal bones below the thumb for about 2 minutes; this is repeated every 20 minutes.

Cystitis

The reflex zones to the solar plexus and the bladder are sedated. The reflex zones to the oronasopharynx are also treated.

Since urinary tract infections tend to recur, it is worthwhile giving the patient the following simple advice on the mechanics of re-infection and the importance of diluting the pool of urine in the bladder.

1. Drink 2 litres of water each 24 hours during the acute phase, and as much clear fluid over and above this as possible. Clear fluids include water, rice or barley water, diluted vegetable or fruit juices. They do not include tea, coffee, alcohol, milky or carbonated (fizzy) drinks.
2. Take as long as is needed to empty the bladder completely, especially the last few drops, and apply pressure over the area just above the symphysis pubis to expel the last ounce of urine.
3. A plastic jug filled with clean lukewarm water is used to douche the genital area every time the bladder has been emptied.
4. Only cotton pants or underpants should be worn and are changed every time the bladder is emptied during the acute phase.
5. Avoid wearing nylon tights at the time of infection.
6. Rest (lying down flat) as much as possible, till all the symptoms have disappeared.
7. Avoid intercourse until the symptoms subside.
8. If toilet paper is used, clean the genital area from front to back. The area is vulnerable to infection from *Escherichia coli* organisms from the bowel which are found round the anus.
9. Recurrent bouts of cystitis should be investigated.
10. Adequate fluid intake should be ensured at all times, particularly in known dehydrating conditions such as flying, centrally heated rooms, and travelling in hot, dry climates.

Premenstrual tension

Either friction or vigorous wringing of the whole area around the wrist joint is applied for at least 2 minutes

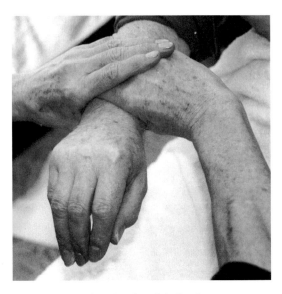

Dry eyes

The complaint is common amongst people taking hypotensive drugs, those suffering from arthritic disease, and in certain occupations such as people working with astringent chemicals.

The reflex zones to the tear ducts are tonified as often as possible during the day.

After amputation

Following amputation of the foot or leg, the opposite foot and both hands can be treated. This helps to relieve pain, particularly when treatment is given to the hand on the same side of the body as the amputation. As well as giving treatment to the whole hand, the reflex zone to the solar plexus should be sedated.

Hair loss following chemotherapy or radiotherapy

Buffing the nails against each other for 5 minutes three times a day stimulates hair growth.

Sleeplessness

Sedating the solar plexus can be done by the patient or nurse. Yin-Yang strokes and a gentle, general treatment to both hands is soothing and relaxing for most people. Firmly pressing and holding the fingertips together helps some people to relax.

Summary

The hands provide an effective surface for treatment, first aid and self-care. Symptoms which do not resolve or recur need to be investigated so that any serious underlying illness which cannot be treated by RZT is not missed.

The contraindications are the same as those for RZT of the feet. Localised or general infection, hyperpyrexia, recent thrombosis, unstable pregnancy in the first trimester, psychotic conditions or loss of skin or tissue make RZT an inappropriate choice of treatment.

Fig. 9.8 *Wringing the wrists for pelvic disorders*

every hour from the time that symptoms are first felt (Fig. 9.8).

This technique is also helpful during the first stage of labour, when the descending head of the baby presses on pelvic structures, impeding venous and lymphatic return (see Ch. 12). Backache in the late stages of pregnancy can be partially relieved by wringing the wrists in this manner.

The therapist should sedate the reflex zone to the sacroiliac joint (where the scaphoid bone articulates with the radius) for backache in late pregnancy, or when the joint has been strained. The lift exercise is recommended (see Appendix III, p. 283).

Poor milk flow

If, after delivery, the breasts fill only slowly with milk, the spaces between the metacarpal bones on the dorsum of both hands should be vigorously tonified every 4–6 hours.

The midwife, a friend or relative can treat the breast area on the hands, as well as those on the feet.

10

The back

Introduction

The back presents a much larger surface for observation and palpation than that of the feet. Its surface is less vulnerable than that of the abdomen, and therefore lends itself to RZT, massage and other therapies.

The functioning capacity of many internal organs is mirrored on the back, and they can be treated through massage, connective tissue massage, neural therapy, shiatsu and lymphatic drainage.

Advantages and disadvantages of treating the back

Advantages

1. The zones are more widely separated than they are on the feet. They are also larger and therefore more easily identifiable. On the feet the reflex zones of the stomach, pancreas, liver and duodenum overlie each other in places, and it is not always easy to distinguish which is the most disordered.

   If RZT of the foot and its reactions have not clarified which organ is weakest, the back may give further clues.

2. The foot or feet may be injured or there may be local infection.

3. There are occasions, usually when the patient is very debilitated, when the feet are too painful to treat.

4. Treatment to date may have provoked reactions which are stronger than expected. When this happens the feet become sensitive even to light touch. An assessment on the back which does not further stimulate an already overexcited ANS, giving frequent effleurage strokes and avoiding deep touch or vigorous treatment, helps to stabilise the patient.

5. Treatment on the back can confirm findings made on the feet and at times amplify the picture of disorder.

6. The patient may be physically or psychologically uncomfortable when lying supine, and prefer the prone position.

7. A plateau may have been reached in treatment, in which a smaller or greater improvement has been obtained, but the pattern of disorder on the feet shows that healing is not yet complete. One or more sessions on the back can give a new stimulus and further improvement.

8. The patient does not usually feel overexposed by having his back bared.

9. If the patient finds difficulty in relaxing and is overtalkative, he is less inclined to converse in the prone position, usually becoming deeply relaxed.

10. The patient may prefer it.

Disadvantages

Not everyone can lie in the prone position, and it may be difficult or impossible if there is or has been:

- strain or injury to the back, particularly the lower spine
- strain or injury to the neck
- surgery to the breasts, sternum or heart
- if the breasts are large, tender or sometimes during the premenstrual stage of the cycle
- if there are any breathing difficulties
- after the first 3 months of pregnancy.

Contraindications for giving treatment on the back

Treatment of the back is contraindicated in the following circumstances:

- in the acute phase of any back injury, i.e. if the patient cannot stand up straight and if the pain is acute
- in deep, chronic pain which comes in waves, waking the patient at night; here a full medical investigation is called for
- where there is a nerve pain down or over bone, especially on the spine
- in febrile conditions
- in psychotic conditions
- after deep vein thrombosis
- when a pregnancy is unstable
- when the patient has cancer and medical treatment is not concluded, unless the therapist is especially qualified to give treatment in this situation; never massage towards the site of an old tumour
- when the intentions of the patient toward the therapist are unclear.

Indications for treatment

The following are indications for treating the back:

- pain in the back, neck or shoulders (but not in the acute stage)
- muscular strain, such as repetitive strain injury, or pain resulting from poor posture

- prolonged and heavy carrying
- stress, especially when it affects the neck and shoulder girdle
- poor respiratory function
- gastrointestinal disorders, especially constipation
- headaches, especially those resulting from disorders of the stomach and duodenum
- insomnia
- difficulty in relaxing, especially if due to overtiredness
- when the SNS has been overstimulated for too long, whether from illness, anxiety, too much noise, movement or flashing lights, or from a daily diet which is overrich in stimulating foods
- where the muscles on one side of the body are used more than those of the other side, e.g. in playing music, hairdressing, and in some sports, such as squash, golf and tennis.

Preparation

Room and equipment

The room should be warmed to a temperature of 20°C (70°F). It must afford quiet and privacy.

The treatment is best performed on a plinth, which should be at a convenient working height for the therapist. Space at the head and on either side is needed so that the back can be approached from any side. A hole for the face is an advantage, otherwise small cushions can be used to support the forehead and keep the face off the bed.

If the patient cannot lie down an armless chair with a high back over which he can rest his arms serves equally well.

The plinth is covered with a fresh washable cotton sheet, cotton or paper towels, newly provided for each patient. A supply of pillows and cushions of differing sizes are useful. A thin pillow can be placed under the abdomen if the patient has a backache or, in women, if the breasts are tender. Smaller cushions can be placed under the ankles, knees, neck and forehead, and to the side of the face to ensure that the neck is not turned too much to one side. The patient must be comfortable.

Coverings or towels with which to cover those areas of the back which have just been treated should be odourless, soft and washable. A small warm blanket or cover is needed for the lower half of the body.

Since massage can be performed with soap and water, French chalk or oil, any or all of these should be to hand. Any good massage oil can be used, but as a growing incidence of intolerance or allergy to nuts and wheat is reported, a bland vegetable-based oil should also be available. Heavily scented oils should be avoided. Some people have a highly developed sense of smell, and women who are pregnant as well as those who are sick become acutely sensitive to smell, often finding strong odours repugnant or nauseating. It is preferable not to add essential oils or any other ingredients at the assessment. If essential oils are added later, care should be taken not to use those which are contraindicated in pregnancy or the patient's particular condition. Women do not always know that they are pregnant, and may come for treatment because they are tired, or nauseated, not suspecting the cause. Therefore a bland base oil is to be preferred.

Treatment cards depicting the zones on the back on which to record the findings should be available (Fig. 10.1).

The patient

The procedure will have been explained to the patient, whose back from the nape of the neck to the buttocks needs to be exposed. Watches, chains, necklaces and earrings should be removed (a small container should be made available) and a sweatband offered to protect the hair from contact with oil.

At least an hour should have elapsed since the last full meal was eaten. The physiological response to food is an increased blood supply to the stomach and digestive tract, under the influence of the PNS. Any treatment (or activity) which competes for a portion of the available blood hinders or even halts the digestive process. RZT to the back increases the blood supply of all treated muscles. Blood needed by the digestive organs has become physiologically unavailable, thus any treatment given at this time is less effective and handicaps or inhibits digestion.

The patient adopts the prone position on the plinth. The therapist needs a good light while looking at the back before she begins treatment, but no direct light should shine onto the patient's face at any time during the session.

The therapist

The arms and hands of the therapist should be free of any metal object which may come into contact with the patient's skin. Sleeves which end at the elbow are more practical than long sleeves, being less likely to tickle the skin or to collect any drops of oil.

The therapist's hands should be warm, and she should feel relaxed and alert. To facilitate easy breathing, constrictive clothing is best avoided.

Treatment method

Principles

A normal treatment time on the back is 20–30 minutes. Treatment for the very young and the very old should be of shorter duration.

Protection for the thoracic and abdominal organs, and support for the spine, is provided by the strong extensor muscles of the back. The vascularisation of muscles and tissues should be achieved slowly, and once the muscles are suffused with blood then more rapid, vigorous and stimulating movements can be made.

All treatment begins with featherlight touch and proceeds with gentle and rhythmical movements. From the slow (but not languorous) and gentle beginning the treatment becomes deeper and more penetrating, then gradually decreases in intensity to resume a quieter tempo before being tailed off completely.

The more rhythmical the movements, the greater their effect. An active movement or treatment on any one area should be followed by a passive movement and a resting phase, and two active movements should not follow each other in close succession. For example, after stretching a muscle it should be allowed to contract. A stimulating percussion movement is followed by a period of rest for the area which has just been treated, and active massage

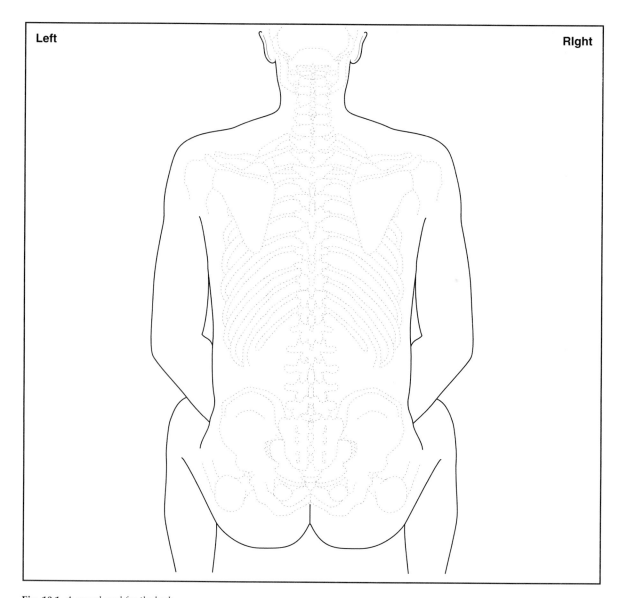

Fig. 10.1 *A record card for the back*

movements are succeeded by light touch or holding. A cyclical variation of activity and rest brings the best results from this treatment.

There should be unbroken skin contact between the patient and the therapist from the beginning of treatment. If one hand is taken off the back to rearrange coverings or for another purpose, the other hand remains on the patient's back, neck or head all the time.

The therapist should not unnecessarily expose any part of the patient's back or body, only that part of the back which is being treated. It is immediately covered again after treatment has been given. The coverings should have been sufficiently warmed that they do not feel cool to the patient's skin. The patient should not be allowed to become cold. The therapist keeps a constant watch on the rate and rhythm of the patient's breathing (which is easy to watch with the rise and fall of the chest wall) throughout the session. Also any changes in skin colour should be noted as the tissues become vascularised, and any muscular contraction which develops. There are instinctive protective mechanisms which come into play when pain or force are anticipated, and if this happens the patient becomes unreceptive to further therapy.

Working from the cervical spine downwards towards the base of the spine generally has a sedative effect, whilst working from the base of the spine upward toward the base of the skull is more stimulating.

Particular care needs to be taken in treating patients with hypertension, as the therapist's movement should neither passively nor actively increase blood flow toward the head, and if a patient develops a headache during a back treatment then long flowing superficial stroking movements directed from the head towards the feet are made until the headache recedes.

In the neck, major arteries, veins and nerves as well as the trachea lie close to the surface of the body. For this reason the neck always feels vulnerable. Any movements which are too quick or any perception of undisciplined strength will cause the muscles of the neck, shoulder girdle and head to tense rapidly, and relaxation is nullified. All movements around the head and neck should be carried out in a carefully measured manner, and the patient must feel that the head and neck are supported at all times.

In RZT palpation is never given to the bony surfaces of the spine — it is the muscular and subcutaneous tissues which are treated.

No vigorous treatment should be given to women while they are pregnant or during menstruation.

Movements and techniques

Initially, palpation is performed with sensitive fingertips as they first indent the skin to note any variations in temperature or texture. The fingertips then flow more deeply into the tissues to perceive the tone and texture of the underlying subcutaneous tissues. Here they can maintain a light but aware touch in the same place, remaining there until any underlying tension is dispersed and there is uniformity of tissue tone beneath the fingers, or little

vibratory movements can be made. Alternatively, the fingers may probe more deeply to release tissue tensions with firmer circular or stroking movements.

It is important in treating tense tissue that all strokes are directed *away from* the 'knot' at the centre of taut tissues. On the other hand, in those areas where the tissues feel flaccid and 'empty', and less resilient to normal touch, the movement is directed *toward* the deficiency.

Any of the movements used in massage may be used on the back. These include the following.

Stroking

Stroking may be either superficial or deep.

Superficial stroking. In this movement the open and relaxed hands of the therapist mould themselves to that part of the body which is being touched, and with light, assured, even and long movements she just strokes the surface of the skin in either a centripetal (toward the heart) or centrifugal direction.

Superficial stroking is the *one* movement to elicit a reflex response only; it has no mechanical effect.

Deep stroking, also called 'effleurage'. The direction of an effleurage stroke is always centripetal, and to be fully effective the muscular system of the whole body should first be relaxed. If necessary, this should be achieved by light stroking before beginning effleurage.

Effleurage has a mechanical effect upon the venous and lymphatic return, which it improves, and it may at the same time also have a reflex response.

Compression movements

These are kneading, friction and petrissage, and skin rolling.

Skin rolling. This is not always done as part of the assessment, but is another method reflecting disorder in particular areas. It is used for tissues which are dense, inelastic and painful to touch. They are frequently found alongside the lumbar spine, over the reflex zones to the kidneys, liver, duodenum, stomach, over the iliac crest and shoulder blades. The therapist should treat over a wide area for several sessions until the tissues become more pliant and less painful.

Although the technique requires a little practice, it is worthwhile persevering until it can be lightly and dexterously performed. Patients often complain that an area of muscular tightness or discomfort remains or recurs, even after the general symptoms have disappeared. When the skin can be freely picked up in folds of little more than 4 mm (1/8 inch) and the pliable skin glides loosely and freely over the subcutaneous tissues, any remaining tautness is relieved.

A fold of skin is first picked up between the thumb and index finger of both hands (Fig. 10.2A); the left thumb then moves slowly along the surface of the skin for a few millimetres, and the index finger rolls over the pad of the thumb (Fig. 10.2B). The fold is picked up by the right thumb and finger and moved forward another few millimetres (Fig. 10.2C), then passed again to the left thumb and finger as before and this alternating pattern of movement is continued as the thumbs and fingers move forward fluidly, creating a wave-like motion in the skin and subcutaneous tissues.

This technique can be used to end a treatment on the back, moving from buttocks to shoulders (or from the spine to the sides of the body) until every part of the skin over the back is easily, or more easily, lifted.

Skin rolling is painful, however, when the underlying tissues are unhealthy. By working first in very small movements and approaching any areas of inelastic tissue slowly and from a wide margin, the therapist causes them to become freer, more pliant and more comfortable. As with all other measures, this should be done only if it relieves pain and frees the tissues.

Skin rolling can be performed on any part of the back, legs, arms or joints such as the shoulder or hip.

Percussion movements ('tapotement')

These movements are more stimulating in nature, and should be used judiciously. Clapping, cupping, beating and hacking movements are all percussive.

Vibration and shaking

The tip of one or more fingers move in a 'vibrato' to bring about a trembling movement in the tissues, either in one place or moving along a track.

In shaking a gentle and rhythmical shaking movement is caused by one slightly cupped but relaxed hand lightly swaying the trunk (in this instance) from one supportive hand to the other.

Assessment

The limbs are covered and the back exposed. If the patient is sitting on an armless chair facing its back, with his arms supported on a pillow, the rest of his body must be adequately covered (Fig. 10.3).

Before any treatment can be given, the back is examined carefully, beginning with the standard observations on:

- the skin
- the bony structure
- the contour of each part
- the temperature of the whole of the back.

The skin inspection

The colour, texture and tone of the skin are inspected. Any variations of texture such as dryness, discoloration or markings are significant, but their location is equally important, since specific areas of the back reflect changes in specific organs.

Bony structure

The shape given to the back by the underlying bony structure is noted, whether long, short, straight or irregular. Disorders of spinal alignment are common, and do not always give rise to symptoms in the early stages, but they give an indication of possible future problems, and frank irregularities show that the spine has become involved in or caused segmental disorder.

Contours

Next the therapist looks closely at the contours, comparing the left half of the back with the right half,

A

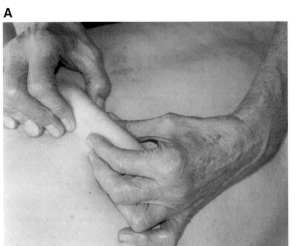

B

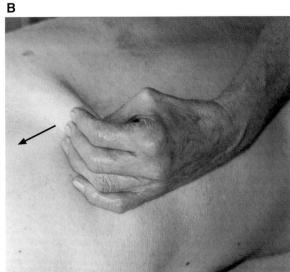

C

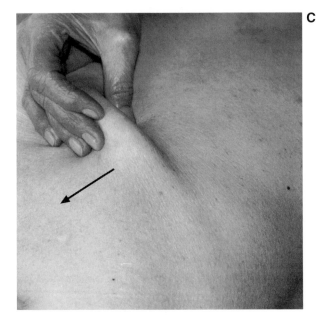

Fig. 10.2 *Skin rolling: **A** a fold of skin and tissue is taken up by both hands; **B** it is glided forward by the left hand; **C** the fold is then taken by the right hand and glided further forward*

the upper half with the lower half, and then in smaller sections, down the length of the spine, over the shoulder blades, waistline and buttocks. Any areas where the tissues are taut, full, or uneven are noted, as are those areas where the tissues are depressed or hollowed and 'empty'.

Temperature

The first contact with the skin is made by placing the warm hands on either side of the spine; either side of C7 is usually a good place to begin. With light but generously long strokes, no more than 10 per minute,

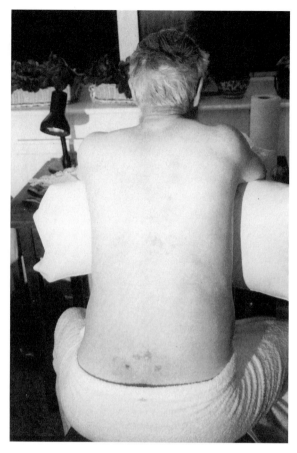

Fig. 10.3 *The sitting position*

the therapist sweeps down towards the buttocks, returning to the starting position of the hands, and then over the whole surface of the back. This allows any variation in temperature to be compared with variations in tissue tone.

Preliminary stretching movements

Placing both ulnar sides of her arms flat against the centre of the patient's back (about T12) the therapist presses down on the back firmly but not heavily (Fig. 10. 4A) and, gradually separating her arms, moves one towards the head and the other towards the buttocks (Fig. 10.4B), without applying undue

pressure and keeping close contact with the skin as the whole spine is stretched (Fig. 10.4C).

Both arms are then laid flat across the spine, again at about T12 and separated in the diagonal, one moving toward the shoulder joint and the other toward the hip joint (Fig. 10.5A–C). The same opening up of the back is repeated on the opposite diagonal. With the palms of the hands on either side of the spine, a firm even pressure is applied as the hands move out toward the lateral borders of the thorax.

If one hand is lifted from the body, the other maintains contact with the skin. Stroking is continued in one or more directions until the patient has started to relax, and the breathing is deep and rhythmical.

The therapist needs to decide whether the assessment is to be conducted from the neck to the base of the spine or vice versa. She should never begin in the area that is most painful or where there is a build-up of muscular tension, but start slowly in the area which both looks and feels least disordered, treating tense muscles later in the session, when there is a deeper state of relaxation: they can be returned to several times if necessary. A few effleurage strokes are directed from the lumbar spine towards the thoracic region.

If there is any muscular contraction, it is necessary to stop and give light stroking movements again until the muscles become relaxed. When treatment is resumed, it should be on another part of the back, and with a less penetrating touch than before.

Assessment and treatment of the reflex zones

The reflex zones of the back are shown in Figure 10.6. Not only are the reflex zones on the back widely separated, it will also be noted that there are six areas (three on each side of the back) which relate to the kidneys, four to the heart, five to the small intestine and four to the gall bladder (all on the right side), as well as the relationship between some of these organs and specific vertebrae.

Each zone needs to be palpated at assessment and, depending on the stage of illness, one or more may

A

B

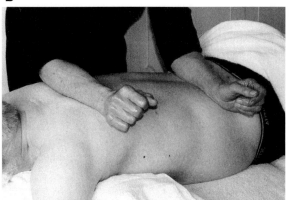

C

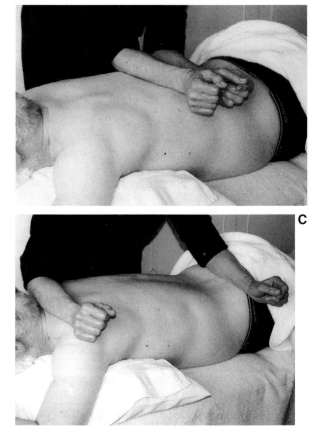

Fig. 10.4 *A–C Stretching the spine*

be found to be painful. In the early stages, there are minimal skin and temperature changes, later followed by disturbances in the colloid state of underlying tissues so that they and the skin become less elastic and flexible, then gradually become more sensitive to touch and pressure. If the illness progresses, the tissues become painful when they are palpated. It is worth noting that skin rolling (see p. 193) causes pain over disordered reflex zones from the earliest stages of disease.

The spine

Using both hands, the tissues on either side of the spine are explored in seamless flowing movements. If the therapist has decided to work from the cervical spine to the coccyx, she starts at C1; if she has decided to work from the base of the spine up to the neck she begins over the coccyx. Alternatively she may decide to treat the whole area of the back except the neck with the patient in the prone position, and then treat the neck and its reflex zones last, the patient turning to lie supine for this section of treatment and the rest period.

The neck

If the choice has been made to begin at the head of the spine, an exploratory palpation of the musculature on either side of the spinous processes is made with one hand on either side of the cervical spine. Light, circular movements are used, and continue to track

A

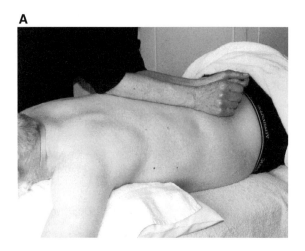

B

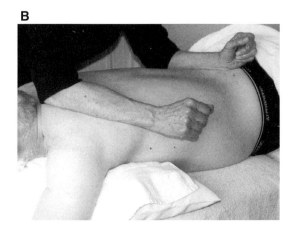

C

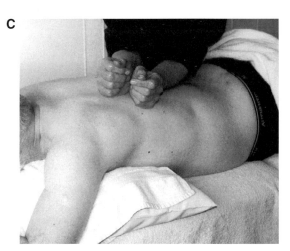

Fig. 10.5 *A–C Diagonal stretching*

from the level of C1 along the base of the skull as far as the mastoid bone, and lightly stretching the muscles here from the medial to the lateral margins. The neck is stroked lightly.

The therapist palpates the reflex zones which relate to:

- the heart, alongside and to the left of the third, fourth and fifth cervical vertebrae on the lateral border of the trapezius muscle (in the posterior triangle of the neck)
- the gall bladder, alongside the third, fourth and fifth cervical vertebrae on the right side of the body

- the kidneys, just below the bony occiput on either side of the first cervical vertebra, using small, smooth and delicate probings to discover whether or not these zones are disordered.

Areas related to endocrine, immune and reproductive systems

Either the thumbs or fingertips can be used to explore the tissue around C7, which has relationships with endocrine, immune and reproductive functions. Where the tissues are tense, taut or knotted, they are

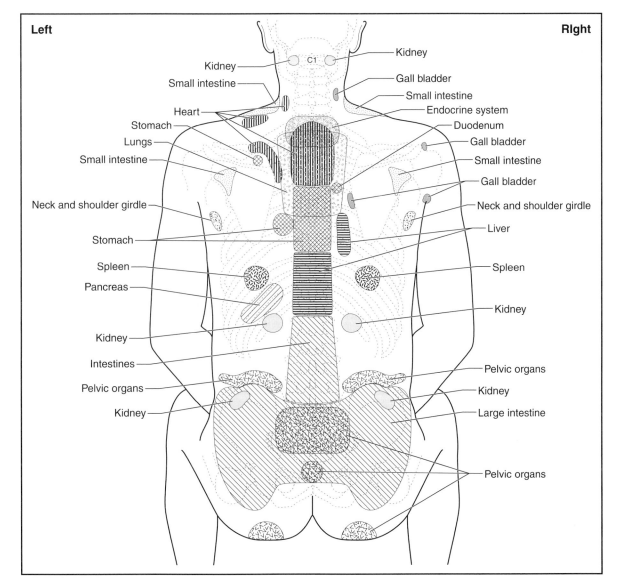

Left

Right

Kidney

Kidney

C1

Small intestine

Gall bladder

Small intestine

Heart

Endocrine system

Stomach

Duodenum

Lungs

Gall bladder

Small intestine

Small intestine

Gall bladder

Neck and shoulder girdle

Neck and shoulder girdle

Stomach

Liver

Spleen

Spleen

Pancreas

Kidney

Kidney

Intestines

Pelvic organs

Pelvic organs

Kidney

Kidney

Large intestine

Pelvic organs

Fig. 10.6 *Relationship of internal organs to surfaces on the back*

stretched and eased in several directions until they are well vascularised, pink and warm.

Separate treatment of the neck

If the neck has not been treated at the same time as the back, the therapist may choose to treat it with the patient lying on his back. No pillows are used but one or both of the therapist's hands support the head

and neck all the time. A small cushion may be placed in the small of the back if this is more comfortable for the patient.

The back

The therapist should make sure that an area at least 2.5 cm (1 inch) on either side of the vertebrae is palpated and, as the lumbar spine is reached, widen the exploration to at least 5 cm (2 inches) on either side of the vertebrae. If there are areas where the resilience within the tissues is raised or diminished, they are treated after the zones along the length of the spine have been assessed, first with more superficial movements and then with deeper palpation. Congestion which feels contained in one area is released by spreading it in a widening arc of movement, and tension is teased away from its centre. With the full surface of the palms close to the skin, several long stroking movements are made from the centre of the back over the entire musculature of the shoulder girdle, and over both shoulder joints.

The skin and subcutaneous tissues overlying and on either side of the:

- thoracic vertebrae 1–4 relate to the heart and lungs
- thoracic vertebrae 5–8 relate to the stomach
- thoracic vertebrae 9–12 relate to the liver
- the lumbar vertebrae relate to the intestines.

With any impairment of function in any of these organs, the related area becomes first sensitive then painful to palpate, the temperature varies from that of the rest of the back, there are textural and colour changes in the skin, and the tissues become first full, congested and taut, and in the later stages of illness they become 'empty'.

The lungs

Treatment over an area some 7.5 cm (3 inches) on either side of the first six thoracic vertebrae has a beneficial effect on lung function, easing respiratory movements when they are distressed, and increasing vital capacity.

The kidneys

The zones which correspond to the kidneys and lie closest to their anatomical position are found some 7.5 cm (3 inches) on either side of the spine at the level of and just below the 12th rib. Since the kidneys are vulnerable organs, protected in the body with a thick layer of perirenal fat, perirenal fascia and by their deep situation, only the lightest of touches is used to assess this zone. If it is painful, the therapist's

(warm) palms should be laid and held over the area until any pain has diminished. All kidney zones should be palpated with much care, and no vigorous or deep palpation or treatment is carried out over this region of the back. If a zone relating to any of the organs which have more than one zone on the back (such as the kidneys) is painful on palpation, the therapist should treat a different organ or system (such as the large intestine) before assessing another potentially painful reflex zone to the kidneys.

A further zone to the kidneys (about 5 cm or 2 inches long) is found over the upper third of the ilium, on an imaginary line running diagonally from the first lumbar vertebra to the greater trochanter of the femur. Light touch is likewise used on these zones for assessment and treatment.

A third reflex zone to the kidneys is found either side of the first cervical vertebrae, just below the bony occiput. Smooth, circular, searching palpatory movements are made. Patients with painful reflex zones here often describe their headaches as beginning in this region and creeping up over the head until they reach the forehead.

Pelvic organs

When one buttock is exposed, the zones relating to the pelvic organs extend along the iliac crest from the sacroiliac joint to about 2.5–5 cm (1–2 inches) from the lateral margins of the back, and palpation should cover this whole area.

The fingertips are moved over a broad band, about 1–8 cm (just over 3 inches) wide, depending on the size of the patient, over the iliac crest. A local hyperaemia should develop over the treated areas. Superficial stroking movements or effleurage are performed at regular intervals, and always when the treated area is painful. Further zones relating to pelvic organs are palpated over the base of the sacrum, over the coccyx and directly under the ischial tuberosities.

A large zone relating the large intestine extends from the sacroiliac joint to the greater trochanter of the femur, and often yields surprising variations in the quality of muscle and tissue tone. This is an area where deeper vibration, kneading, petrissage and frictions can be used to good effect. These zones are, however, often painful on palpation, and deep and vigorous touch is alternated with light stroking and effleurage as needed. Once a good hyperaemia has been achieved, the tissues feel uniform and the reflex zones are less painful, the same area on the opposite buttock can be similarly treated.

The pancreas

The zone which relates to the pancreas is found at the level of the 10th and 11th ribs, extending over approximately three-fifths of this area of the left side of the back, and is treated here. The pancreas is a 'silent' organ, difficult or impossible to palpate in the body, and specific symptoms often appear only in the late stages of disease. Since it is not always possible to distinguish the reflex zone to the pancreas from that of the stomach, liver or small intestine on the feet, palpation here gives an indication of its state of health. There is, however, a caveat. Any local underlying disease of the lungs or pleura refer pain to this area, which must not be confused with a painful reflex zone to the pancreas. Nor should the possibility be dismissed that there may be disease in both the lungs and the pancreas. Reflex zones which are disordered or painful and which do not improve with treatment show that disease is already well established — a finding that does not, however, clarify the nature of the illness.

If during a series of treatments the tissues begin to return to normal, the pain is reducing and the symptoms are abating, therapy can be continued and has been effective. If, on the other hand, the tissues remain congested and painful and symptoms persist, further medical investigation is needed.

The spleen

This lies underneath the 10th rib, over the third and fourth body zones, on the left side. It is treated over this area and a corresponding area on the right.

The stomach

One zone to the stomach is located midway between the seventh thoracic vertebra and the medial aspect of the scapula. It is sensitive in any gastric disorder. Dense, knotted or empty, seemingly hollow tissues are treated accordingly.

Another zone related to the stomach lies across the surface of and is bounded by the superior angle of the scapula. It is palpated with thumbs or fingertips. If the patient lies with his hands under his forehead, shoulders, or alongside his body, the therapist releases and extends his left arm, placing it at right angles to the body (or the elbow may be at an angle with the forearm and rest on the plinth). Palpation of the scapula and attached musculature is now easier. If the patient has limited movement of the shoulder joint, the most comfortable position should be found in which to rest his arm.

The heart

One zone which is connected to the heart curves round the superior angle of the left scapula. The border of the scapula and its neighbouring tissues should be probed delicately with the fingertips. The therapist uses only that depth of touch necessary to discover whether the musculature is supple and elastic, and whether there is any increased sensitivity to touch, palpating around the borders of the triangular scapula. The many muscular attachments of the shoulder girdle and upper arm to this bone develop changes in tone and tension when injury or disease of the related zones is present.

Because it has a wider range of movements than other joints, and the articulating surface of the head of the humerus with the clavicle and scapula are so shallow, the shoulder joint is subject to many complex injuries. Any limitation of movement and pain which does not respond after four sessions with an experienced therapist should be referred to a physiotherapist or orthopaedic surgeon.

At the same time the shoulder is a joint to which pain is frequently referred by several internal organs whose function becomes impaired. Chief amongst these are the gall bladder, small intestine, heart and lungs.

A further zone connected to the heart lies over the trapezius muscle, almost at the angle formed by the neck and shoulder. Palpation of this area takes the fingers from the back over the shoulder towards the clavicle. When these areas have been treated and the whole back warmly covered, a few stroking movements are made up and down the neck.

Alongside the third, fourth and fifth cervical vertebrae on the lateral border of the trapezius muscle (in the posterior triangle) lies a third reflex zone to the heart. As has already been mentioned, care needs to be exercised when palpating the reflex zones which lie in the neck. It is also possible to treat these zones at the same time as those of the cervical spine when the patient is lying on his back toward the end of the session.

The small intestine

Zones to the small intestine are found on the upper lateral triangle of the scapula, and at the angles of the neck and shoulder girdle, and are treated here.

The neck and shoulder girdle

Lateral to the inferior angle of the scapula over the latissimus dorsi on both left and right sides of the back is an area relating to the neck and shoulder girdle. It is frequently found to be dense and taut when the neck does not have free movement.

The liver

The area which relates to the liver lies to the right of the sixth, seventh, eighth and ninth thoracic vertebrae over an area approximately 3 cm (1 inch) in diameter and 9–10 cm (4 inches) in length, although this varies according to the patient's size and shape. With the tips of the fingers probe the length and breadth of this zone. Persistent discomfort indicates impairment of function, for which the cause should be sought. Toxicity from chemicals external to the body or toxicity arising from faulty metabolism and requiring a period of chemical rest for the liver need to be distinguished one from another.

The duodenum

To the right of the fourth or fifth thoracic vertebra (allowing for differences in anatomy) is an area related to the duodenum. It usually lies midway between the bony vertebrae and the medial border of the scapula. This reflex zone reflects many disorders in the first part of the small intestine, and is, at times, exquisitely painful when palpated. It is regularly found to be a primarily disordered reflex zone in patients with migraine headaches. The area is usually quite small and well defined, and the subcutaneous tissues can feel as taut as a drum to the palpating fingers.

The gall bladder

To the right of the fifth–sixth thoracic vertebrae, along the medial margin of the scapula, is found a zone relating to the gall bladder, about 3 cm (1 inch) in length. This area is palpated with the customary light but searching fingertips. The therapist should palpate around the borders and over the surface of the scapula, as was done on the left half of the back when treating the heart zones.

A further zone which is well known to relate to the gall bladder lies just medial to the superior angle of the scapula, on the right shoulder. Inflammation of the gall bladder, or the presence of gall stones, classically gives rise to sharp pain at the tip of the right shoulder.

Yet another reflex zone relating to the gall bladder lies in the latissimus dorsi just above the armpit.

Alongside the third, fourth and fifth cervical vertebrae on the right side of the neck is a fourth reflex zone to the gall bladder, which is more lightly palpated than those on the back. Light stroking movements are repeated after palpating this zone, which may also be treated at the same time as the neck.

General treatment procedure

Long, even stroking movements, which may be deep or superficial, are made at regular intervals over the shoulder girdle, as well as in a figure of eight, and up and down the spine and back. They are made whenever reflex zones are painful, or if the patient has experienced palpation as being too deep or strong, and are used to bring the treatment on the back to a close.

Reactions to treatment

The therapist should remain alert to:

- the patient's breathing becoming faster, shallower or less rhythmical
- muscular contractions in any part of the body
- the patient complaining of heat or feeling cold; the session is brought to a close if he begins to shiver, and he must be warmed with footbaths and, if necessary, hot water bottles before leaving the premises
- pallor of the skin
- the patient beginning to perspire, however slightly.

In this event, he should be warmly covered and the palms of both hands placed over the spine. With no pressure other than that of the lightly positioned hands, a steady, warm and calm attentive contact is maintained until the breathing returns to normal. Another restorative measure is for the therapist to rock the trunk lightly and slowly between her two cradled hands.

Repeated light stroking from neck to sacrum and from the midline spine towards the sides of the trunk (following the direction of the ribs) stabilises the patient.

Finishing the session

Stroking the cervical spine

The sides of the neck are stroked from shoulder to occiput with first one hand then the other to renew contact. If the head and neck are stiff, the therapist continues with the stroking movements until the muscles relax. She should not try to overcome any stiffness in the neck; calming but deft movements are sufficient to encourage relaxation. Supporting the occiput in the palms of both hands, she takes the weight of the head into the right hand and strokes lightly with the left hand, keeping an even contact between the palm of the hand and the skin. Broad sweeping strokes are made from the ear to the shoulder, while the head is allowed to rotate gently to the left, but only to the extent to which rotation is free. Both hands now support the head, which is gently rotated to the left and supported on the left hand. The right hand sweeps broadly from ear to shoulder several times.

The reflex zones to the kidneys, heart and gall bladder should be treated (see pp. 198–199).

Finishing the session

To finish, the therapist notes the patient's breathing and the degree to which he is relaxed as the treatment draws to a close.

The therapist's touch becomes lighter and lighter as the final stroking movements are made. No stimulating movements are given towards the end of any treatment.

Both hands may stroke in the same direction simultaneously, or one hand may follow the other in an unbroken rhythm, each stroke lighter than the last, until the patient is barely aware that touch has ceased.

The alignment of the head, neck and spine must be maintained. Two small cushions can be placed on either side of the head to maintain support, or, if desired, the patient is given a pillow. The patient is left comfortable, warmly covered and undisturbed for 20 minutes.

At the end of the rest period the patient should roll over onto one side before sitting up, and should be discouraged from moving directly from the supine position to a sitting position.

Records

At the end of each session the therapist records her observations and the treatment which has been given.

Summary

If treatment (whether on the back, the hands or the feet) is to be beneficial there must be steady progress in the patient, no matter how slight. Intervention which does not lead to improvement should be halted, and the therapist must question why it is ineffective.

Treatment to muscles which are taut and tense and zones which relate to parts of the body whose function is imperfect are painful on palpation and feel disordered to light touch. The patient may have been unaware of discomfort in some part of the body until touched by the therapist, and this discomfort may continue for a few sessions of treatment, but should not be given undue importance if the symptoms are improving.

Reactions may be a consequence of treatment on the back, as on the feet. There may be slight tenderness in some previously tense muscles which become relaxed during treatment, but no other zones of the back should be painful once the patient leaves the treatment room.

The best therapy is given when the therapist uses the lightest touch, probing or palpation to achieve the greatest possible improvement. Neither physical nor muscular strength are necessary to achieve this desired result. It is more the result of skill exercised by sensitive fingertips combined with knowledge and experience.

The usual immediate effects of a treatment on the back are of a loose-limbed freedom of movement and deep relaxation.

11

The oronasopharynx and teeth

Introduction

When assessing the reflex zones to the head and face, therapists frequently find disordered reflex zones to one or more teeth, or to their sockets within the maxilla or mandible. These may be to teeth which have been filled, capped or extracted, sometimes many years beforehand.

Discomfort in the reflex zones provoked by palpation, or SNS reactions such as cooling and sweating, are also commonly found in patients who are unaware of any dental problems, who attend regularly for dental appointments, and whose teeth appear to be in good condition. Yet such patients may respond to light touch on a disordered reflex zone with strong reactions, such as shivering.

Treating the oronasopharynx

The whole of the oronasopharynx is capable of reflecting changes which are happening or which have taken place elsewhere, in the same way as do the skin, hands, the feet and the back. Very small areas of the mucous membranes within the buccal cavity, including the upper and lower surfaces of the tongue, and the nasopharynx, mirror the condition of organs and structures throughout the body. Drs Voltolini (1883) and Fliess (1893) were the first to record changes in the mucous membranes of the nose during pregnancy in their writings at the end of the last century. Drs Fitzgerald (Fitzgerald & Bowers

1917) and Starr White (1926) later described the energy field of the nose, mouth, tongue and pharynx, and found that pressure or manipulation when applied to specific areas within the mouth had an effect on other parts of the body lying within the same zone. They also described how pressure or contact on the dorsal surface of each zone on the tongue affected anterior parts of the body within the same zone, whilst the underside of the tongue related to the posterior part of the body. Dr Fitzgerald wrote 'One of the most significant facts in connection with zone therapy is the intimate relation between morbid dental conditions and pain or even pathological changes in practically every section of the body' (Fitzgerald & Bowers 1917). He observed that infection of the third molar was frequently associated with the pain of sciatica. Furthermore, pressure applied to the mucocutaneal margins of the nose resulted in analgesia similar to that obtained in nerve bloc in the related body zones. Drs Voll (1974) and Kramer (1979) of the International Society for Electro-Acupuncture in Germany, and their dentist colleague Dr Adler (1983), have over the past five decades identified which parts of the body are related to each of the 32 individual adult teeth (see Fig 11.2, p. 209). Their work has shown a connection between patients' symptoms and illnesses and those teeth which have suffered either developmental, infective, traumatic or degenerative change.

Most recently, Gleditsch (1981) has discovered a remarkable correlation between the work of Drs Voll and Kramer and his own on the oronasopharynx. Gleditsch described a collection of points on the oral and buccal mucosa, near the teeth, and in the upper and lower lips which, if they are found to be sensitive to pressure and hyperalgesic, are associated with dysfunction in organs and joints. These points and their relationship to other parts of the body correspond closely to those of the odontones and their relationships first described by Drs Voll and Kramer. They are treated with neural therapy.

Painful and/or disordered reflex zones are often (but not always) found reflecting teeth which are apparently sound as well as in those which have been reconstructed. Yet not every tooth which has been filled or extracted provokes disorder in its corresponding reflex zones. The same phenomenon is seen when areas relating to some (but not all) scars are found to be painful when their reflex zones are palpated.

Furthermore, responses to treatment in the form of reactions in the oronasopharynx are regularly observed. Small, temporary blisters or boils may appear in the gums around one or more teeth, and apparently sound teeth can become more sensitive to heat, cold and touch, or even become painful for short periods.

The tonsils, teeth and paranasal sinuses are the commonest sites in the whole body in which an interference field is found. An understanding of interference fields helps the therapist to decide whether RZT is appropriate and likely to be beneficial, and whether it should be combined with or substituted by neural therapy (Dosch 1984; see also Ch. 2, p. 34). Certain dental conditions such as an unerupted tooth are reflected in disordered reflex zones, and respond only minimally or not at all to RZT. If an interference field results from the resulting impaction in the jaw, and causes symptoms at distant sites such as in a joint or an organ, the patient will not be helped by RZT. As there are concavities in tooth dentine which contain the basic elements of connective tissue, terminal autonomic fibres and capillary and lymphatic vessels, the arena is set in which disturbances in the GRS can arise.

A careful assessment of the zones of the teeth and jaw also provide help in deciding which disorders are primary (and therefore most in need of treatment), and which are secondary (which often improve with little therapy once the primary disorders have been identified and are being treated). The relationship between each tooth and several corresponding parts of the body also allows disorders in areas which do not have reflex zones on the hands, feet or back to be identified and treated. While reflex zones to the upper arms and elbows, thighs and knees are well described, those to the lower arms and hands and those to the lower legs and feet are not. Such areas can be treated via the reciprocal reflexes, as well as through disordered reflex zones to the teeth.

It is the province of the dentist to examine, treat and make a diagnosis on the health or otherwise of the teeth and gums. All that a good therapist can do is to make a careful examination of the reflex zones on the feet and observe the patient's response to treatment. Reflex zones to teeth which do not improve with treatment and are associated with ongoing symptoms call for further investigation by an informed dentist.

The therapist who is aware of the significance of interference fields is able to avoid some certain failures in treatment. If he suspects that an interference field is present, and the patient does not respond to treatment within a few sessions, he will not continue with treatment which he knows to be ineffective, and will direct the patient toward more appropriate help.

Causes of interference fields in the teeth

There are many possible reasons why an interference field may arise in one of the zones of the teeth. Not only the dentine or pulp of the tooth have to be considered, but its entire field of socket within the containing bone of maxilla or mandible, the nerve supply to the tooth, any of those cranial nerves whose branches meander into intimate contact with the roots of the teeth, and the fleshy gums which surround each tooth.

Infective causes

Infective causes include recent or old healed or imperfectly healed infection or granulomata (usually when incomplete healing has taken place). Infection may also be present within the jawbone, the root canal or the gums. Antibiotic cover for extractions is a common practice, but many people have been found to have a residual osteitis afterwards.

Trauma

Trauma in the form of a blow or a fall may lead to dislocation, chipping or breaking of one or more teeth. The protein present in dentine can decay, releasing one of its constituents, mercaptan, which is a known neural irritant, into surrounding tissues. This then spreads neurally via the GRS. Teeth which are used as a support for bridgework have an extra strain imposed on them, and often give rise to disordered reflex zones.

Foreign bodies

Foreign bodies such as splinters of bone, tooth or amalgam and other assorted filling materials, gravel or threads of fabric can become encapsulated within the tissues.

Scars

Scars arise from trauma, extraction and from poorly fitting dentures. Poor dental hygiene leads to food residues becoming lodged under dentures. This is an irritant to the mucous membranes, which if not removed may lead to the formation of a scar or an ulcer.

Developmental causes

Common developmental causes of an interference field include teeth which are impacted or semi-impacted, or those with an abnormal lie, projecting either into the mouth or toward the gums, and teeth which are recessed or lying at an angle to their neighbours.

Position of the teeth in the mouth

Each tooth is numbered according to its position in the mouth (Fig. 11.1). The buccal cavity is divided into right and left halves and lower and upper halves. There are eight teeth in each of the upper quadrants of both the right and left halves of the body, and eight teeth in each of the lower quadrants on the left and right.

Each tooth is numbered according to:

- the quadrant in which it lies, and
- its position within that quadrant.

Teeth lying in the upper right quadrant are identified by bearing '1' as their first number. The first number for teeth in the upper left quadrant is 2. The first number for teeth in the lower left quadrant is 3. The first number for teeth in the lower right quadrant is 4.

The next number locates each tooth within its quadrant. Tooth 1 lies closest to the midline and tooth 8 is the most lateral.

Reflex zones to the teeth are palpated on the dorsal aspect of the big toe, distal and medial to the interphalangeal joint space. They are also palpated on the dorsal, medial and plantar aspects of the second, third and fourth toes, and on the dorsal, medial and plantar aspects of the fifth toe (see Ch. 8, p. 146). The relationship which has been found to exist between each tooth and the various organs and structures of the body is seen in Figure 11.2.

Example

As an example of this relationship, take tooth 13 — the canine in the right upper quadrant. This tooth is related to:

- the posterior lobe of the pituitary (its endocrine connection)
- the organs of the gall bladder and liver
- the vertebrae T9 and T10
- the spinal cord segments T8, T9 and T10 (a spinal cord segment is a defined area of skin and muscle, the nerve supply to which emerges from a recognised spinal cord level; e.g. usually either the whole or part of segment Th5 or Th6 is affected by the herpes virus (shingles), becoming painfully inflamed when the virus attacks either of these nerve roots)
- The right hip and posterior knee joints and the right foot; and to the right eye.

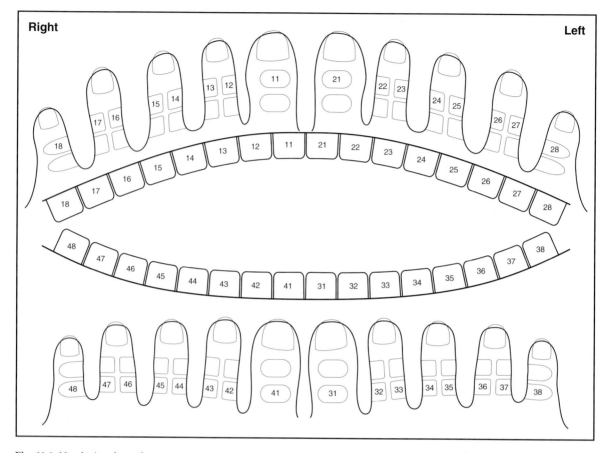

Fig. 11.1 *Numbering the teeth*

In practice

As an example of this relationship in practice, suppose a patient comes for treatment because she has pain in the right hip. At the first visit she describes the symptoms, and the therapist assesses the degree of movement in the joint and determines which movements cause pain.

The feet are visually and palpably assessed. During assessment, the reflex zone to tooth 13 (lying third from the midline in the upper right quadrant) is found to have altered skin or tissue tone. Discomfort is experienced when the zone is palpated. The remaining reflex zones to the teeth are normal.

The reflex zones to the liver, gall bladder, hips, posterior knee and vertebrae T9 and T10 (all of which relate to tooth 13) are carefully examined at

assessment. All the findings are recorded, and any teeth whose reflex zones are disordered are noted separately on the treatment card.

At subsequent sessions, the therapist watches to see whether there are any changes taking place in the disordered reflex zones, considers any reactions reported by the patient and those noticed by himself.

At every visit all disordered reflex zones, including that to tooth 13, are treated. Each zone is palpated for 20–30 seconds at least twice and preferably three times until there is no further discomfort, and the overlying skin and underlying tissues are normal.

The therapist should become suspicious if, after two or three treatment sessions, there is:

- no change in sensation in disordered reflex zones

Fig. 11.2 relationship chart (upper teeth, from R to L):

	8	7	6	5 (V)	4 (IV), 3 (III), 2 (II), 1 (I)	1 (I), 2 (II), 3 (III), 4 (IV)	5 (V)	6	7	8
SENSE ORGANS	Inner ear	Maxillary sinus	Ethmoid cells	Eye	Frontal sinus	Frontal sinus	Eye	Ethmoid cells	Maxillary sinus	Inner ear
JOINTS	Shoulder, Elbow	Jaws	Shoulder, Elbow	Back of knee — Hip	Back of knee — Sacrococcyx	Back of knee — Sacrococcyx	Back of knee — Hip	Shoulder, Elbow	Jaws	Shoulder, Elbow
JOINTS	Hand ulnar, Foot plantar, Toes, sacro-iliac joint	Front of knee	Hand radial, Foot, Big toe	Foot	Foot	Foot	Foot	Hand radial, Foot, Big toe	Front of knee	Hand ulnar, Foot plantar, Toes, sacro-iliac joint
SPINAL SEGMENTS	C8, T1 T5 T6 T7, S1 S2 S3	T11, T12, L1	C5 C6 C7, T2 T3 T4, L4 L5	T8, T9, T10	L2 L3, S4 S5, Coccyx	L2 L3, S4 S5, Coccyx	T8, T9, T10	C5 C6 C7, T2 T3 T4, L4 L5	T11, T12, L1	C8, T1 T5 T6 T7, S1 S2 S3
VERTEBRAE	C7, T1 T5 T6, S1 S2	T11, T12, L1	C5 C6 C7, T3 T4, L4 L5	T9, T10	L2 L3, S3 S4 S5, Coccyx	L2 L3, S3 S4 S5, Coccyx	T9, T10	C5 C6 C7, T3 T4, L4 L5	T11, T12, L1	C7, T1 T5 T6, S1 S2
ORGANS	Heart rt	Pancreas	Lung rt	Liver rt	Kidney rt	Kidney lt	Liver lt	Lung lt	Spleen	Heart lt
ORGANS	Duodenum	Stomach rt	Large intestine rt	Gall bladder	Bladder rt, Urogenital area	Bladder lt, Urogenital area	Bile ducts lt	Large intestine lt	Stomach lt	Jejunum ileum
ENDOCRINE GLANDS	Ant. lobe of pituitary	Para-thyroid, Thyroid	Thymus	Post. lobe of pituitary	Pineal gland	Pineal gland	Post. lobe of pituitary	Thymus	Thyroid, Para-thyroid	Ant. lobe of pituitary
OTHERS	CNS, Psyche	Mammary gland rt							Mammary gland lt	CNS, Psyche

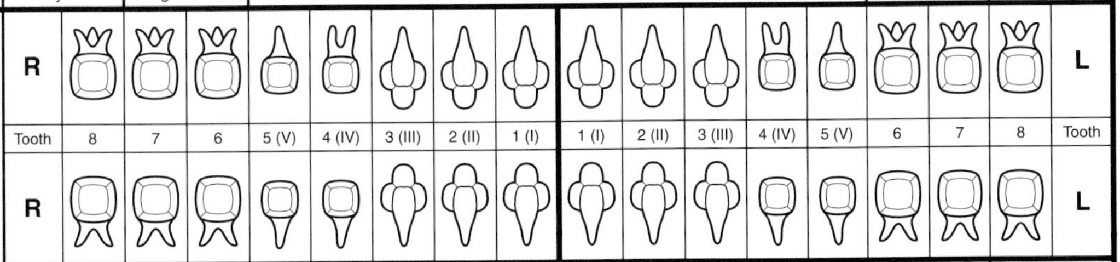

R [upper tooth diagrams] L

Tooth: 8 | 7 | 6 | 5 (V) | 4 (IV) | 3 (III) | 2 (II) | 1 (I) || 1 (I) | 2 (II) | 3 (III) | 4 (IV) | 5 (V) | 6 | 7 | 8

R [lower tooth diagrams] L

Fig. 11.2 relationship chart (lower teeth, from R to L):

	8	7	6	5 (V)	4 (IV), 3 (III), 2 (II), 1 (I)	1 (I), 2 (II), 3 (III), 4 (IV)	5 (V)	6	7	8
OTHERS	Energy metabolism		Mammary gland rt					Mammary gland lt		Energy metabolism
ENDOCRINE GLDS TISSUE SYSTEMS	Peripheral nervous system	Arteries, Veins	Lymph vessels	Gonad	Suprarenal gld	Suprarenal gld	Gonad	Lymph vessels	Veins, Arteries	Peripheral nervous system
ORGANS	Ileum rt	Large intestine rt	Stomach rt, Pylorus	Gall bladder	Bladder rt, Urogenital area	Bladder lt, Urogenital area	Bile ducts lt	Stomach lt	Large intestine lt	Jejunum Ileum lt
ORGANS	Ileocaecal region									
ORGANS	Heart rt	Lung rt	Pancreas	Liver rt	Kidney rt	Kidney lt	Liver lt	Spleen	Lung lt	Heart lt
VERTEBRAE	C7, T1 T5 T6, S1 S2	C5 C6 C7, T3 T4, L4 L5	T11, T12, L1	T9, T10	L2 L3, S3 S4 S5, Coccyx	L2 L3, S3 S4 S5, Coccyx	T9, T10	T11, T12, L1	C5 C6 C7, T3 T4, L4 L5	C7, T1 T5 T6, S1 S2
SPINAL SEGMENTS	C8, T1 T5 T6 T7, S1 S2 S3	C5 C6 C7, T2 T3 T4, L4 L5	T11, T12, L1	T8, T9, T10	L2 L3, S4 S5, Coccyx	L2 L3, S4 S5, Coccyx	T8, T9, T10	T11, T12, L1	C5 C6 C7, T2 T3 T4, L4 L5	C8, T1 T5 T6 T7, S1 S2 S3
JOINTS	Shoulder and elbow	Shoulder and elbow	Front of knee	Back of knee — Hip	Back of knee — Sacrococcyx	Back of knee — Sacrococcyx	Back of knee — Hip	Front of knee	Shoulder and elbow	Shoulder and elbow
JOINTS	Hand ulnar, Foot plantar, Toes, sacro-iliac joint	Hand radial, Foot, Big toe	Jaws	Foot	Foot	Foot	Foot	Jaws	Hand radial, Foot, Big toe	Hand ulnar, Foot plantar, Toes, sacro-iliac joint
SENSE ORGANS	Ear	Ethmoid cells	Maxillary sinus	Eye	Frontal sinus	Frontal sinus	Eye	Maxillary sinus	Ethmoid cells	Ear

Fig. 11.2 *Relationships between the teeth and organs and structures in the body (From Dr R. Voll, with kind permission)*

- no alleviation, however slight, of the symptoms
- no lasting sense of relaxation after a treatment and
- no reactions.

At this stage he must ask whether there has been any injury, infection or dentistry to this tooth at any time in the past. If a tooth is malpositioned, altered in shape or colour (either lighter or darker), used to buttress a bridge, chipped, broken or filled, it is likely that there is an associated interference field. The patient often complains that such a tooth 'feels dead', is sensitive to very hot or cold foods or fluids, or is at times painful.

Distinguishing the source of a problem

It is not always clear from assessment whether the primary problem lies within the tooth or the hip, and in doubtful situations the patient should be referred to a knowledgeable dentist. If one or more reflex zones improve with each session, however slowly, and if the patient responds to RZT by becoming less stressed, and increasingly relaxed, with diminished pain and increased mobility, and if she has any reactions, treatment is continued. The presence of an established interference field in and around a tooth can and often does block the appearance of reactions and the possibility of improvement.

If the reflex zones to the hip improve while the reflex zone to the tooth does not, at the end of a course of treatment the impression remains that the tooth is the site of the primary disorder. If the reflex zone to the tooth improves while that to the hip remains disordered, the impression is that the primary disorder lies in the hip, and this has been mirrored in the teeth and the feet. Thus it may be possible to distinguish primary and secondary disordered zones from the teeth. If there is no improvement in the patient's symptoms and all other avenues of RZT have been explored, then treatment must be discontinued. It should be explained to the patient that RZT is unlikely or unable to improve her condition. Neural or some other therapy may be more helpful to her, and she should be referred appropriately.

Treatment of interference fields in the teeth

Interference fields are nearly always reflected in the reflex zones on the feet. They may be small and weak, or large and strong. A weak interference field in any of the teeth can often be eliminated with a series of treatments. A larger and stronger field indicates that a substantial part of the GRS has become weakened, and it will therefore take longer for the interference field to be eradicated. It also indicates that the patient has to participate considerably in restoring the GRS to health and function. Sometimes changes in long-established but deleterious habits with regard to nutrition, mastication, rest, exercise, breathing and work are called for wherever possible. Chewing is important for the health of the teeth and gums, as well as for the digestion of food, and a healthy mix of food textures and variety of foods which need chewing should be eaten, not only those foods which are bland and easily chewable.

An established interference field which has chronically degraded the health of the patient poses an urgent question for patient and therapist. Any unnecessary stresses on the GRS should be relieved as soon as possible. RZT is supportive of the patient, the GRS and its functions, but inadequate by itself to restore health to a GRS whose function is being continually eroded, from whatever cause.

When symptoms have not responded to treatment within four to six sessions the therapist must try to discover what factors in the treatment, the illness, the therapist or the patient are responsible for the impasse.

Before it is decided to stop therapy, the therapist should:

- make a careful examination of all the reflex zones to the face, the teeth and the oronaso-pharynx, and reassess all the zones on the feet (or hands or back)
- treat all scars which are reflected as disordered reflex zones on the feet
- give relevant and concise practical advice on diet, breathing, relaxation (within his sphere of competence), which it is suggested the patient should write down for herself. This gives her the opportunity to think about what is being suggested while she is writing, to ask questions and seek clarification if necessary. It can also be referred to in the future, prevents any misconception and engages her in the treatment process.

A well-established interference field in one or more teeth puts limitations on what can be achieved through RZT. Recognising this limitation spares patient and therapist from ineffective sessions.

Two examples of this situation are detailed in Case study 11.1.

CASE STUDY 11.1

1

A physiotherapist learning reflex zone therapy was responsible for mobilising an elderly woman who had just had a revision hip replacement. She was frail and tired after the operation, and had developed an infection in the wound which was not responding to the prescribed antibiotics. As the patient found it too difficult and painful to stand, the physiotherapist decided to treat her with RZT. At assessment tooth 48 (the right lower wisdom tooth) was very painful, causing the patient to flinch on palpation and provoking immediate sweating and cooling of the feet. A carious tooth was discovered and reported to the consultant. The tooth was extracted, after which the woman made a straightforward recovery, the infection subsided and she was able to be mobilised.

2

A 50-year-old woman came for treatment complaining of tiredness as a result of much travel. She did not complain of any other symptoms. While she was recounting her history, the therapist noticed that her left upper front tooth was darkened and its surface roughened. She was questioned about past genitourinary disorders, and replied that she had had several serious bouts of cystitis years ago. These she had learned to prevent by taking adequate fluids and careful hygiene. The change in colour and texture of her tooth dated from that time, but had stabilised as the urinary infections subsided. The reflex zones on her feet showed some change in skin texture over the area of the bladder; there was minor discomfort in the reflex zones of tooth 21, the left kidney, ureter and bladder on both feet. Other disordered reflex zones were to the endocrine and lymphatic systems. After six sessions all reflex zones were free of any discomfort.

Summary

- The teeth are an energy field as are the feet, back or hands.
- They are related to other parts of the body.

- Disorders of the teeth or jaw may block the effects of any other treatment.
- They provide a platform for treating areas for which there are no reflex zones.
- They support the findings of disordered reflex zones in the feet.

References

Adler E 1983 Allgemein Erkrankungen durch Storfelder (Trigeminusbereich), 3rd edn. Verlag für Medizin Dr Ewald Fischer GmbH, Heidelberg

Dosch P 1984 Manual of neural therapy according to Huneke, 11th German edn. Karl F. Haug Verlag, Heidelberg (1st English edn transl. Lindsay A 1984)

Fitzgerald W H, Bowers E F 1917 Zone therapy. I W Long, Columbus, OH

Fliess W 1893 Die nasale Reflexneurose. Bergman, Wiesbaden

Gleditsch J M 1981 Mundakupunktur Biologische-Medizinische. Verlagsgeschellschaft, Schorndorf

Kramer F 1979 Lehrbuch der Elektroakupunktur. Karl F. Haug Verlag, Heidelberg

Starr White G 1926 Lecture course to physicians. Health Research. Mokelumne Hill, CA

Voll R 1974 Wechzelbeziehungen von Odontomen zu Organen und Gewebessystem. In: Dosch P Freudenstadter Vortrage, Band 2. Karl F. Haug Verlag, Heidelberg pp 136–139

Voltolini R 1883 Etwas über die Nase. Monatschrift für Ohrenheilkunde

RZT in different groups

12

RZT in pregnancy

Introduction

The care of women during pregnancy is the province of the midwife and obstetrician. If there is any doubt about the well-being and safety of the mother or baby, or if any unusual features are detected during treatment, she should be advised to see either of these, but always the therapist should consult with the midwife.

There are many commonly occurring minor ailments and discomforts of pregnancy which respond to simple measures. For example, elevating the legs helps to reduce physiological swelling of the ankles. If, however, the swelling exceeds what is normal, as in sudden, severe swelling of feet, ankles, face or elsewhere in the body, it is the task of the midwife to interpret the signs and decide whether further treatment is necessary.

Normal pregnancy is a healthy state, and many women feel radiantly well for some or all of the months of their pregnancies and little intervention is required. But sometimes women who are sick become pregnant, and sometimes women who are pregnant become sick. There are also those physiological changes and strains occurring in a woman's body (such as backache) which regular or intermittent RZT can alleviate while supporting the general health of mother and child.

The definition of a midwife adopted by the World Health Organization is as follows:

■ *"A midwife is a person who, having been regularly admitted to a midwifery educational programme, duly recognised in the country in which it is located, has successfully completed the prescribed course of studies in midwifery and has aquired the requisite qualifications to be registered and/or legally licensed to practise midwifery."*

Within her practice:

■ *"She must be able to give the necessary supervision, care and advice to women during pregnancy, labour and the postpartum period, to conduct deliveries on her own responsibility and to care for the newborn and the infant. This care includes preventative measures, the detection of abnormal conditions in mother and child, the procurement of medical assistance and the execution of emergency measures in the absence of medical help. She has an important task in health counselling and education, not only for the women, but also within the family and the community. The work should involve antenatal education and preparation for parenthood and extends to certain areas of gynaecology, family planning and child care." (UKCC 1998)*

Pregnancy and childbirth were hazardous all over the world one and a half centuries ago, and remain so in many parts of the world to this day. That much of the risk has been eliminated is a tribute to the training and practice of midwives over the past century.

In the UK the law states that the practice of midwifery may be conducted only by an appropriately qualified person. All matters pertaining to (a) the expectant mother at the time of pregnancy, labour, the puerperium and (b) the care of the infant for the first 10 days of his life are attended to and supervised by the midwife. It is the duty of any therapist to cooperate with the midwife, whose decisions about the care of the mother and baby are final.

Contraindications — when not to use RZT

Those contraindications which have been stated in Chapter 5 apply in all situations, but there are certain conditions found only in pregnancy. These are:

- placenta praevia
- pre-eclampsia
- antepartum haemorrhage
- postpartum haemorrhage
- pelvic infection
- deep vein thrombosis
- bleeding or cramps
- when a Shirodkar suture has been inserted
- unstable pregnancy in the first trimester (3 months of the pregnancy)
- marked instability at any time during the pregnancy
- threatened abortion
- preterm labour (before 34 weeks of the pregnancy are complete)
- if the mother does not want treatment.

Midwives with many years of experience and practice, and who are familiar also with the effects of RZT, may choose to use some calming and sedating strokes or movements on the feet or hands in one of the above situations. Such a decision can only be made in the given situation and the midwife decides what is clinically in the best interest of mother and infant. A therapist who is not a midwife and not experienced should not use RZT in any of the above circumstances. If the therapist does not know how to recognise any of these circumstances she should refrain from giving treatment when a pregnant woman is unwell and the cause is unknown.

Assessment

When a pregnant woman wishes to have RZT, the same procedure is followed at the first visit as for any other person. The woman should indicate why she wants treatment, and the therapist describes RZT briefly with special reference to pregnancy, a careful history is taken followed by visual assessment, palpation, and this is followed by 20 minutes of rest.

Usual reasons for seeking RZT during pregnancy

General

Pregnant women may generally seek RZT for the following reasons:

- for relaxation
- for prophylactic assessment and to prevent as far as is possible any disorders which may develop
- because previous treatment has resulted in a sense of well-being.

Related to pregnancy

Reasons relating to the pregnancy include:

- for tiredness
- for treatment for one of the minor ailments of pregnancy.

For gynaecological complaints

Reasons relating to gynaecological complaints include:

- urinary incontinence
- stress incontinence
- laxity of the pelvic floor or any of its possible complications such as a threatening prolapse of the bladder, vagina or rectum

- dysmenorrhoea
- irregular menstruation
- menorrhagia
- metrorrhagia: any woman suffering with metrorrhagia should be referred to her doctor without delay for further investigation.

Treatment

Treatment can be given twice a week or every 4 or 5 days. All disordered reflex zones and all reacting systems are treated at each visit until the tissues become normal to touch once more.

The therapist should keep in mind that both mother and baby are being treated at each session.

Reflex zones to pelvic supports

Women who are pregnant or suffer from gynaecological complaints often require treatment to the reflex zones of specific pelvic supports.

The pelvic basin is formed by the bones of the pelvis (Fig. 12.1) in which lie the pelvic organs (Figs 12.2 and 12.3). It is closed inferiorly by a muscular sheet called the pelvic floor or pelvic diaphragm (Fig. 12.4). This consists of two muscles, the larger levator ani and the smaller coccygeus, which is perforated in the midline to allow space for the urethra toward the front, and the anal canal towards the back, with the female vagina between these two openings. The nerve supply to the levator ani is from the third and fourth sacral nerves. The pelvic viscera of bladder, uterus and rectum are supported by the levator ani muscle, whose posterior fibres (the puborectalis) help form the anal sphincter and canal and encircle the wall of the vagina.

The pelvic floor may be weakend by childbirth, prolonged labour, multiple pregnancies, long hours of standing, heavy lifting, constipation, pelvic surgery, lack of oestrogen, some drugs and generalised loss of muscle tone due to inherited faulty collagen production. When the levator ani of the pelvic floor is weakened there may be prolapse of the bladder or rectum. If the cervical ligaments (those which support the cervix) are ruptured during pregnancy, surgery, or weakened by an incompetent levator ani, the uterus may prolapse.

The uterus is held in position by:

- the levator ani, which has its origin in the pubis and the side walls of the pelvis as far round as the spine of the ischium; it is inserted into the perineal body (which lies just in front of the anal canal) and held in place by the perineal muscles
- three ligamentous slings (all formed from peritoneum), which are attached to the cervix and the side walls of the pelvis (see Fig. 12.1):
  — the pubocervical ligaments lie anteriorly
  — the transverse cervical ligaments lie laterally
  — the uterosacral ligaments lie posteriorly
- the minor support of the round ligament, which runs laterally through the inguinal canal to the labia majorus.

The reflex zones to the pelvic support structures are shown in Figure 12.5.

Treatment for specific circumstances

The following are guidelines for treatment only. Although the physiological changes which take place in pregnancy can be described, and although they follow a similar pattern, no two pregnancies have the same physiological and emotional effects upon any two women. Each RZT session must be tailored to suit the individual recipient. These patterns have been found to be beneficial over the years, but there will always be variations in women's responses to therapy, just as responses to medicines vary. (For illustrations of specific reflex zones on the foot, refer to Chapter 8.)

First aid treatment

First aid can be given in the form of treatment to a specific reflex zone, such as to the iliosacral joint for backache in late pregnancy or during the first stage of labour, to the diaphragm to assist with relaxation, to

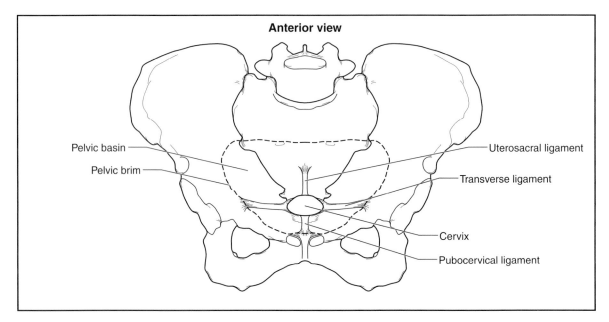

Anterior view

Pelvic basin

Pelvic brim

Uterosacral ligament

Transverse ligament

Cervix

Pubocervical ligament

Fig. 12.1 *The pelvic basin*

the bladder and solar plexus for urinary retention, or a combination of these. Otherwise a full assessment should be made.

Harmonising hold

The most comforting and stabilising harmonising hold, which is preferred by almost all pregnant and parturient women, is a cupping of the therapist's hands over both of the woman's heels (Fig. 12.6). Keeping the hands in this position for a minute or two whilst observing the breathing and colour gives her a respite and restores a measure of equilibrium to the ANS.

Traction

A gentle traction (starting with slight leverage only) applied to the length of the spine (see Fig. 6.7, p. 105) also helps to regularise breathing if it has become faster and shallower in rhythm. The therapist holds both heels in the palms of the hands and, keeping the fingers flat against the medial aspects of both heels, engages her whole spine in gradually extending the woman's spine. (The therapist should lean backwards

using her whole body weight to *gently* stretch the hips and spine from the heels to the base of the skull, rather than using her shoulder girdle just to pull the legs.)

Preconceptual care

When the woman wishes to prepare for a pregnancy, or if she is having difficulty in conceiving, a full assessment is made, followed by treatment to any disordered reflex zones which are found.

Twice weekly treatments should be given until the disorders of skin and tissue tone are no longer present, and all reactions have ceased.

Supplementary care. A diet high in folic acid and folic acid supplements is advisable for any woman planning to become pregnant. There is evidence that folic acid lessens the risk of neural tube defects.

Infertility

True infertility is an irreversible condition in both men and women, and RZT cannot alter the situation.

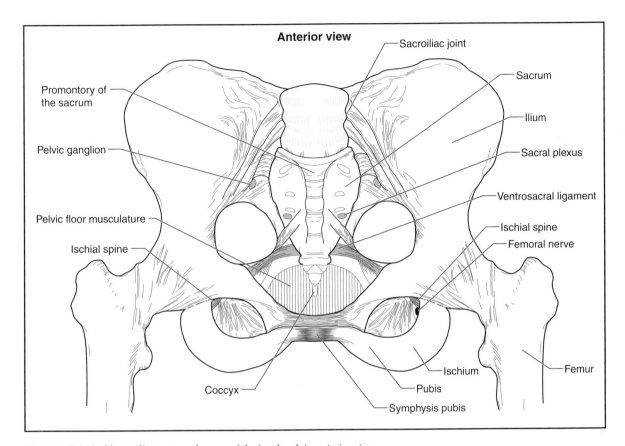

Fig. 12.2 *Principal bones, ligaments and nerves of the female pelvis: anterior view*

No false hope should be given to anyone seeking a cure for infertility. RZT may be given for as long as necessary to strengthen the GRS and because it is emotionally calming, and for as long as there are painful or disordered reflex zones which respond to treatment.

Subfertility

An assessment is made and followed by treatment twice a week for 6 weeks during which there should be no sexual intercourse. This gives a respite to both partners and allows the changes in body chemistry which take place through the improvement in ground regulating function to be consolidated.

Supplementary care. The therapist should ensure that nutrition, exercise, attitude and technique are optimum for conception to take place, also that no unnecessary medicines are being taken, and advise with tact where necessary. A diet high in folic acid and folic acid supplements is recommended (see above). Where possible, it is preferable for both partners to participate in any investigation and treatment.

Pregnancy

In pregnancy the increased circulating blood volume and weight make for greater physiological demands on the expectant mother's circulatory system. It is suggested that the following general indications for treatment be adopted for any of the common but troublesome minor ailments associated with pregnancy. Additional treatment is given (for example to teeth or scars) where the history or

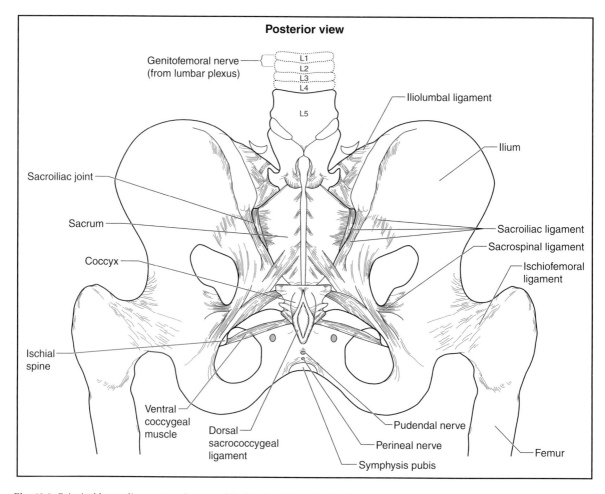

Fig. 12.3 *Principal bones, ligaments and nerves of the female pelvis: posterior view*

palpable findings dictate. Obstetric referral is essential if the expectant mother develops abdominal cramps, bleeding, or if there are any indications that the pregnancy is abnormal or is at risk.

Threatened abortion

The therapist should not treat with RZT, but refer the expectant mother immediately to her midwife or general practitioner.

Inevitable abortion

Once the inevitability of the miscarriage has been established, light treatment is given as follows:

- first the endocrine system
- the pelvic organs and pelvic lymphatics
- the urinary system and the small intestine
- stimulation (but not sedation) of the pelvic lymphatic system
- sedation of the solar plexus.

After a miscarriage or termination

An assessment is made, and all the disordered reflex zones are treated. Specific treatment is as follows:

- stimulation of the urinary system
- the small intestine

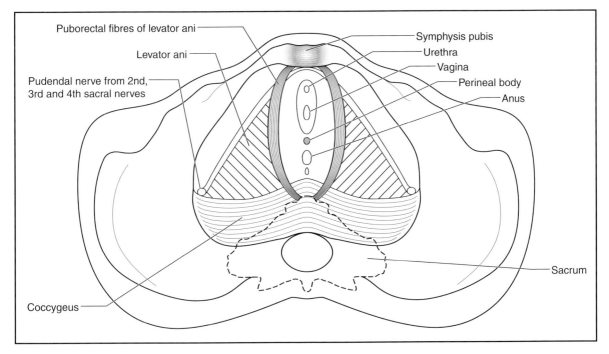

Fig. 12.4 *Muscles of the pelvic floor*

- the spleen
- the lymphatic system and
- the endocrine system, particularly the pituitary (which is usually found to be in need of treatment)
- normal treatment on the pelvic organs
- sedation of the solar plexus and adrenals.

Supplementary care. The therapist should advise the woman to wring her wrists frequently to stimulate pelvic lymphatic drainage.

Morning sickness

A standard assessment is made. Specific treatment is as follows:

- repeated sedation of the solar plexus
- the diaphragm
- the stomach and
- the thoracic spine
- sedation of the solar plexus, but for no longer than 20 seconds at any one time, as this may lead to the opposite effect from that which is intended

(if the woman becomes anxious and restless rather than calm and relaxed, the therapist should lightly stimulate the solar plexus)
- frequent calm stroking movements to encourage deep breathing
- treatment of the shoulder and pelvic girdles, to relax them
- light measured treatment to the whole of the endocrine system
- supplementary treatment to the reflex zones of the stomach and solar plexus on the hands.

Supplementary care. The leaves of the raspberry plant contain an active principle called fragrine, whose effect is most marked on the female reproductive organs, and one of its most important effects is to tone the uterus. It can be taken throughout pregnancy and the puerperium, and is often helpful in morning sickness. If, however, a rash develops around the waistline, the recommended dose has been exceeded. An infusion of some 250 ml on waking, before eating or drinking anything else in the morning is recommended. As dried herbs are

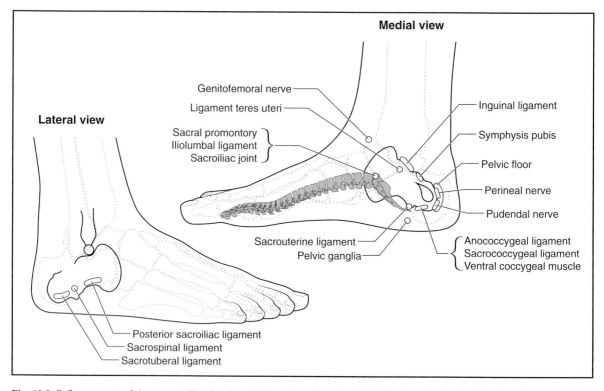

Fig. 12.5 *Reflex zones to pelvic supports (Developed by W. Froneberg. Reproduced with kind permission of N. Gosch and A. Froneberg)*

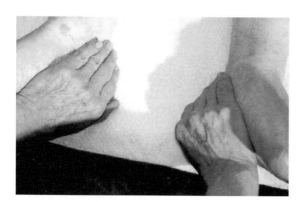

Fig. 12.6 *Cupping the heels*

stronger than the fresh leaves, the woman should be careful not to exceed the stated dose.

Although infusions can be prepared in many ways, the following satisfactory method has long been used and recommended by herbalists. The water should have been brought to the boil, but should not be boiling when it is poured over the herb and allowed to stand (covered) for 3 minutes. A pinch

of the dried herb, that is, as much as can be held between the thumb and forefinger, is the amount needed for 250 ml of water.

Hyperemesis gravidarum

In this debilitating and often persistent illness, in which no food or fluids are able to be retained, obstetric referral is essential. A period of time in hospital may be necessary. The endocrine system is usually grossly disordered, and the excessive vomiting is usually the cause of painfully disordered zones in the stomach, spleen and small intestine. All the emphasis in treatment is on measures which calm the expectant mother, and frequent rhythmical stroking movements which are light but which the woman also finds relaxing are repeated many times over.

No stimulating movements are made at all. Specific treatment is as follows:

- normal palpation on the endocrine system and
- all other disordered reflex zones as above

- sedation of the stomach and
- the solar plexus.

The midwife and doctor are best able to decide which measures are helpful in this complex illness. RZT can be given because of its globally supportive effect, to help relieve the nausea and vomiting, and to promote rest.

Incompetent cervix

As the expectant mother has to spend long periods resting or in many instances remain completely bedfast, regular treatments to all disordered reflex zones are given in order to detect disorders before they give rise to signs and symptoms, and to prevent any of the complications (such as renal calculi, loss of muscle tone) which are associated with prolonged bedrest. No vigorous or stimulating treatment is given in the pelvic region.

Specific treatment is as follows:

- the musculature of the pelvic floor
- the urinary system and
- the spine. (The parasympathetic nerve supply to the cervix is from the inferior hypogastric plexus (sacral) and an extension of the inferior hypogastric plexus lying at the base of the broad ligament — there called the uterovaginal plexus. The outflow is from the last thoracic and first lumbar segments of the cord. Efferent fibres run down the vaginal artery directly to the cervix.)

Backache

The therapist should calm (sedate) those reflex zones which are most painful along the spine. (This is usually the sacroiliac joint or some part of the lumbar spine, often accompanied by compensatory pain in the neck or shoulder girdle due to muscle spasm and the rigid position in which the spine is protectively held.)

Specific treatment is as follows:

- sedation of the solar plexus and adrenal glands
- relaxation of the shoulder girdle by circumduction of the heads of the metatarsal bones one against each other; with the thumb of one hand on the plantar head and the fingers of the same hand on the dorsal head of the first

metatarsal, and the thumb of the other hand on the plantar head and the fingers on the dorsal head of the second metatarsal, one hand gently rotates clockwise and the other counter-clockwise (see Fig. 6.3D, p. 101); this is repeated on each of the other articulations at the mtp joint line

- relaxation of the pelvic girdle by slow rotation of the ankle joint
- treatment of the musculature of the abdominal wall over the tarsal bones on the dorsum of the foot
- the hips and symphysis pubis
- the lower thoracic spine (see Ch. 8, p. 148), which is often painful as the enlarging breasts exert an unaccustomed forward pull on the whole musculature of the shoulder girdle and thoracic spine, and
- the whole of the small and large intestines.

Supplementary care. The woman can be shown how to relieve pain by sedating pressure on disordered reflex zones on the hands. Appropriate advice on posture (using a lumbar roll), exercise and rest should be given. The manuals 'Treat your own back' and 'Treat your own neck' by Robin McKenzie are invaluable.

An example of the use of RZT for backache and pain during pregnancy is detailed in Case study 12.1.

Frequency of urine

Frequency is a physiological response in the early and late months of pregnancy as the enlarging uterus compresses the bladder. The urethra is stretched in the second half of pregnancy and the nerves associated with micturition become irritable. As infection in the urinary tract is also common during pregnancy the therapist should ensure that any frequency is not due to infection.

Specific treatment is as follows:

- stimulation of the kidney zones as the increasing blood volume places more demand on the kidneys
- treatment of the bladder zones (to maintain the muscle tone)
- the bladder

CASE STUDY 12.1

A healthy 28-year-old primiparous schoolteacher (at 27 weeks' gestation) presented at an antenatal clinic complaining of low backache in the sacroiliac region and bilateral pain in the buttocks along the sciatic nerve. The pain had gradually become worse and had failed to benefit from physiotherapy. She was tearful and distressed, in part because of the pain and in part because she was still working.

Inspection revealed an exaggerated curve to the lateral aspect of the feet. There was no callus. The tone in the feet was slightly diminished on palpation.

1st treatment. Sedation was given to the lower back, lumbar and sacral regions, the pelvic ligaments and the solar plexus. Frequent Yin-Yang strokes were made.

The outcome was that 3 days later the woman was cheerful and pain free. She had seemingly made a good recovery.

2nd treatment. Eleven weeks later, at 39 weeks, gestation, she returned for further treatment because the backache had recurred, less severe than previously, but limiting and painful. The baby's head was engaged in the pelvis.

Inspection revealed pallor over the sacroiliac joint zones. On palpation the pelvic ligaments were slightly tender, and the reflex zones of the lumbar and sacral spine were painful.

Sedation was given to the solar plexus, lower spine and pelvic ligaments. Stimulation was given to the cervical and thoracic spine, also rotation of the big toe, and gentle pelvic rotation. Yin and Yang stroking was given. She was advised to rest more. The outcome was that she was pain free for 4–5 days.

- the anal sphincter and
- the pelvic floor musculature
- sedation of the solar plexus and diaphragm.

Cystitis

If any urinary infection persists the woman should see her midwife or doctor.

Specific treatment is as follows:

- sedation of the solar plexus
- treatment of the oronasopharynx
- the whole lymphatic system
- the lower thoracic and lumbar spine and
- the kidneys and bladder, taking care not to irritate the reflex zones of the enlarging uterus.

Supplementary care. Proper attention must be given to fluid intake, hygiene and rest. If proteinuria, haematuria or glycosuria are suspected or detected on urine testing, an obstetric referral is necessary.

Constipation

Specific treatment is as follows:

- the reflex zones to the spine, especially the lumbar region

- the small and large intestines
- all sphincters
- the liver and gall bladder
- the abdominal wall and
- any other disordered reflex zones; care should be taken not to irritate the reflex zones to the uterus
- sedation of the solar plexus and diaphragm.

Supplementary care. The hands should be treated twice daily by the expectant mother. Attention should be paid to the diet. Adequate clear fluids should be taken over every 24 hours, of which plain water is the best (and for which tea, coffee, canned and bottled drinks are no substitute). A diet which has sufficient fibre, fruit and vegetables and adequate exercise is recommended. Sitz baths can be helpful (see Appendix IV, p. 287).

Varicose veins

The increased weight load and hypervolaemia of pregnancy usually exacerbate existing or developing varicose veins. The extent to which RZT is helpful depends on whether there is a congenital weakness of the valves in the vein, or the degree to which valves have become incompetent as a result of long hours of standing or carrying heavy weights.

The most effective (and cheapest) way to relieve excessive back pressure on the veins is to lie down with the feet elevated above the height of the hips, and to keep them elevated for 20 minutes at least twice a day. The hips should not be so acutely flexed (no more than 45°) that there is an obstruction there to the free passage of fluid. To relieve the pressure on valves the veins need to empty passively as gravity drains the viscous blood from the lower limbs and prevents venous stasis there.

Specific treatment is as follows:

- stimulation of the reflex zones to the liver and gall bladder
- the small and large intestines
- the kidneys
- the bladder and
- the lymphatic system, particularly the lymphatic drainage of the thighs and pelvis.

Supplementary care. Alternate hot and cold sponging, and cool or cold showering of the legs after bathing, also help with the pain and discomfort. Sitz baths (see Appendix IV, p. 287) are recommended to stimulate circulation in the lower limbs.

Haemorrhoids

Specific treatment is as follows:

- the small and large intestines
- the liver and gall bladder
- the lymphatic system and
- sedation of the pelvic floor and anal region without irritating the uterus and
- the solar plexus.

Supplementary care. Simple measures such as drinking enough water, regular meal times, chewing all food properly, eating only when sitting down, a daily intake of fruit and vegetables (preferably those which are in season), adequate exercise, avoiding constipation and gentle massage of the abdominal wall are all helpful. Reducing the amount of treated wheat (that is, wheat to which too many non-nutritive substances have been added) can be helpful for both constipation and haemorrhoids. The hands

should be treated twice a day. Sitz baths (see Appendix IV, p. 287) are also recommended.

Oedema

Most women experience a degree of oedema (usually of the ankles) during pregnancy, especially during the later months. The midwife will monitor any fluid retention to see that it does not become excessive and that there are no signs of pre-eclampsia. RZT is most beneficial in helping to reduce oedema.

Specific treatment is as follows:

- the kidneys
- the heart
- the lymphatic system
- the liver and
- the small intestine
- frequent stroking movements and effleurage of the feet and lower legs are both relaxing and reduce pooling of fluid.

Supplementary care. Resting with the legs elevated is advised, as are relaxation techniques (diaphragmatic breathing, yoga, relaxation classes, recreation) and exercise. If the daily consumption of salt is high it should be reduced and salty foods should be avoided.

Cramp

Always check that there is no deep vein thrombosis.
Specific treatment is as follows:

- the thyroid and parathyroid glands
- the kidneys and
- any other disordered reflex zones
- sedation of the solar plexus and diaphragm.

Supplementary care. The therapist should discuss nutrition, and advise that salt should be reduced or avoided. Tonic water contains quinine, which is an effective remedy for reducing cramp. The expectant mother is advised to drink at least one glass of tonic water a day. Elevating the foot of the bed, and foot and leg exercises, are helpful. Relaxed abdominal breathing should be taught and encouraged. The expectant mother should also be encouraged to breathe out (and not hold her breath) during an attack of cramp. As the growing uterus presses on the diaphragm, there may be less expansion of the lungs, with a consequent build-up of carbon dioxide in the bloodstream. Shallow breathing and hyperventilation may be factors responsible for cramp.

Pathological laxity of the symphysis pubis

Specific treatment is as follows:

- the symphysis pubis
- the lower spine
- the adductor muscle group
- the sacroiliac joint
- the abdominal musculature and
- the lateral and medial uterine supports
- any other disordered reflex zones.

Supplementary care. Sedation on the painful reflex zones of the hands helps to relieve this painful condition.

Hypertension

As the causes of hypertension are so many and varied, an assessment is essential. The therapist should start with frequent Yin-Yang strokes. Specific treatment is as follows:

- sedation of the adrenals repeatedly for short periods (up to 20 seconds with each palpation) and
- the solar plexus and diaphragm
- treatment of all disordered reflex zones
- the liver
- the small and large intestines
- the endocrine system and
- stimulation of the kidneys and bladder
- relaxation of the shoulder girdle, neck and sternum.

Supplementary care. No salt should be added to food during cooking, and salty foods should be avoided. Relaxed breathing should be encouraged. The solar plexus on the hands can be regularly sedated by the patient.

Malaise

A general treatment is given from the 6th month onwards, or when poor sleep, restlessness, pain, frequent Braxton-Hicks contractions, breathlessness, or a taut and heavy abdomen in an otherwise straightforward pregnancy cause the expectant mother discomfort.

The woman should be comfortably supported with several pillows, and have a support in the small of the back. The reflex zones to the uterus enlarge in accordance with the stage of pregnancy, as do those of the fetus within, who also responds to any touch. The therapist should start with harmonising and Yin-Yang strokes.

Specific treatment is as follows:

- quiet sedation of the uterine supports
- relaxation of all the musculature of the shoulder girdle until the mother's breathing becomes deep and rhythmical
- sedation of the solar plexus
- treatment of the diaphragm
- the lower spine
- the abdominal and pelvic musculature
- the lymphatic system
- the urinary system and
- any other disordered reflex zones.

Monitoring of the scanner during RZT shows that calming the expectant mother has an equal and simultaneous effect on the fetus. Treatment is best given at intervals which meet the needs of the woman. If there are no complications, sessions once every 3 weeks, then every 2 weeks, then weekly in the last month, cover most needs. Repeated light stroking and sedation on the solar plexus are relaxing in most instances.

Labour

It is advisable for midwives to be experienced in all aspects of midwifery before adding RZT to their practice. At the Frauenspital in Berne midwives do not learn RZT until they have been qualified for a year. The midwife is expected to know when she should choose to use or refrain from using RZT, and when complications are developing in either pregnancy or labour.

As expectant mothers prefer not to be surrounded by any more apparatus than is essential for the safety and well-being of their babies and themselves, RZT can be used for pain relief during the first stage of labour. The endorphins produced by touch on appropriate reflex zones (see Ch. 2, p. 31) helps to reduce pain to a tolerable level for many women. The midwife retains the option of giving pain-relieving drugs if required, and decides to do so whenever she deems it necessary.

Unlike a normal RZT session, which lasts for approximately 30 minutes, treatment during labour may be intermittent over many hours. The therapist, if she is not the midwife, should always work in cooperation with the midwife, and must not counteract any of her instructions.

The guiding principle for the therapist is to start all assessment, treatment and first aid with the lightest therapeutic touch, to deliver the smallest stimulus at the beginning of any treatment, and to build up depth and intensity of her palpation in small steps if this is needed. If too much stimulation or sedation is given to a reflex zone, or if there is an unexpected and strong reaction in the patient, the therapist should do the opposite of what she has just done, and slow the breathing. Yin-Yang strokes or light stroking movements diminish autonomic imbalance.

If a sedation hold on the solar plexus is maintained for too long (or is too deep) and the patient becomes distressed, restless, breathless or complains of palpitations, the adrenals should be sedated and the solar plexus lightly stimulated.

Note: Medication alters the internal milieu, and the responses to RZT after taking or being given drugs may be faster or slower than usual. This also happens when there is sensory deprivation of any kind. For this reason it is inadvisable to use RZT at the same time as epidural anaesthesia. A very fine judgement is needed when treating those who are heavily medicated.

Preterm labour — from 34 weeks' gestation

Obstetric advice must be sought. Complete bedrest is necessary for the mother, and it is usual for the necessary observations to be carried out in the antenatal ward. The therapist can start with gentle, rhythmic and light harmonising and Yin-Yang strokes.

Specific treatment is as follows:

- sedation to the solar plexus is all that can be given while waiting for the midwife
- if RZT is deemed appropriate, the midwife sedates the solar plexus, adrenal and pituitary glands
- the lower spine, uterus, ovaries and uterine supports
- the endocrine and lymphatic systems are lightly treated.

Early rupture of membranes

This usually requires admission to the maternity ward. Harmonising and calming strokes are all that may be given at this time.

Postmaturity induction of labour

The decision to induce labour is an obstetric one. The midwife decides whether and when RZT should be given.

Specific treatment is as follows:

- light stimulation of the pituitary, thyroid and ovaries
- the lumbar and sacral spines and
- the small and large intestines
- treatment of the abdominal wall
- light treatment of the reflex zones to the uterus
- sedation of the solar plexus.

If there are indications that the woman is going into labour, this pattern is repeated every 2 to 3 hours, but she should not be overstimulated by spending more than 10 minutes on the feet at each time.

The first stage of labour

Treatment is directed at inducing deep rhythmical breathing between contractions, and relieving backache, cramp, and easing the pain of contractions.

Specific treatment is as follows:

- an even sustained hold of up to 2 minutes on the reflex zone to the solar plexus of the feet is the first choice for pain relief; if the woman is up and about the hands can be treated; long, generous stroking movements or Yin-Yang strokes help to compose the woman between contractions

- relaxation of the musculature of the shoulder girdle and of the diaphragm with even, undulating palpation of these zones; and circumduction of the heads of mtp joints 1 and 2 (see p. 223, also Fig. 6.3D, p. 101)
- relaxation also of the thoracic and lumbar spines and
- the hip joints
- sedation of the reflex zone to the sacroiliac joint if there is low backache (repeat as necessary)
- for cramp and tingling, encouragement of expiration and treatment of the reflex zones of the diaphragm, solar plexus, lungs and shoulder girdle
- the therapist should keep her hands in contact with the feet during the whole of a contraction, lightly sedating the solar plexus, then lightly holding the reflex zone of the uterus.

Being present and attentive is reassuring to the mother, who is constantly given encouragement and support.

Incoordinate uterine action. If there is incoordinate uterine action, the therapist should give calming and Yin-Yang strokes, and encourage relaxed breathing by the following:

- treatment of the lungs, diaphragm and shoulder girdle
- sedation of the solar plexus
- treatment of the endocrine system, beginning with the pituitary; treat the thyroid, the adrenals, pancreas, ovaries and
- the uterus.

Tonic uterine contractions. If there are tonic uterine contractions, the therapist should give calming and Yin-Yang strokes, and then treatment specifically as follows:

- sedation of the ovaries
- the thyroid
- the uterus and
- the solar plexus.

Slow labour. If progress in labour is slow, the therapist should give calming strokes, then the following specific treatment:

- stimulation, with care, first of the lower spine
- the small and large intestines
- the pituitary
- the ovaries
- the abdominal wall and
- the uterus.

Fetal distress. If there is fetal distress, no RZT should be given other than light stroking while the midwife or obstetrician decide how to proceed.

Towards the end of the first stage of labour the mother's toes dorsiflex, and light relaxation of the shoulder girdle is helpful before the second stage begins.

The second stage of labour

RZT is not used unless there is delay in the second stage, but if so the therapist should give the following treatment:

- sedation of the solar plexus and
- light stimulation of the pituitary gland.

The third stage of labour

Non-separation of placenta. If the cervix closes and the placenta does not separate, the therapist gives the following treatment:

- sedation of the solar plexus and
- all the pelvic organs (briefly)
- stimulation (lightly at first until the response is clear) of the pituitary and
- the ovaries and uterus.

After the birth

Flaccid uterus

If the uterus remains flaccid after delivery and there is a seeping blood loss, the therapist gives the following treatment:

- sedation of the solar plexus
- light stimulation of the uterus
- sedation of the ganglion pelvinium (see Fig. 12.5).

Cramps and shivering

For cramps and shivering after the birth, a warm footbath will soothe, warm and relax the mother. She should not be allowed to get cold again, and is given warm socks for her feet.

The puerperium

If possible the mother is treated daily for the first week of the puerperium to reduce fluid retention, establish lactation and stimulate involution of the uterus. The therapist starts by giving frequent harmonising strokes.

Specific treatment is as follows:

- stimulation of the urinary system
- treatment of the lymphatic system
- the breasts
- the lower spine
- the pelvic organs and
- the abdominal wall
- sedation of the solar plexus and
- any bruised perineal areas.

RZT is continued twice a week, reducing to once a week until the milk flow is well established, the uterus involuted, and the lochia has ceased.

Pains after birth

The uterus should remain well contracted after delivery, and should not be oversedated. If, however, the pains are very strong the therapist should give the following treatment:

- sedation of the solar plexus
- light sedation at frequent intervals (for a few seconds only) to the uterus.

Subinvolution of the uterus

Specific treatment is as follows:

- stimulation of the uterus
- the bladder
- the small intestine
- the lower spine
- the pituitary and
- the musculature of the abdominal wall
- treatment of the solar plexus and diaphragm.

The hands are treated twice a day, especially the pelvic lymphatics around the wrist.

Dysuria

Specific treatment is as follows:

- sedation of the solar plexus
- stimulation of the bladder and lumbar spine. (This is repeated every 5 minutes until the bladder is empty, and then every 4 hours until normal urinary output and muscle tone have been re-established.)

Bruised perineum

Specific treatment is as follows:

- the lymphatic drainage of the pelvis
- sedation of the zones which correspond to the bruised perineal areas.

Supplementary care. The addition of 10–15 drops of tea tree oil (a natural antiseptic) to the water when having a bath reduces bruising and discomfort after a tear, episiotomy or when the perineum is bruised. The bruised areas can be painted with arnica, and bathing the perineum regularly with a warm mixture of 1 teaspoonful of witch hazel with a quarter cup of (boiled) water relieves pain and bruising. A jug can be used to douche the area each time the bladder or bowels are emptied, but it is better to make up the remedy freshly for each use.

The area can be bathed in lavender oil hip baths twice a day and lavender compresses applied.

Painful coccyx and sacrum

Specific treatment is as follows:

- sedation of the solar plexus and
- the disordered reflex zones on the lower spine

- the painful zones can also be sedated on the hands.

After an epidural anaesthetic

The reflex zones to the spine are almost always very painful after an epidural. Too strong a touch over this region often causes a 'lightning-like' surge of pain through the foot and up the leg. Consequently all treatment of the reflex zones of the spine should begin with light touch.

Specific treatment is as follows:

- sedation of the reflex zone to the site of the epidural
- treatment of the reflex zones to the spine with smoothly regular, light palpation, starting from the coccyx and moving up towards the neck.

After an episiotomy

Painful reflex zones are found over the musculature of the pelvic floor on both the medial and lateral aspects of the heel at the back of the malleoli and either side of the Achilles' tendon, also over the lumbar and sacral spines.

Specific treatment is as follows:

- gentle sedation of the painful reflex zones and
- the solar plexus
- treatment of the pelvix lymphatics
- sedation of the painful zones on the hand can be performed as often as needed.

After caesarian section

It is preferable to assess the reflex zones first, otherwise the therapist treats the reflex zones which are most often found to be disordered after a caesarian section.

Specific treatment is as follows:

- sedation of the solar plexus
- stimulation of the urinary system
- the lymphatic system
- the liver
- the lungs (postanaesthetic) and
- the lumbar spine

- treatment of the musculature of the abdominal wall
- the reflex zone of the scar on the feet and
- the splenic flexure of the large intestine (usually helpful in relieving 'wind' pains).

After a forceps delivery

Specific treatment is as follows:

- sedation of the solar plexus
- the painful reflex zones to the perineum and
- the ganglion pelvinium
- stimulation of the urinary system
- the lymphatic system
- the sacrum, coccyx, symphysis pubis and
- the uterine supports
- treatment of any other painful reflex zones.

After prolonged labour

The therapist should start with Yin-Yang and harmonising strokes, and cupping the heels. Specific treatment is as follows:

- gentle treatment to the spine
- the abdominal wall and
- the endocrine system
- sedation of the solar plexus
- treatment of the diaphragm.

Supplementary care. Support, rest and reassurance should be given to the mother.

Retention with overflow

Treatment is given for 3 to 4 minutes every half hour. The medial heel is usually discoloured and the tissues oedematous. Specific treatment is as follows:

- sedation of the solar plexus
- stimulation of the lumbar spine, sacrum and coccyx and
- the bladder.

The therapist should continue treating these areas frequently until the bladder is completely empty and has regained its tone.

CASE STUDY 12.2

A healthy 30-year-old woman was 2 days post delivery (after a Ventouse extraction) of a 4.3 kg baby. The uterus was lax instead of well contracted, she had perineal pain and she lacked milk for the infant.

On inspection, both feet were oedematous, especially over the dorsum and around the ankles. The tissue tone was tense and palpation was uncomfortable.

Treatment given was vigorous stimulation of the uterus, also stimulation of the urinary system, pelvic lymphatics, large and small intestine, pituitary gland and breast reflex zones. Sedation was given to the perineal area.

The following day the uterus was half-way involuted and well contracted. The lochia was diminished. The woman had passed urine every 2 hours, the volume had increased and was satisfactory. Oedema of the feet was lessening. The treatment was repeated.

On day 3 the lochia was much reduced. The perineum was less painful, breastfeeding was established and the baby was satisfied. The woman made a good recovery and felt that she had been greatly helped by RZT.

Abnormal lochia

If the mother is at home, the midwife should be informed. A complete assessment is made and treatment given to all disordered reflex zones.

Specific treatment is as follows:

- the reflex zones to the uterus are usually very tender and full (the therapist should start with light touch, and if this is tolerated well then as follows)
- stimulation of the area of the enlarged postgravid uterus and
- the urinary and lymphatic systems
- sedation of the solar plexus.

An example of the use of RZT for urine retention and abnormal lochia is detailed in Case study 12.2.

If the breasts are slow to fill with milk

Specific treatment is as follows:

- stimulation of the breast reflexes (on the hands and feet for 5 minutes every 4 hours) and
- the pituitary gland
- sedation of the solar plexus
- treatment of the cervical spine reflexes, especially C2, C3 and C4, the thoracic spine, the neck and
- the endocrine system on the feet.

Supplementary care. Gentle massage can be given on either side of the vertebrae C2, C3, C4 and C7 and the thoracic vertebrae every 3–4 hours.

If there is too much milk

Specific treatment is as follows:

- stimulation of the urinary and lymphatic systems
- sedation of the solar plexus
- treatment of the neck and shoulder girdle.

The therapist should avoid touching the reflex zones to the breasts on feet or hands.

Engorgement of the breasts

Specific treatment is as follows:

- the urinary and lymphatic systems
- the small intestine
- vertebrae C7 and T1–7
- sedation of the sternum and solar plexus
- the entire breast area on the feet should be covered with a steady hold.

(The therapist should not treat or touch the reflex zones of the breasts other than with a sedating hold.)

To help suppress lactation

In this situation, the therapist should not stimulate or treat the breasts or the pituitary. Specific treatment is as follows:

- the lymphatic system, particularly the axillary lymphatics and
- the spleen
- stimulation of the urinary system
- treatment of any other disordered reflex zones.

Laxity of the pelvic floor and weakened uterine supports

A very careful assessment of all the reflex zones of the pelvic organs, pelvic floor and uterine supports on medial and lateral heels is made as part of a full general assessment.

Specific treatment is as follows:

- all disordered reflex zones
- the pelvic floor
- the pelvic supports
- the pelvic organs
- the endocrine system
- the abdominal musculature and
- any scars.

Supplementary care. It usually takes 3 months of regular pelvic floor exercise to strengthen these muscles, so patience and persistence are needed. The mother should be shown how to do them, and if she is able to halt her urinary flow in midstream she is contracting the right muscles.

References

McKenzie R 1993 Treat your own neck. Spinal Publications New Zealand Ltd, Waikane

McKenzie R 1997 Treat your own back, 5th edn. New Zealand University Press, Price Milburn

UKCC 1998 Midwives' rules and code of practice — 1998. United Kingdom Central Council for Nursing, Midwifery and Health Visiting, London

13

RZT for children

Introduction

There are very few children who do not enjoy and benefit from RZT from their earliest days onwards. A natural interest in their own bodies and events taking place around them, coupled with an immediate perception of what is pleasing and a leaping vitality, make them willing participants in treatment. Equally, their responses are instantaneous and usually undisguised by convention, giving useful indications as to how treatment should proceed.

It is quite possible for many children growing up in large cities in the Western world to be sensorily deprived. Their feet are always shod and they walk largely on floors and concrete. The tendency to smaller families with the loss of a large extended family in many cases, combined with concerns about safety, frequently mean that there is less physical contact between people outside of the close family, less playful sport, less walking or cycling and more travelling by car. The variety of textures, odours and diverse substances with which they come into contact is diminishing, as more of the artefacts which they handle are made of plastic and paper. RZT offers touch which is neither too threatening nor too intimate, provides a diversity of sensations, does not last for too long, and takes place in a controlled situation. The quiet cosseting that involves soothing physical touch is appreciated by nearly all sick children.

Neonates

Neonatal development

The neonatal period extends from birth to the first 30 days of life. The fit infant born at term (after 38–40 weeks of intrauterine life), although capable of breathing, sucking and discharging waste products, is nevertheless immature in many ways. The immune system contains no antibodies to environmental pathogens; the liver, though large, cannot break down many animal proteins or drugs, and is unable to cope with solid foods for the first 6 months of life; the bladder has not descended into the pelvis and lies under the diaphragm; the sphincters are not closed and are not yet under voluntary control and the adult benign gut flora have not yet colonised the intestinal tract.

Many nerve fibres are unmyelinated. Corticospinal tract myelinisation is not completed until 2 years of age, when the infant has gained motor control. The optic nerve is also not yet covered by its myelin sheath, nor yet are many other nervous structures, which need the stimulus of sound, movement, colour and shapes over the next 6 months before the baby acquires these perceptions, as well as those of height and depth. Although speech appears to be programmed within us, it is learned through long exposure to voices.

The infant foot is pronated at birth and is wider and fatter than in later life. There is seldom a distinct longitudinal arch, the muscular tone is poor and all tendons are softer than in an active 1-year-old baby. Calcification shows first at 2 weeks in the cuboid bone, appears in the lateral cuneiform bone at 4 months, in the big toe at 9 months in the female infant and 1 year 4 months in the male, and continues until full stature and bony growth have been achieved, usually between 18 and 20 years. The big toes of the feet begin to unite at between $12\frac{1}{2}$–13 years in girls and 14–$14\frac{1}{2}$ years in boys, and is completed when the tibia and fibula fuse towards the age of 20 years. The bony formation of a baby's foot is incomplete at birth, with the arch forming at about the age of 3 years when standing and walking are finished accomplishments.

Although all the structures are in place and quite perfectly developed for the baby's age, they are immature in the sense that they have to be tested in the new environment, and must adapt to life outside the womb. If the adaptations are learned one after another, and march in time with normal developmental stages, all is usually well.

There are, conversely, tissues valuable to the infant which will regress with maturity:

- brown fat, particularly round the head, neck and back; this is slowly metabolised to produce heat, as the shivering response is not yet present
- a large, retrosternal thymus gland to produce T cell lymphocytes, as liver, spleen and lymphatics have yet to mature.

Also essential for survival, the sucking reflex, the grip reflex and the Moro reflex (see Fig. 13.1, p. 236) are all present.

A baby who is born at term, that is after 40 weeks of intrauterine life, is ready to lead an independent physiological life, but remains dependent on those around her for the satisfaction of all her physical, mental and emotional needs for a long time.

A baby is at its most vulnerable for the first month of her life. From a stable and protected environment she must become accustomed to breathing, drinking and excreting for herself, to people, touch, noise, temperature and humidity changes, to handling and to light. These activities provide essential stimulation, but a nervous system not yet completely developed is easily overstimulated, and the infant must be protected from too much exposure to noise, bright light and restless activity.

Indications and contraindications for treatment

RZT can be given to a healthy baby as a form of positive touch, in order to support the natural developmental progress, or to treat minor ailments. It may be combined with massage, and given as part of a daily routine, or at regular intervals. The importance of touch for premature and sick babies as well as for those who are healthy is increasingly being recognised in Western culture, although it has been an inseparable part of child care in most other cultures.

RZT can be given to the hands, the feet and the back, and, depending on the infant's needs and responses, treatment may be varied from one surface to another.

The contraindications for giving RZT are as follows. Treatment should not be given if the baby:

- has a high temperature (over 39°C)
- has an inflammation of the venous or lymphatic system
- is asleep
- becomes manifestly more distressed with what is being done to her
- has a local infection on the feet.

The therapist should also avoid treating if he does not know what is the matter and suspects that the baby may be seriously ill or in a medical or surgical emergency.

Preparation

A quiet, warm and draught-free room is desirable. The light should not be too bright, with no direct light shining onto the baby's face. Loud noise is startling to an infant, and is best avoided.

The baby lies in the most comfortable position, warmly covered, except for the area under observation. This can be on the mother's lap, against her chest if the back is being treated or in her cot. Lying close to the mother's skin the baby has the reassuringly familiar smell of her skin and the sound of her heartbeat and breathing for comfort. If the baby lies in a large open space like a bed, her outline should be surrounded with a folded blanket arranged round her in a circular fashion to ensure that she feels secure within an enclosed boundary.

Assessment

The therapist should first be sitting in a comfortable and relaxed position. He should take a few deep breaths, since this is calming and imparts receptivity to the hands. Now he should attentively try to learn as much as possible about the baby from the reflex zones. He speaks softly to the infant, who will begin to associate the sound of his voice, the words that he uses and his smell with comfort. The eyes of a newly born baby focus quite clearly at some 17–30 cm (7–12 inches) away from the face, so he should approach the baby's face slowly and allow eye contact to be made.

The therapist's hands must be warm, and any jewellery or watches which might be cold or contact the baby's skin should be removed. Assessment in the infant consists of tracking across the plantar, dorsal, medial and lateral surfaces of the foot, rather than palpating system by system. If there are areas which feel disordered or cause the baby to withdraw the foot, the reflex zone and system to which it belongs must be identified.

Observation

The therapist should spend the first few minutes really looking at the baby, noting the colour of her skin, the expression on her face, the position in which she lies, her breathing pattern and any movements that she makes.

The infant has to make her needs known through crying, movement, gestures and facial expressions, which later become the vehicle for expressing pleasure, recognition and delight. A mother who has regular close physical contact with her baby learns to recognise when she is contented or otherwise, well or ill, through the 'feel' of her body and limbs, as well as by knowing the baby's normal colour, cry and gestures, and looking at every one of her parts and features, including her feet.

The therapist should look at the outline and position of the feet, and the condition of the skin. Babies very quickly develop a dry skin if they are dehydrated. Their feet become swollen just as rapidly if they are retaining fluid. The fullness or otherwise of the tissues should be noted (see Ch. 4, p. 63). These observations can be corroborated by checking the fontanelles. Taking both feet gently into both his hands, the therapist keeps quite still whilst registering the temperature of the feet and the response of the baby. A warm, sure and attentive hold generally allows the baby to relax. If her colour or breathing changes, if her fists clench or, most importantly, if the big toe becomes dorsiflexed or plantarflexed, or if she is startled, the therapist should wait until she is calm again before proceeding.

Palpation

Each system is palpated very gently, paying attention to the visual aspect of the feet. There may be colour changes in reflex zones before or after they have been palpated. There may also be changes in the texture of the tissues. For instance, mild congenital dislocation of the hip produces a perceptibly loose, flaccid tissue in the reflex zone to the affected hip joint.

The therapist watches the baby closely for the whole of his time with her. Reflex zones which are disordered evoke the previously described changes of autonomic imbalance — the hands and feet may sweat, the breathing rhythm may change, the body may become tense with evident distress, and she may either change position or cry as a response. Holding the feet or performing any of those movements which have been observed to be calming to the infant should be done until the tension lessens and the SNS reactions disappear.

Palpating the back. The therapist exposes the back but keeps the rest of the infant warmly covered. His hands should be warm, still and lightly oiled before being placed over the infant's back. He should observe the temperature and colour of the skin and any surface variations there may be (e.g. it may be pallid in some areas), whether it is dry and sweaty in patches or overall, whether the body is tense or flaccid, and the character of the baby's breathing.

Gently but with sure hands the therapist palpates on either side of the spine and then each of the reflex zones of the back to see whether discomfort is elicited over any area.

Note: The therapist should try to ensure consistent physical conditions for the assessment and all subsequent treatment so that no unnecessary nervous energy has to be expended anticipating the unknown, from which babies and children suffer more acutely than do most adults.

Assessing the sick or premature baby

The therapist needs to be acquainted with the birth and subsequent history before treating a sick child. If her child is sick, it is helpful if the mother keeps a diary in which she records the daily routine and the baby's reactions. Notes on how much she drinks at each feed, whether she posits or vomits, and the nature and frequency of any vomiting, how many wet nappies she has had, and whether they were very wet or just damp, what was the colour of the urine, how many stools are passed each day and what is their colour and consistency, whether the temperature is raised, whether the baby perspires or has a dry skin, whether she cries, is restless or listless, sleeps or is wakeful, and for how long, give useful information and clarify whether the baby is sickening or getting better.

General observations. In premature baby units and children's intensive care units it is noticeable that, from the smallest baby to the teenage adolescent, the feet reflect the stresses and strains of illness more quickly than do the hands. For example, nearly all premature babies are born with a markedly prominent thyroid area on the plantar feet. This is usually more pallid in colour than the surrounding skin but may be more flushed, depending on the infant's condition, and whatever essential drugs and interventions have been prescribed. If the baby is immature or sick, she may not be seeing as well as she should, and in this case the rest of her environment needs to be stable. Movement is more perceptible when the eyes are closed, and people may shut their eyes to diminish the impact of visual and other stimuli when they have a headache or wish to

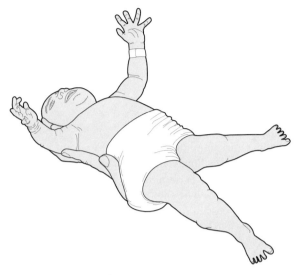

Fig. 13.1 *The Moro reflex*

concentrate. A sick person whose energy and attention are inwardly focused is acutely aware of every change in his environment, as is the baby.

Sick babies, like sick people, do not want to be disturbed. And babies sometimes want to be left alone, a response which must be respected. They have only two ways of expressing themselves, by crying and through their body language. They show quite individual likes and dislikes and expressions of pleasure and annoyance. The therapist should try to observe the baby's cues and what she is trying to express through them. For example, some babies prefer to have their backs rubbed in the morning, and some show a clear preference for the afternoon. Generally they show their dislikes by:

- tensing up their limbs
- clasping their arms across their chests
- displaying the Moro (or startle) reflex (Fig. 13.1): if a normal baby is startled by a sudden or jarring movement or noise, or if her head is allowed to drop backwards slightly when she is supported in a supine position, classical reflexes come into play — the neck becomes slightly flexed, the legs are drawn up, the arms are simultaneously extended and abducted at right angles to the trunk, the hands open wide, with the fingers splayed to begin with after which they become clenched, and the baby then flexes

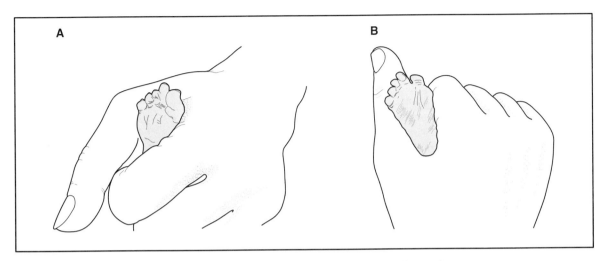

Fig. 13.2 *A The contented baby's foot; **B** dorsiflexion of the big toe when the baby becomes distressed*

her arms toward the midline; a baby who has permanently adopted the Moro position, however, is or has been very ill and this position is a feature of infants who have been hospitalised for a long time
- dorsiflexion of the big toe (Fig. 13.2B)
- plantar flexion of the big toe, which is an indication of neurological damage; babies suffering any neurological deficit draw their toes down towards the sole of the feet
- yawning, in a sick baby
- screaming.

Palpation. As many of the procedures to which very sick or previously hospitalised infants have been subjected were not physically comforting, they are quickly and easily startled and defensive, and it may take a little while for them to learn that touch can be reassuring. Frequent heel pricks may have been necessary in order to collect blood samples, and monitors and infusions are also often attached to the feet, so that the baby's trust has to be earned by first 'still holding' on hands or tummy, or anywhere where there has been least intervention. Very small and very sick babies do not like too many stroking movements. They respond better to smaller strokes and small movements and to 'still holding'.

There is security for a baby in being held and cuddled, the more so when they are sick, but their greatest need is for physical and chemical rest, and respite from unnecessary disturbances.

Treatment decisions

The therapist needs to decide whether he is going to treat the hands, feet or back.

The back

The back is a good choice in babies who are suffering from chest infections, those with heart conditions, who are being nursed in the prone position, who have had infusions and many heel pricks, who are vomiting and also any baby who is unsettled and wishes to be close to her mother's chest and heartbeat.

The feet

The feet are a good choice when a sick baby has become accustomed to the therapist's touch and some of the associations of the feet with pain have been erased.

The hands

The hands are a good choice in the baby who is closely swaddled, has to be nursed on her back, or has had many interventions on her feet.

Treatment

Enough time should be allowed to:

- spend the first few minutes observing the baby before each session; this is as important in healthy as in sick babes, whose condition can change, improve or deteriorate with startling rapidity
- give full attention to the session
- observe the effects of treatment for a few minutes afterwards.

It is preferable not to treat a baby immediately after a full feed, nor when a nappy change is due, nor if she is just drifting off to sleep, and a baby should never be wakened from sleep for a treatment.

The healthy baby

Movements should be gentle, quiet and unhurried, and if the infant becomes distressed then the therapist should stop what he is doing and hold her until she is calm again.

Although treatment touch needs to be gentle, too light a touch is irritating for most babies, while the infant winces and moves her limbs away if the touch is too heavy.

Stopping frequently and holding the feet or back gives the infant 'breathing' and relaxing spaces during treatment.

The therapist should keep his attention as wide as possible during the session. Babies react rapidly to all stimuli, and the therapist should watchfully observe the infant's response to treatment. Changes in the skin colour, texture or tissue can occur several times a day in a healthy baby, and even more in a sick one.

One or both hands are kept on the infant until the session is over, and then the hands are lifted lightly off the feet or back, with the transition from touch to release being smooth and effortless.

The sick baby

If possible the treatments should be arranged so that they fit in as well as possible with the baby's routine. Small, regular stimuli are preferable to irregular and longer sessions. If the mother or the carers wish to participate, clear directions can be given on how to give small, specifically directed stimuli.

The first session may take anything from a few minutes up to 20 minutes if much time is spent holding the feet. At the end of the session the therapist lightens his touch and lifts his hands gently away. The featherlight strokes with which most treatments are brought to an end in adults are, in general, irritating to a very sick, small baby.

Treatment may be given daily for a few minutes or every other day. Very sick children may be treated two or three times a day for short periods of no more than 2 minutes each time. The infant should be warmly wrapped after a treatment and allowed to rest quietly.

Case study 13.1 details the RZT treatment of a premature baby.

First aid treatment

These treatments should be given only in the short term. If the symptoms are unexplained, persistent or worsen the infant must be referred for specialised help.

CASE STUDY 13.1

A baby born 2 weeks prematurely was severely jaundiced and drowsy at birth. He was slow to feed and gain weight. With the consent of and under the continuing supervision of the general practitioner, RZT assessment was made in the form of gentle palpation over the dorsal, plantar, medial and lateral surfaces of the feet, but no perceptible changes in tissue tone were noted. The skin was yellow but otherwise healthy. The reflex zones of the liver, small and large intestines, adrenals and solar plexus were treated for approximately 3–5 minutes at approximately 4-hourly intervals, and tolerated well by the baby. The jaundice subsided rapidly without any noticeable reactions, and within a week the skin was normal in appearance and the infant was responding normally to his surroundings and feeding well.

RZT can be used as first aid in the following conditions.

Constipation. First the abdomen should be examined to see if it is tense and protuberant. Illness, dehydration, too high a sugar content in artificial feeding, which may as yet be poorly tolerated, and some medicines affect small and large bowel function.
The following specific treatment is given:

- the reflex zones to the small and large intestines on the feet, moving in steps of a millimetre each across the area of the small of the foot.

Supplementary advice. Circling the legs gently in a wide arc in a clockwise direction over the tummy is also a useful manoeuvre. The therapist should ensure the infant is drinking enough plain water, and the mother avoids giving all sugar filled prepared drinks and reduces the amount of sugar in feeds or foods. (Checking the labels of all prepared foods and tins for their sugar content will show which should be avoided.)

Wind and colic. After quietly holding the feet, the therapist treats the following reflex zones:

- the stomach
- the small and large intestines, particularly the hepatic and splenic flexures and
- the liver, tracking across the arches of the feet in small steps
- light still holding of the solar plexus on the feet, 'sheltering' the solar plexus on the abdomen with the other hand at the same time
- massage of either side of the 12th thoracic vertebra to the sacral spine in small, circular movements every 4–5 hours.

Supplementary advice. The baby's hips are flexed and the upper legs are delicately coaxed against the abdomen and held there. Rotating the legs in a wide arc may also help to relieve colic by indirectly massaging the musculature of the large intestine in a peristaltic direction, as mentioned above.

Vomiting or excessive positing. Common causes of vomiting or positing are: drinking too fast, swallowing too much wind, the baby being overstimulated by noise and movement, or when the mother has eaten something which is difficult for the baby's immature gut and liver to metabolise.
Specific treatment is given as follows:

- firm but gentle sedation of the reflex zones to the solar plexus
- the stomach
- the liver and
- the small intestine in turn.

Supplementary advice. The mother should allow 20 minutes for a full feeding time and, if the baby is bottle fed, the hole in the teat should not be too large (nor so small that she becomes frustrated). The feed should be interrupted several times to hold the baby upright so that any wind trapped in the pyloric antrum can more easily be brought up. A note should be made of the nature of the vomited material and the frequency with which it occurs. If the baby has a projectile vomit (a seemingly effortless fountain-like vomit) and the pitch of her cry becomes higher, or if she develops a rash which does not blanch on pressure, she needs immediate medical care.

Inability to pass urine. This may be a consequence of fever or of some medicines. The following specific treatment is given:

- gentle treatment of the reflex zones to the kidneys, ureter and bladder
- holding of the solar plexus
- stimulation of the small intestine.

Supplementary advice. The baby should be encouraged to drink as much fluid as she wants, and as much plain water as possible. Persistent difficulties with micturition need investigation in case there is a mechanical cause such as a kinked ureter.

Restlessness. The following specific treatment is given:

- holding of the solar plexus
- treatment of the whole foot (in a quiet atmosphere if possible).

Sticky eyes. Specific treatment is given to the following reflex zones:

CASE STUDY 13.2

A 20-day-old baby had 'sticky eyes' which were responding slowly if at all to local antibiotic treatment. At assessment, during which the infant lay contentedly still, there was a very faint pink flush over the reflex zones to the eyes, and a slight fullness over those to the kidneys on both feet. These reflex zones were treated daily for no more than 3 minutes by the physiotherapist and by the mother every 4 hours. The infection cleared within 48 hours, after which the reflex zones to the eyes and kidneys were indistinguishable from all others in colour and tone. There were no other observable reactions.

- the eyes on both dorsal and plantar surfaces of the second and third toes, as well as those on the dorsum of the big toe and
- the urinary system.

Supplementary care. RZT is an effective and simple remedy for sticky eyes. Mother can be shown how to treat the appropriate reflex zones every 4 hours during the day, but the midwife needs to be told of this potentially serious condition in a neonate. Case study 13.2 gives an example of the RZT treatment of sticky eyes.

Diarrhoea. The following specific treatment is given:

- holding then light treatment of the reflex zones to the stomach, cardia and pylorus
- the solar plexus and
- the small and large intestines.

Supplementary advice. The therapist should check whether the mother has changed her diet if the infant is being breastfed (it is normal for a breastfed baby to have soft or liquid stools). Otherwise any new additions to the infant's foods should be noted. The therapist should look for a rash, which may be due to allergy or any developing illness. The commonest causes of diarrhoea are infection, too high a sugar concentration in the feed, allergy, antibiotics and, for some babies, the composition of prepared formula feeds, or some food intolerances. It is necessary to watch to see that the baby does not become dehydrated and she is given lots of extra, plain water. Continuing diarrhoea needs investigation.

Treating the back

If the breathing is distressed the therapist should make small, slow, circular movements on either side of the thoracic vertebrae and, with the palms held flat against the back, move outwards from the spine toward the lateral chest wall.

If there is cardiac embarrassment the same small, slow circular movement is made on either side of the thoracic vertebrae, with particular emphasis alongside the fourth, fifth and sixth vertebrae. The reflex zones to the stomach, heart, the left shoulder and the upper left arm are treated.

The baby's breathing and colour should be watched all the time. If she becomes flushed or pallid, or if her breathing becomes more rapid or shallower, she needs smaller stimuli. The therapist wraps his hands quietly around her until she recovers.

If there is intestinal malfunction small, slow circular movements should be used to treat on both sides of the lumbar vetebrae, the buttocks, the upper parts of the legs, the reflex zone to the liver, and any other areas which appear or feel disordered.

Oils

Because of the rising incidence of food intolerance and allergy, even in tiny babies it is advisable for the therapist to avoid using wheatgerm or any nut-based oil should he decide to treat the infant's back. A bland, plant-based oil such as safflower is less likely to cause any sensitivity reactions. Nor should any scented oils be used. Babies have a finely tuned sense of smell to recognise the scent of their mothers and carers, and scented oils interfere with this capacity. Babies and children can spike very high temperatures when they are sick, and lose fluid and heat rapidly through the relatively huge surface area of their skin. Scented oils quickly turn pungent when combined with the acidity of a febrile sweat and add to the baby's malaise.

Completing the session

The baby should be dressed and covered warmly when the therapist has finished. The temperature-regulating mechanism is immature in babies and they lose heat rapidly. The head should be covered as there is greater heat loss from here than from any other part of the body.

Infants up to 2–3 years of age

Infant development

Infancy is defined as the period of complete dependency before one is able to walk, talk and feed oneself, and is usually considered to last for the first 2–3 years of human life. During this time of unprecedented learning, as the infant adapts to an external environment and becomes independent, her nervous system matures as the pathways which allow for movement and speech are laid down. Looking, listening and responding become more acute, the alimentary tract has matured sufficiently to digest solid foods, and the cues for likes and dislikes become easier to read and more pronounced. By the time the healthy infant is 2 she is boundlessly curious, energetic and engaged in all she does. Her immune system responds rapidly to any invasion, as do the alimentary and endocrine systems.

Signs and symptoms

Malaise, fatigue, nausea, vomiting, fever, excessive irritability, skin rashes and mucous discharges from the nose and throat or ears indicate that a child is not well. If the symptoms persist, and do not respond to rest, a higher fluid intake and only light nourishment, the cause of such changes should be looked for before the infant becomes debilitated and a chronic pattern of illness sets in. The infant is affected by changes in her social scene as much as by inappropriate nutrition or by infection.

In general, infants do not want to eat when they are sick. As their recuperative mechanisms are strong and resilient they mend most quickly if they are ensured quiet and rest, and given copious clear fluids to drink (clear fluids include water, diluted vegetable soups or home-prepared diluted fruit juices without any added sugar, colouring or preservatives).

Common reasons for seeking treatment in this age group are chest, ear, throat and urinary infections, infantile eczema and teething and digestive upsets. If there are repeated infections, it is best for an assessment to take place during a remission, when the visual and palpable abnormalities on the feet are less obscured by the changes which result from infection. At a time of acute infection the feet are usually hypersensitive, with redness or pallor of the zones which are involved in the symptom picture.

Parental responsibility

In the United Kingdom a parent or guardian is legally obliged to provide adequate medical care for any child who is not yet 16 years old. Other therapies are not discouraged, but may be given only after such medical care has been sought. RZT can be given alongside allopathic medicine, which it should enhance, or on its own for an infant who is not seriously ill and for whom the right medical provision has been made.

Preparation

It is best to choose a treatment time which does not conflict with meal or napping routines. There should be a warm room available and some toys appropriate to the child's age. One ploy which works well is to provide a doll or teddy bear on whose feet or paws the infant can give attention similar to that which she is getting.

Assessment

History

Unless the therapist is giving first aid before seeking specialist help, a careful history of the present complaint is taken and recorded. This should include the length of time the infant has been unwell, her temperature, whether she is eating, sleeping and behaving normally, whether she is crying more or less than usual, the nature of her bladder and bowel function, whether she is vomiting or coughing, and whether her cry is any different to normal, also the position she adopts when lying and sitting. This teasing out of as accurate a picture as possible helps both the mother and the therapist to draw a baseline against which any future changes can be compared and, should the infant not improve, provides essential information for the doctor.

Observation

The therapist focuses his attention on the child and observes her for a while before the session begins. A note should be made of her colour, breathing rhythm, brightness or dullness of her eyes, demeanor, vitality and interest in what is going on. The therapist should also talk to her, and may care to use the doll's feet to show to her what he is about to do.

Palpation procedure

When the therapist has had a chance to look at the shape, structure, skin and tissues of the feet, he should start stroking the feet, with warm hands, in the direction of the flow of Yin and Yang pathways (see Ch. 5, p. 104). The infant is generally happier with stroking movements than is the neonate. An assessment should be made of all the reflex zones on the feet, and a record of visual and palpable observations put on her chart. Coolness, sweating, chilling, restlessness, change in breathing pattern or colour are indications that the reflex zones being palpated are disordered and these should be noted together with the reaction they provoke.

Treatment

Ten minutes is the longest that should normally be spent on treatment time on an infant, though this time may be extended if several minutes are spent on stroking or holding of her feet. But the treatment time is always going to be dictated by the response of the child. If signs of autonomic imbalance become apparent early in the treatment and are slow to subside, only 2 or 3 minutes should be given for the first few sessions, and treatment time increased only as her tolerance permits. There will always be those for whom less treatment time will have the same effect as a longer time spent treating another person.

The healthy infant

If the infant is healthy, RZT can be given from time to time as a way of supporting and maintaining her, as well as being another way to monitor her well-being. Any developing functional change can often be observed in its early stages on the feet.

The sick infant

RZT can be given two or three times a week to the sick infant, concentrating on those reflex zones which are visibly and palpably disordered and on the reacting systems. If, for example, the infant begins to cough up a copious quantity of mucous-laden phlegm, then the whole of the respiratory system as well as all other disordered reflex zones should be included in treatment for as long as such reactions continue. If on the other hand there is a discharge from the ears, these areas should be treated at each visit and continued for as long as the discharge persists. Even if the symptoms subside and the infant is apparently normal, the feet should be treated for as long as there is any palpable disorder in the reflex zones, or for as long as there are physical or other reactions. When colour, tone and touch sensation in the feet and behaviour return to normal, the regular sessions are no longer needed, but it is advisable to arrange a follow-up after 4 to 6 weeks to ensure that recovery has been consolidated.

Common patterns of treatment for infants, toddlers and children

If the child is fretful and does not seem happy to have her feet or back bared, the first few sessions can be given over socks or a thin covering to allow her to become accustomed to the procedure and the therapist's touch.

Respiratory infections. Treatment is given to all the reflex zones which are disordered (i.e. where the tissue tone of the small intestine becomes perceptibly altered, being either full or empty in tone, and there are skin changes over the area); their reflex zones are in most cases more painful than those of the symptom zones. The following specific treatment is given:

- the spleen and lymphatic system

- the urinary system
- if they are disordered, the respiratory system on both dorsum and sole and
- the diaphragm.

Supplementary advice. The body chemistry of many of these infants is such that they have difficulty in digesting starchy foods, which should be reduced, while the alkaline content of the diet is increased. This can be done by giving diluted soups and juices made from alkaline fruits and vegetables. The bodies of babies and children need both chemical and physical rest when they are sick. If the chemical challenge to the as yet weak liver and alimentary tract is lessened the infant becomes stronger. Some small children have difficulty in metabolising large amounts of dairy produce. Some of these evident differences in body chemistry can be partly explained by the differing nutritional backgrounds of modern families and cross-cultural intermarriage. For example, some cultures (particularly the Scandinavian and north European) have for generations consumed dairy foods daily; their climate is cold and the butter, cheese and milk produced by their herds of cattle keeps well over the long winters, when fat is needed for warmth. Over the generations their digestive systems have developed an efficient enzyme system for metabolising dairy products. In other cultures (such as those around the Mediterranean and in South-East Asia), because of higher population density, religious conviction and the relative expense of animal proteins, very small quantities of dairy produce are consumed daily and the bulk of the diet is derived from locally grown staple carbohydrate. Consequently they do not have such an efficient enzyme system for digesting large quantities of dairy foods. Two infants from one set of parents may have quite different enzyme systems and need a different balance of foodstuffs.

Antibiotics and hormones are given to animals regularly in some countries (Sweden being a notable exception in the West), and their residues in the food chain contribute to thrush and many other digestive disorders. A source of plain, nutritious, organic food which has had as little added to it as possible is the only antidote to denatured foodstuffs.

The mother can be shown how to massage the back gently on either side of the spine and over the area of the lungs (always working from the midline to the lateral edges, and from the base of the lungs towards the apices).

The therapist should check that the child is not confined in too hot and dry an atmosphere for too long. The mother can boil a steam kettle or have a nebuliser in the room to help the child's breathing.

Case study 13.3 gives an example of RZT for respiratory disorder.

Ear infections. In this condition the primary disorder is often found in the reflex zones of:

- the stomach and small intestine
- the secondary disorder is often in the ears.

Supplementary advice. If the daily intake of complex carbohydrate is reduced until the gut has strengthened and all infection subsided, the infant recovers. In some children the dairy content of the diet may need to be reduced.

Urinary infections. The disorder is often reflected in the reflex zones of:

- the liver
- the intestines
- the spleen
- the urinary system
- sometimes the oronasopharynx.

Treatment is given to all disordered reflex zones.

Supplementary advice. The therapist should ensure that the child is given copious amounts of water and diluted alkaline fluids. All fizzy, concentrated, sweetened and chemicalised drinks and foods should be avoided until she is well again, and then given only in moderation. The genital area should be douched frequently and kept as dry as possible.

Teething and digestive disorders. If these happen frequently the mother should be asked to keep a food and drink diary to try and identify which foodstuffs may be responsible. The primary disorder usually lies in:

- the small intestine
- the adrenals
- the liver
- the spleen and
- the thyroid glands if they are painful.

CASE STUDY 13.3

A boy, nearly 2 years old, who had sustained mild cerebral damage at birth, suffered from a chronic running nose, snuffles, sinusitis, cough and chestiness, and was behind in reaching his developmental milestones. His vision and gait were particularly disturbed. A series of twice-weekly treatments was arranged. On first inspection the feet were cold, the colour pallid throughout, and the shape narrow and elongated, with no arch showing or developing. The tissue tone was full over the dorsum of both feet, and appeared 'ballooned out' over the surface of the metatarsal bones (corresponding to the lungs) on the dorsum of both feet. On palpation the impression was that of touching a taut balloon overfilled with water.

The infant was interested and allowed a 3 minute partial assessment, but then rapidly became cool and sweaty, and the rest of the assessment was left for the next visit. Some 12 hours later he became quiet, perspired profusely, spiked a temperature, and vomited a large quantity of mucous. He recovered after 2 hours, and was cheerful the following day.

At the next session the assessment was completed but, because of the strong reactions he had experienced after the first visit, treatment time on the feet was no longer than 2 minutes. Twelve hours later he had the same reactions as after the first visit, and increased mucous secretions for a further 12 hours.

In view of this, it was decided that treatment would be given only once a week. No more than 2 minutes of very gentle palpation to the areas of the small intestine, lungs and endocrines was given, interspersed with holding and stroking, and there was no increased tolerance for longer treatment. The boy was cheerful, and his mother noticed a slight improvement in his gait and vision. For each of the eight succeeding sessions the same reactions were reported — a mucousy, projectile vomit, sweating during the night after therapy, and increased mucous secretions from lungs and nose. At the same time his gait became more stable and the acuity of his vision improved.

Nine months after the sessions had ended he had not had a recurrence of his rhinitis, cough, sinusitis and chronic low grade respiratory infection. The mother's opinion was that the child was now more robust and alert, and the small improvement in his cerebral function had been maintained.

Supplementary advice. As the infant seldom wants to eat, she should not be pressed to do so, but it should be ensured that she drinks plenty of water and clear fluids. A good, safe, nutritious and alkaline drink for all sick children is plain boiled barley or rice water. Hippocrates said of barley gruel some 2300 years ago (Lloyd 1978):

■ *"Barley-gruel seems to have been correctly selected as the most suitable cereal to give in these acute diseases and I have a high opinion of those who selected it. Its gluten is smooth, consistent and soothing; it is slippery and fairly soft; it is thirst quenching and easily got rid of in case this be necessary. It contains nothing to produce constipation or serious rumbling, nor does it swell up in the stomach for during cooking it swells up to its maximum bulk."*

The barley or rice is boiled for 20 minutes in plenty of water, then the fluid is strained off to drink. It is preferable not to add sugar, salt or any other flavouring as strong tastes are not well tolerated by the sick.

Acid urine burns, and is painful to void. In a urinary tract infection, a larger volume of alkaline fluids are needed to diminish the acidity of the urine and also to provide a buffer, which gives acid waste a carrier facilitating its excretion. Most illness causes metabolic acidosis, the acid having to be excreted through the kidneys on the back of a buffer substance. The lungs and skin act as accessory organs of excretion when the acidosis becomes too great, but they can only assist the kidneys and cannot take over their function.

The eczemas. Specific treatment is given to the reflex zones to:

- the stomach and small intestine
- the spleen
- the liver
- the urinary system and
- the endocrine system.

Supplementary care. Since some article in the diet may be a contributory factor to this complex condition, it is as well to look at the infant's food intake. Sugars, chemicals and additives are best avoided, as is too much protein and fat, and a diet more weighted towards alkaline food will often bring some relief.

RZT for children over 2 years

Child development

The foundations of health are laid down in childhood. Affection, playfulness, a certain stability, some adventure combined with sound nutrition, shelter, physical and mental stimulus, exercise, social cohesion and a confident developing sense of self give any child the best chance of healthy development. It has to be emphasised that many children grow up to be physically, mentally and emotionally healthy and sturdy even though they have not had the benefit of these advantages, and that overcoming challenges and difficulties is also necessary for our development.

From the moment of conception there are multiple feedback mechanisms at work in us. In illness, a chain of events is linked one to another as the result of failure of one particular function. If food is taken as an example, it is broken down into digestible parts and absorbed through the lining of the small intestine, detoxified and refined in the liver, circulated to every cell in the body and its end result, waste, is excreted through the kidneys. This process can take minutes, as in an anaesthetic or poisonous substance, or build up over months, years, or a whole lifetime as the function of the GRS is eroded. The whole lining of the alimentary tract is a body surface reflecting the integrity of its function, or otherwise, through its reflex zones.

The recuperative capabilities of children are vital and strong, their hold on life tenacious, and they respond gratefully to care.

Presenting conditions

Ear, nose and throat infections, recurring chest and urinary infections, digestive disturbances, certain food intolerances, asthma, sleep and skin disorders, delay in reaching their developmental milestones and behavioural changes are the usual reasons which concern parents and for which treatment is sought.

Assessment

After the age of 2–3 years, children are more active participators in events, and able to say what they do and don't like. For toddlers a doll can be used, and for older children an amusingly shaped animal whistle or toy, to let the therapist know when they feel discomfort; this is usually a great game if a child is shy at the outset.

By this age children are more resilient, they are able to tolerate up to 10 minutes of palpation on their feet, and their responses are spontaneous and simple. By the time they are running around at 3 years their feet are fully developed for weight bearing, the foot arch has formed, and there is more definition of any disordered reflex zones. The young child is given the choice as to whether she would like to lie down or sit up during assessment. By this age each system can be assessed individually.

By the age of 10 years, some 15–20 minutes are generally well tolerated.

Treatment

RZT can be given at regular but widely separated intervals in the healthy child for support and maintenance. As there are wide differences in the constitutional make-up of each child, the therapist looks for the system which is most disordered and, while visual clues are important, at the moment of treatment it is the disorders of tissue tonus which dictate treatment. This is always given to whichever system is weakest. Some children need more treatment to the endocrine system, some to the urinary system and some to the alimentary tract.

In the sick child two or three sessions a week are the norm, the emphasis being placed on whichever systems show up as constitutionally weaker, those which lie in the background but are responsible for the presenting symptoms and, in the foreground, the symptomatically painful zones.

After the age of 7 years, the hormones which are responsible for the development of secondary sex characteristics begin to be produced. Care should be taken not to overstimulate the endocrine system from this age until after puberty, and during menstruation in an adolescent. The older child who is able to speak for herself and familiar with therapy may want to be alone during treatment.

The therapist should be able to put the child at her ease, and to keep the balance between giving the necessary treatment to painful and disordered reflex zones without breaching the child's pain threshold. This leaves her with an improved sense of well-being at the end of the session and makes therapy a positive experience.

Many illnesses in children are self-limiting, as a healthy immune system builds up resistance to organisms through exposure. The therapist must be able to recognise when serious illness threatens to overwhelm normal defence mechanisms and immediate medical care is essential. Appearance and behaviour need to be weighed against the severity of any symptoms. A child who does not drink, eat, play, display her normal interest, is excessively drowsy, dehydrated, has excessive vomiting or diarrhoea, has blood in her urine or stools, has laboured respirations or is hyperventilating, is pale, mottled or cyanosed, has opisthotonis, severe photophobia, a high-pitched cry, oliguria or anuria needs urgent investigation and treatment.

Asthma. The following specific treatment is given:

- vigorous treatment of the large intestine, particularly the ileocaecal valve and appendix on plantar, lateral and dorsal aspects
- the small intestine
- the abdominal wall
- the rectum and anus
- sedation of the adrenals and solar plexus
- treatment of the urinary system
- the spleen
- the diaphragm and
- all disordered zones
- sedation of the respiratory system if the child is wheezing; no stimulating movements are made over reflex zones to lungs until the attacks are less frequent and less severe
- holding of the webs between the second and third toes firmly between finger and thumb for

2 minutes as soon as the child starts to wheeze, or for up to 4 minutes if respiration remains distressed.

Supplementary care. So many factors may contribute to this disabling illness in children and all should be given careful consideration. Diet may be a contributory factor; any known allergens are to be avoided. Substitutes (soya milk, goat's milk or cheese) should be tried for those children who do not tolerate dairy food well. Chemicals and colorants in foods should be avoided, as should a smoky atmosphere.

Mother should be shown how to apply alternately hot and cold packs to the spine, which should be a nightly routine until the attacks are less severe, and these can be applied at any time respiration becomes distressed.

Moderate, regular exercise is to be encouraged.

The atmosphere around the child should be kept calm during an attack; too much fussing is usually counterproductive. The therapist should ensure and oversee that the inhaler is being used properly.

There should be an attempt to try to discover and address the child's fears.

Ear infections. Specific treatment is given as follows:

- sedation of the reflex zones to the ears and eustachian tube on the big toe, fourth and fifth toes on both feet
- sedation then treatment of zones relating to teeth 18, 28, 38, 48 (whether they have erupted or not)
- treatment of the stomach and small intestine
- the urinary system
- the adrenals
- the liver
- the spleen
- the oronasopharynx
- the lymphatic drainage of the head and neck and
- all disordered zones.

Supplementary care. The patient should avoid draughts, keep the neck and ears covered in cold weather, pay attention to nutrition, and be given plenty of fluids.

Recurring respiratory infections. Specific treatment is given as follows:

- tonifying treatment to the stomach and small intestine
- the urinary system
- the entire lymphatic system
- the adrenals
- the abdominal wall, shoulder girdle, thoracic spine and
- the respiratory system.

Supplementary care. Massage is given along the length of the thoracic spine nightly, either in the bath with soap or before bed. The therapist should teach and oversee relaxed abdominal breathing when the child is old enough, plus 'the lift' exercise for chest expansion (see Appendix III, p. 283). Dry, overheated atmospheres should be avoided. The patient should be encouraged to take clear fluids, and eat a nutritious, well-balanced diet.

Recurrent urinary tract infections. Specific treatment is given as follows:

- the oronasopharynx
- the liver
- the spleen
- the small intestine
- the lumbar and sacral spine
- the adrenals
- the urinary system and
- any disordered teeth, particularly 11, 12, 21, 22, 31, 32, 41, 42.

Sleep disorders. Specific treatment is given to all disordered zones, using many soothing and stroking movements.

Supplementary care. A nightly routine needs to be established, with a regular bedtime and quiet activities for an hour before going to bed. Lots of soothing strokes to feet and hands should be given once the child is in bed, and the mother should hold the area over the solar plexus. The child's fears need to be addressed.

Skin disorders. Specific treatment is given as follows:

- the respiratory system
- the urinary system
- the gastrointestinal tract

- the urinary system
- the liver
- the endocrine system
- the spleen and
- any disordered zones.

Supplementary care. As some children are affected by environmental factors such as constituents in certain soaps, washing powders, dyes and chemical additives to food, or have particular food intolerances, a very careful history is needed, and it is helpful if the mother keeps a diary of all eruptions to try and identify provocative factors.

Behavioural changes. The therapist should try to discover whether there is any physical cause. He then performs a full assessment and treatment of all disordered zones, or refers as necessary for appropriate help, as the example given in Case study 13.4 illustrates.

Summary

- First a full assessment is completed.
- All disordered reflex zones are treated.
- Treatment is concentrated on the disordered reflex zones which form the background to the illness.
- Painful reflex zones relating to symptoms are treated to give relief but receive less emphasis than those in the background.
- Parents or carers are informed about possible reactions and asked to report their occurrence.
- The nutritional, environmental, family, social and psychological factors involved in this child's care are considered.
- The child and parents should be involved in the plan of care, which should be realistic and achievable.
- Both child and parents should be encouraged and complimented on their progress.
- If in doubt about findings or slow progress, the therapist should seek help.
- The therapist should do and say nothing to alarm parents unnecessarily.
- The therapist should not overstep the boundaries of his training.

CASE STUDY 13.4

A mother of a 12-year-old boy sought help for his torticollis, which had not responded well to painkillers and had caused him to have 2 to 3 days away from school on several occasions over the past 6 months. The lad had enjoyed very good health generally in the past, but presently seemed a little tense at times.

On assessment the feet were neither warm nor cold, shapely, the arches were good, the skin uniform in colour with no corns or callus. There was good healthy tissue tone, though tight to touch over the neck and shoulder area.

On palpation there was sharp pain, graded to a 5, over the reflex zones of the neck and shoulder girdle and the cervical spine, which was more pronounced on the right side. There was marked tenderness over the reflex zones to the lymphatics of the groin.

After the first treatment, the neck pain and stiffness was greatly relieved by rotating the large toes and working over the corresponding reflex areas of the neck, shoulders and spine. After a second session the pain and stiffness of the neck and shoulders were completely relieved, but the reflex zones to the lymphatics of the groin remained painful, and an appointment to see the general practitioner was recommended. Shortly afterwards a circumcision was performed for a phimosis.

At a follow-up visit for RZT all reflex zones were painless and his neck and shoulders had remained free of pain.

Table 13.1 *Summary of general treatment procedures*

Years	Infants (0–1 years)	Toddlers (1–3 years)	Small children (3–5 years)	Children (5–12 years)	Adolescents (12–16 years)
Position	Sitting or lying	Sitting or lying	Sitting or lying	Lying down	Lying down
Assessment	Track over dorsal, medial plantar feet	Track over dorsal, medial plantar feet	Each system	Each system	Each system
Harmonising holds	More holding, small strokes	Holding and stroking	Stroking	Stroking	Stroking
Treatment time (min)	1–5 with holding	2–7	5–10	5–15	10–20
Treatment time (acute illness)	Daily to 3 times a week	Daily to 3 times a week	Daily to 3 times a week	Daily to 3 times a week	2–3 times a week
Treatment time (chronic illness)	2–3 times a week	2–3 times a week	Twice a week	Twice a week	Twice a week
Maintenance till recovery	Weekly	Fortnightly	Fortnightly	Monthly	Monthly
Treat	All visibly and palpably disordered reflex zones and reacting systems				
Watch for	Dorsiflexion or plantar flexion of big toes				
	Cooling, sweating and withdrawal				
Avoid	Overstimulation				
			Endocrine overstimulation		

Reference

Lloyd G E R 1978 Hippocratic writings. Penguin, Harmondsworth, p 188. First published 1950, Blackwell, Oxford

14

RZT for elderly people

Introduction

Elderly people usually like RZT. They do not have to expend too much effort in order to receive treatment, the physical contact between themselves and the therapist is not threatening, and its effect is not dependent on their ability to describe their complaints. Treatments are given at planned intervals, they do not last for too long, and the touch is pleasing. It is easy for elderly people to become socially isolated and for their lives to become more circumscribed as they become less mobile, less robust and more anxious, particularly if hearing, sight or balance begin to fail.

The infirmities of old age are eased by RZT, which is remarkably effective in relieving pain and stiffness in their joints and muscles, constipation, indigestion in its many guises, lapses in concentration and memory, and respiratory difficulties. Sleep improves, lassitude is lifted, and, for those immobilised in home or bed, it is a welcome break in the monotony of a confined existence. The spectrum of need for treatment in the elderly is wide. At 80 one may be mobile and have all one's faculties intact, and want treatment for an attack of bronchitis. Others with fewer years are less mobile and have lost their mental agility, yet for all there are incontrovertible physiological, mental and psychological processes in progress after the sixth decade.

Physiological changes of ageing

Maturity is that period during which adults reproduce and raise their young, after which the vigour of many metabolic processes gradually declines.

Hormonal changes

In women, the biological reproductive functions begin to decrease at about the age of 50 years, and ovulation gradually ceases. Comparable changes occur in men a few years later. The physiological changes of age include a fall in the basal metabolic rate and a slowing down of endocrine function. Reproductive functions cease, as does the capacity to replace mineral in bones and hair, while cardioprotective oestrogen levels fall in women.

Tissue changes

There are losses of subcutaneous fat, water from tissues and elasticity in all connective tissues, including that of the dermis of the skin.

Elastic fibres are impregnated over time with mineral salts, so that they become harder and less tensile. These changes and endothelial plaque formation are responsible for atherosclerosis in arterial walls, whether in main, smaller or cerebral vessels.

Proteoglycans, the small protein protectors surrounding the neurovascular bundles which perforate the fascia just beneath the skin, begin to decrease in number after the age of 62 in both men and women. This leaves all supporting connective tissue more vulnerable to infection and injuries, which then take longer to heal. The protective response of the immune system takes longer to be mobilised and there is growing fragility of the red blood corpuscles, with ready bruising.

All bones become lighter, less dense and more brittle as their mineral content becomes reduced over the years, consequently they break more easily, particularly if there is a decrease in mobility.

Hyaline cartilage of the body, especially in costal cartilages, becomes calcified and many fibrous and cartilagenous joints become ossified.

Changes in sensitivity

The very old, like the very young, are acutely sensitive and responsive to all physical changes of temperature, draught, noise, barometric pressure, humidity, activity and smell which take place around them.

There is less physiological tolerance for noise, excessive stimulation, extremes of temperature, change, physical exertion, and less resilience against hunger, thirst, infection and injury. Body heat (most loss occurring from the skin covering the head) and fluid can be lost rapidly in the elderly, who need to be protected from cold and dehydration. The physiological need for simplicity reasserts itself, smaller and simpler meals better suiting the digestive, metabolic and chemical processes at this age.

While an active and fulfilled life is enjoyed by many people after the sixth decade, others find increasing limitations being placed on their mobility, sight, hearing, digestion and energy reserves — the common infirmities of old age.

Psychological changes

Also notable is a changed perception of time, which assumes a different psychological importance. The old can make such delightful companions for the young because both share a timescale in which tomorrow is filled with uncertainties. Immediate events are more important than those planned for the future. There is often a clear recall of certain events and an immediacy to living which is heightened by the imminence of its ending. It is usual for people to become more reflective in old age, while their interests generally become more circumscribed.

It is unusual for the very old to have unrealistic expectations about their treatment, and their appraisals are often refreshingly forthright.

Benefits and limitations of RZT in the elderly

If the matrix regulation is still resilient and functioning well, RZT is straightforward to give and evokes an uncomplicated response, which is often surprisingly rapid. The symptoms recede, reactions are moderate and a sense of renewed energy and well-being ensues.

If, on the other hand, the attrition of long years of illness, poor mobility, emotional exhaustion, excessive exposure to heat, cold or damp, heavy labour, poor nutrition and a weakened biochemistry of the body have degraded or weakened the basic matrix of connective tissue and its functions, the response to RZT is modified in accord with the history. The possibility of full recovery from an acute illness or a fracture becomes limited, reactions may be more labile, and a longer course of treatment is needed. Imaginative solutions must be sought to cope with attention to nutrition, mobility and social intercourse in which the person is able to participate. RZT is none the less an effective form of therapy, if judged by the extent to which drugs and medicines can be avoided and freedom from discomfort maximised.

Many elderly people living alone feel deprived of physical and social contact. Touch is often limited to the hairdresser or the chiropodist. For them, the benefits are shared equally beween RZT, the one-to-one contact, the continuity of the same therapist, the half hour of undivided attention and the physical touch.

Preparation

The room should not be overheated in winter, but sufficient coverings are needed and the bed should have been warmed beforehand.

As with the very young, very light but warm coverings are needed, and during RZT most elderly people like to be cocooned (like small babies) so that they can feel the boundary of their skin in contact with the blanket or duvet. Many very old people (and those of some other cultures) like to have a covering for their head.

If it is difficult for the patient to lie down, pillows should be provided to support him in a reclining or sitting position. The therapist should ensure that stiffened joints are not hyperextended (they should ideally be in slight flexion), adducted or at too great an angle of external rotation. With the imaginative use of a variety of small cushions it is possible to find a position which is both comfortable and gives good support to areas where it is needed. These are mostly the small of the back, painful shoulders, hips and knees, in the elderly frail.

For those who are bedfast and can only lie on their sides the therapist can support the separated legs on pillows.

If treatment is taking place in a domestic setting, and the bed is low, the feet should be elevated on one or more pillows or two foam wedges, and rolled-up towels used for small cushions. The patient's breathing should be unrestricted.

Assessment

General

A simple and clear explanation of what is going to be done must be given by the therapist before starting *any session*, more especially so if the patient's memory is failing, and this may need to be repeated before each session. If an elderly person is dependent on family or carers, the therapy is explained to them, the effects which are anticipated, and their cooperation enlisted in noting the appearance of any reactions.

It needs to be established at the outset what is desired from RZT. Elderly people may have quite different wishes and expectations from those caring for them. The therapist should try to discover before beginning an assessment what help would be most valued, and from which complaint the *patient* would like to be relieved. People with quite serious illnesses often complain more than might be thought of pain or discomfort in the back, knee, hip or shoulder than of their illness.

If the patient is confused and there is little history available, the therapist is reliant on her palpation and any changes taking place in the tissues of the feet from one treatment to another. Consulting with the family or carers at each visit gives an opportunity both to exchange information and to assess progress.

It is a courtesy to the old to remember that the values of a younger generation may not be those of the older, and that not everyone in previous generations was raised in an atmosphere of open speech and discussion on every topic, nor with the easy familiarity of touch and assumed intimacy which is now prevalent.

Palpation

Where possible, the first session consists of a complete assessment of the reflex zones of the feet, and should take no longer than half an hour.

The elderly are sensitive to weight, therefore coverings should be warm and loose. The hands of the therapist hold the feet supportively, and she should avoid resting any weight on them or holding them in an unnatural position.

Because of the heightened responsiveness to any stimulus which occurs at both extremes of age, the touch is kept light and soft at first, becoming firmer according to the wish or responsiveness of the patient. Reflex zones should be palpated only for as long as is tolerable for the patient, and the therapist should take account of any SNS reactions.

The loss of tone which is often seen in the feet of the elderly occurs in part as a result of the physiological changes within the connective tissue, and in part from debility of the GRS concomitant to an illness. In those who are chair- or bedbound there is further loss of tone and muscle mass because of derangement of normal gravity-adapted physiological mechanisms.

Diminished sensation may occur when there are circulatory disturbances, or when ingestion of many medicines has altered the internal milieu, from peripheral neuropathies and vitamin or nutritional deficiencies.

Multifactorial influences in disease

Many factors combine to cause and further the advance of disease. Failing function in one organ sooner or later affects others. Changes occurring when organic disease is no longer confined to one organ or system of the body are usually visibly and palpably reflected in the feet, where many systems are shown to be disorganised.

For example, the patient may arrive complaining of shortness of breath and with a known coronary insufficiency. Palpation reveals disordered reflex zones to the kidneys and the liver, as well as to the heart. The functioning capacity of the liver or the kidneys has been overwhelmed by the biochemical load placed on them by dietary, environmental, occupational, congenital or other factors. In order to provide an adequate supply of oxygenated and chemically pure blood to all vital organs, the heart responds and its action increases. If the load is not lifted, over a period of time and, despite pumping at its peak response, it becomes impossible for the heart to provide a pure enough blood flow to all organs (including the heart itself). The urgent need here is for rest, physical and chemical, so that the liver can fulfil its functions of metabolism and detoxification, and the kidneys do not have to excrete excessive products of catabolism. Improved function in these organs improves the purification and oxygen-carrying capacity of blood, unburdening the heart. The same holds true in many other disease states. People cope, from necessity, until they are no longer able to, and seek treatment when the illness has ramified to involve other organs and systems.

In trauma and the very early stages of an illness pain and disorder in the reflex zones are palpable in a limited number of zones, and may at this stage be confined to one system. In the later stages of disease many systems have become affected via one or more

of the body's feedback mechanisms, and this spread is matched in the many disorders apparent in the reflex zones, so that the first impression on many occasions is that all the reflex zones are disordered. They may be, but not all to the same degree. With discriminating palpation the therapist can discover which are the most discomposed, and they will receive more treatment.

Completing the session

If the elderly person has difficulty in bending to wash his feet, a warm footbath and wash can be given at the *end* of the session.

Referrals to a chiropodist may need to be made (see Ch. 5, p. 84).

Treatment

RZT can be given at weekly or twice weekly intervals. In acute illness or for symptomatic pain relief (such as a sore shoulder) it can be given for short sessions for a few minutes every day. While it is important to treat all disordered reflex zones on the feet, hands or back, paying particular attention to the patient's principal discomfort affords immediate relief. The therapist can concentrate on the underlying causes once he is more comfortable. Immediate aims are more relevant to the elderly (and to the sick) than the promise of relief in weeks to come.

A longer period of time is set aside for the first few sessions, accommodating for any slowness of speech, comprehension and mobility. Enough time should be allowed to answer the patient's questions and for him to comment on how the treatment is affecting him.

Even when briefly giving first aid one should allow enough time for an explanation, and not rush the treatment. The elderly sometimes need conversation as much as therapy. If they are on their own for long periods, the dictum of not speaking more than is necessary during a session is relaxed. Since the actions in RZT both soothe and relax, as well as heal, quiet concentration often ensues once the session gets under way. Otherwise the stimulus of human communication in these circumstances adds to the benefit of RZT.

Treating the back

The most comfortable position for an elderly person is to sit sideways on a chair and rest the arms and head on cushions on a table. As it becomes more difficult to reach behind the back, many elderly people both enjoy and benefit from a treatment on this area, particularly if they have pain in the spine, shoulders or the hips, or if they have long-standing cardiorespiratory complaints. Treatment can be alternated between the back and the feet, and, where possible, the patient should make the choice.

Because there can be such a rapid loss of body heat, the room needs to be warm and free of draughts, and adequate light but warm coverings available.

The therapist should take particular care not to work on the bony surfaces of the spine, especially if there has been wasting of muscle and subcutaneous tissue. Since the bones may be brittle and frail, the joints less free in their movement, and the capillaries fragile, a delicate and light touch is all that is needed. Warm contact comes from the palms of the hands making light stretching movements from the sides of the spine to the lateral edges of the rib cage to expand the lungs, and stretching of the spine from the neck to the coccyx also to assist breathing. These preparatory stretching movements are made before treating the painful reflex zones. If there is fluid in the lungs, movements directed upwards from the base of the lungs towards the apices, and gentle tapping at the bases of the lungs encourages expectoration.

The therapist should assess the length of time that needs to be spent on the back by the colour, expression, temperature, breathing and comfort of the recipient, and remember that elderly people tire easily in unaccustomed positions.

Completing the session

A longer rest period may be needed for the elderly, who often sleep deeply for an hour or two after a session of RZT. This is usually a restorative sleep during which time they are best left undisturbed.

Supplementary advice

Practical recommendations are the only ones worth making. The lift is an exercise which the frailest person can do, either standing up or lying in bed. It improves breathing, helps to prevent stiffness, uses all muscles and relieves much back and neck ache (see Appendix III, p. 283). (Any suggestions which are difficult or impossible to carry out increase the patient's sense of impotence and dependence on others.)

Treatment of acute, degenerative or chronic illness

Acute illness

In any acute illness recovery depends upon the physical capacity of the patient, the maintenance of appropriate fluid intake, food, rest, hygiene, as well as freedom from anxiety and physical care — the psychological aspect of recovery.

RZT is given to all disordered zones to enhance rest and relaxation, to relieve symptoms and promote recovery. The patient's immunity and the care he receives determine in large measure the outcome.

Degenerative illnesses

In degenerative illnesses there is a permanent need for physical care and support. The degree to which: (a) the matrix connective tissue functions have been compromised, and (b) the person's vitality continues to be eroded by internal or external factors influence the outcome, and a more extended course of RZT needs to be given.

Although human beings have in this century travelled in space and looked down electron microscopes, our lifespan is still largely determined by genes and luck. Growing life expectancy in the West has become for a significant number of people an extended period of frailty. The aim of care for them is to maintain, as far as is possible, independence, comfort and normal physiological activities. RZT is given because it supports such activities, and is a form of communication often lacking for this group. Treatment is directed toward maintaining respiratory, digestive, urinary and cardiac function, at keeping the patient as comfortable as possible, and providing a form of touch which is not directed solely at functional activities such as washing, feeding, dressing, etc.

If there is some long-standing impairment such as a weakness of the pelvic floor, stress incontinence or constipation, RZT is given to these specific areas needing treatment once an assessment has been made.

RZT can be given two or three times a week, and 20 to 30 minutes is an appropriate time to spend on palpation, with emphasis on warming, passive movements of all joints, holding and harmonising movements.

Regular sessions should be continued until a plateau is reached, and there are no further changes in the tissues. None the less, if it is evident that there is a place for further treatment (because, for example, sleep is more restful, or because the treatment is reassuring) it can be continued for the human contact and not because it is going to restore physical capacity. It may also be given to check that no new ailment (such as cystitis) is developing, particularly for those who find it difficult to complain, or cannnot easily express themselves.

The matrix regulating system gradually becomes more depleted after the sixth decade; reactions may be exaggerated or labile when treatment begins. The therapist should reduce the time spent on palpation and give more harmonising strokes and a warm footbath.

Almost more than any other age group, elderly people are agitated by and dislike haste. Movements and palpation are more effective if they are measured and rhythmical, without probing too deeply into the tissues. Rapid treatment will quickly lead to sympathetic overstimulation.

Chronic and long-standing illness

Here also the functions and resilience of the ground system have been largely eroded. RZT is valuable in so far as it relieves joint pains, stiffness, loss of continence, constipation and similar discomforts. The calming and reassuring physical contact which is able to relieve aches and pains affords the patient some respite.

Treatment of specific disorders

The bedfast

When the spine and joints become fixed in positions of flexion, and if the legs are adducted (scissored) making it difficult to sit up, change clothing and to wash the legs and pubic area, gentle but sustained sedative pressure on the reflex zones to the adductor and abductor muscle groups relieves muscular spasm, and can be given before any of these activities. A few minutes' sedation is often all that is required.

Constipation

This is perhaps the most common disorder to afflict the elderly, and probably the one about which they most complain.

Treatment should include:

- sedation of reflex zones to the cardia, pyloric sphincter, ileocaecal valve and anus
- stimulation of the stomach, the small and large intestines on the plantar and lateral aspects
- stimulation of the musculature of the abdominal wall on the dorsum and the lumbar spine medially.

Supplementary care. Constipation is a side-effect of many medicines, and the elderly frequently have many drugs prescribed for them. The therapist should check that no unnecessary drugs are being taken. The elderly are often unaware of hunger or thirst, and may need encouragement to drink enough fluid. Keeping a record of what they drink and how much urine they pass for 48 hours will show up any deficiency, and a concentrated or deficient urinary output is potentially dangerous. Some change in the composition of the diet may have to be made; however, it is better for the elderly and the sick to eat a little of something that they like than nothing, however nutritionally sound it may be, of what they do not like.

Stress incontinence

Assessment includes a careful and precise assessment of all reflex zones in the pelvic areas.

Specific treatment is as follows:

- treatment of the urinary system
- the lumbar and sacral spine, the pelvic floor and the supporting structures of the pelvis
- treatment also of the related teeth zones, oronasopharynx and solar plexus.

Retention with overflow

It is easy for this condition to develop in men if there is prostatic enlargement, and in men and women with cardiac insufficiency. Its presence should be suspected if frequent small amounts or driblets of urine are passed, either with urgency or incontinently.

Treatment is as follows:

- stimulation of the bladder and ureters, the lumbar and sacral spine
- treatment of the prostate gland (in men)
- sedation of the diaphragm and solar plexus for 3–5 minutes every 2 hours until the bladder is empty, then every 4 hours until a satisfactory flow is established and some bladder tone has returned
- treatment of all disordered reflex zones in the pelvic area, the pelvic floor, and all disordered reflex zones, of which the heart will be one.

Treatment should be given two or three times a week until improvement is sufficiently established to reduce treatment to once weekly and then fortnightly. RZT may need to be given regularly to stimulate bladder tone, usually once every 7–21 days.

Hypertension

There are many causes of this complex disorder, commonly renal and endocrine diseases, and a raised systolic measurement is common in old age as the arteries become less elastic. RZT is helpful in reducing anxiety and inducing relaxation and is indicated. Blood pressure readings should be taken before and after each session in the early stages of treatment. Because there may be more than one provocative factor causing raised blood pressure in the elderly, an assessment is essential and all

disordered reflex zones need to be treated, combined with frequent harmonising and stroking movements. Specific treatment is as follows:

- sedation of the solar plexus and diaphragm
- sedation of the adrenal glands.

Supplementary advice. Salt intake should be reduced.

Stiff neck

Treatment is as follows:

- gentle rotation of the big toes every few hours or
- sedation of the reflex zones to the neck on the hand
- treatment of the musculature of the neck and shoulder girdle, and the TMJ, the sternum and the cleidomastoid muscle on toes or thumbs as first aid
- treatment of the liver and gall bladder, because of their segmental relationship to the right side of the neck and right shoulder girdle
- treatment also of the heart for its segmental relationship to the left side of the neck and left shoulder girdle
- circumduction of the heads of the metatarsals, one against each other, may also be used, and may be sufficient in itself if the pain is caused by injury or stiffness of the shoulder or shoulder girdle, or from long hours of sitting or lying in one position.

Back ache

The causes of back pain are numerous and varied. It may originate in the kidneys, any part of the alimentary tract or the reproductive organs. It may result from poor posture, trauma to or degeneration of the bones or joints of the spine itself, be part of generalised disease in any other part of the body, or have a psychosomatic origin. It should never be dismissed in the elderly as being one of the concomitants of old age, and, while first aid may be given to relieve acute pain, this should be followed as soon as possible by a full assessment.

Specific treatment is as follows:

- for symptomatic relief, treatment of the painful reflex zones of the spine, the abdominal musculature on the dorsum of feet or hands
- on the back, treatment of the reflex zones which indicate the origin of the pain; this is particularly successful in treating sciatic pain which accompanies a bowel disorder (commonly constipation); the reflex zones in the buttocks feel 'knotted' and the muscles on either side of the lumbar spine are 'taut'.

Pressure sores

There is usually some change in the colour and texture of the skin in the area of the foot corresponding to the site of a developing bedsore, which becomes more pronounced once the skin has broken down, and the reflex zones are painful. As well as regular turning to relieve the pressure on the area, the reflex zones are treated for a few minutes every 4 hours. As debilitation is a major factor in the development of pressure sores, an assessment and course of treatment is recommended.

Case study 14.1 gives an example of RZT in the elderly.

Summary

Regular sessions are valuable for elderly people, especially if they are uncomplaining or have difficulties in communication. Developing eye or urinary tract infections, for example, can be detected and treated early, before their symptoms become apparent. Consequently they are less likely to further weaken the patient, and discomfort is minimised.

- All symptoms such as back ache, constipation and loss of weight in the elderly need investigation. Assessment is followed by treatment, and if there is no improvement in the symptoms or the reflex zones after six sessions the patient should be referred to the doctor.
- The therapist should address the need expressed by the elderly person as to what troubles him most.
- Treatment to relieve symptoms is acceptable, but the therapist has to be alert that no other illness or complication is developing. An assessment should be conducted from time to time to monitor the situation.

CASE STUDY 14.1

An elderly man came for treatment complaining of abdominal discomfort, bloating and pain which was not confined to one specific area, but extended across the whole of the abdominal wall. It had worsened over the past month.

An assessment was made. Painful reflex zones were found to the left inguinal canal and pelvic lymphatics (level 4), the left kidney, the adrenals, the small and large intestines and the abdominal wall on the left, the left thigh, teeth 36, 37, 24, 17 and 48, the lumbar and sacral spine and the right shoulder.

At the second visit the pain was confined to the left side of the abdomen; reactions of diuresis and frequent

bowel movements had been noted. Reflex zones to the inguinal canal and pelvic lymphatics provoked SNS reactions of sweating and dry mouth.

At the third visit the pain had localised in the lower left quadrant of the abdomen. Reflex zones to the left groin remained at level 4, whilst other reflex zones were less painful on palpation. He was still having a slight diuresis. His sleep and appetite had improved, and he was feeling better within himself.

It was suspected that this man was developing an early inguinal hernia, which was confirmed when he visited his general practitioner. Surgery was recommended.

- When a course of treatment is started and improvement follows, the therapist should check with the doctor whether any medicines which the patient is taking need to be reduced.
- The therapist should be clear about her treatment objectives and monitor whether they are being met. If they are not, she should question whether the treatment is appropriate.

- Treatment time and frequency of sessions should be graduated according to the tolerance, reactions and progress. Just as medicines have a more potent effect in an older person than in a fit, healthy young adult, so too does RZT.
- A warm footbath and stroking the feet or harmonising strokes help the frail elderly to sleep.

15

Treating people with cancer, life-threatening and degenerative diseases

Introduction

All illness is stressful. Fear of hospitals, medicine, surgery, technology and the eventual outcome accompany all episodes of ill health. In spite of public health measures, preventative X-rays and smear programmes, and the availability of information, there are terrors *peculiar* to a diagnosis of cancer. It is, not always correctly, associated with pain, rapid death, fear and a conspiracy of silence among embarrassed friends, family and colleagues.

Advances in technology have imposed their own stresses on doctors and patients alike. Better diagnosis and longer survival, often after daring interventions, have necessitated new support groups to help patients, carers and relatives. The help may be emotional, social or informative, and includes the newer therapies such as RZT, aromatherapy, relaxation, creative visualisation (or mental imagery) and healing, either singly or in combination.

RZT, used in hospices, is gradually being introduced into the oncology wards of NHS hospitals. RZT is supplementary to conventional treatments for cancer, and is one of a range that can be given at all stages of disease for both physical and psychological support, to encourage attitudes of hopefulness and to strengthen trust in the medical team. As positive attitudes of hope and personal beliefs, which do not have to be a part of any formalised religion, bolster the immune system, they play an important part in recovery from any illness. As has already been stated, RZT makes no diagnosis and offers no total cure, but it can lessen and ameliorate pain and distress when skilfully performed.

The many technological advances in medicine over the past decades have allowed people with cancers once thought untreatable to survive and resume normal or near normal life. Yet the same life-saving technologies which are used in diagnosis, surgery and treatment at the same time make new and heavy demands on the psychological and physical capacities of the patient. The invasiveness of treatments and their side-effects are an added burden to the ongoing nature of the illness.

The fact that the enormous and impressive expenditure of energy and resources used in their diagnosis and treatment can also fail to cure them often adds to a general feeling of impotence in the face of any incurable illness. Patients have to mobilise every inner resource they have when given such a diagnosis. They commonly say that they feel subsumed by it, as though everything else about themselves, their abilities, relationships, the roles they fill in life and their achievements easily become insignificant to others, that they feel reduced to being nothing more than a cancer, multiple sclerosis or AIDS patient, and that their sense of self and identity is seriously threatened.

Patients are transient visitors in hospital; their lives revolve around their families, homes, work and communities. Of necessity, the atmosphere in hospitals is busy and often impersonal, even though perceptive doctors and other staff are aware of the way in which illness impinges on every aspect of their patients' lives, and RZT can be used to counterbalance the impersonality of a hospital stay, and bring a sense of peace and relaxation to such patients.

Merits of RZT

Reflex zone therapy is given to the person and not to the diagnosis. Each treatment is tailored and adapted at each session to the needs of the person being treated.

The purpose of RZT is to:

- buttress whatever treatment the patient is receiving
- fortify the compromised immune system through its effect upon the GRS
- help relieve pain
- relieve symptoms, the most common of which are nausea, vomiting, muscle weakness, constipation, diarrhoea, painful coughing, dyspnoea, fitful sleep, hiccoughs, lethargy, pain and retention of urine
- promote relaxation
- give respite.

RZT is valuable alongside conventional treatment because:

1. Many patients experience a feeling of distaste arising from the changes which have taken place in their bodies as a result of disease, the treatment, or both. Family members and friends may be experiencing and embarrassed by the same feelings. The therapist, through his touch, whether to the hands, feet or back, conveys to the patient that she has not become 'untouchable'. Thus a sense of body image which has been corroded can be helped to be restored.
2. Touch is a form of communication which does not depend on speech. The patient is spared from speaking unless she wishes to, and the patient who has difficulty with her speech or cannot speak is reassured by the intention transmitted through the therapist's touch. The patient can communicate without words with the therapist through her responses.
3. The patient has some choice. She may have treatment on her hands, feet or back.
4. Privacy remains intact. The body does not have to be exposed unless the patient chooses to have treatment on her back, and such exposure can be limited.

5. It is not invasive.
6. It is a quiet activity. The movements are rhythmical and systematic. It provides a period of sanctioned rest, free from interruptions or demands.
7. The patient retains control of the session. She can ask for the treatment to end, to be extended, and for movements and holding which have previously been soothing or pain relieving to be repeated.
8. It is relaxing.
9. It provides continuity of care if the patient sees the same therapist at each visit, and it is therefore easier to establish a relationship. It saves the patient the burden of explaining her symptoms and reactions anew at each session.

    By being able to compare small changes taking place on the feet with previous observations the therapist is able to assess more accurately the effects of RZT in combination with other treatment.
10. It does not take place at or near the site of the tumour, operation or radiotherapy. It is perceived by almost all patients as a time when they 'forget they are ill, and feel like a person again'.
11. The hands can be used to complement treatment. The patient can learn how to apply pressure to appropriate zones of her hands to relieve pain and symptoms. She has something positive to do, and is not entirely dependent on others.

These are small things on their own, but put together their effect is gratifying for the patient. The therapist who is able to amalgamate as many of these aspects as possible into one session provides a prerequisite of all recovery — healing rest. RZT derives its validity from its capacity to relieve pain and symptoms. Convalescence and recovery frequently impose some changes in lifestyle: there is a need for rest, some foods may be less well tolerated, and some movements may be restricted. The patient should be given helpful, structured and proven advice on how to cope with the effects of illness and treatment. No suggestions should be made that are too difficult to comply with; a light approach which seeks to find ways round difficulties and constant encouragement are more helpful in the long run.

Factors influencing treatment

Location

Private practice

In private practice regular sessions can be given at whatever intervals are judged most appropriate by the therapist. This may be once, twice or three times a week, depending on the stage and severity of the illness, and take place in the practice or in the patient's home. Many patients having radiotherapy prefer to have RZT on the same day to reduce the nausea and lassitude from which they often suffer afterwards.

There is a certain amount of latitude in altering appointments to suit the patient, who may want extra sessions from time to time, or to extend the intervals between sessions.

If the therapist is in private practice a brief letter should be sent to the general practitioner when a course of RZT is begun and when it is completed, noting any significant findings.

Hospices

In hospices, staff members who are trained therapists are able to give treatment as required.

A therapist visiting a hospice regularly will be directed by the staff. He is able to share useful first aid techniques with staff members, as well as the patient's family and close friends participating in her care.

Support groups

It is usual for therapists, patients and carers to attend regularly on given days, providing continuity of care. Patients are usually able to make choices about how their time is spent at such centres, but the therapist may need to see many people in one day. The setting is usually semiprivate and, although a quiet environment may be difficult to achieve, it should be as private and as peaceful as possible.

Within the NHS

The NHS is a large, busy, well-established and hierarchical institution, responsible for many activities and functions. Treatment must be fitted into a complex mosaic of care involving many other patients and professional staff. All treatment is authorised, overseen and dovetailed into a regime by the consultant in charge. The therapist must be prepared to liaise with nursing and medical staff and to be flexible. Hospital records must be completed and kept up to date, and the therapist may wish to keep his own personal documentation as well. A quiet, private and separate environment is not always available but the need for it is increasingly being recognised and provided for.

As a matter of courtesy and professionalism the therapist works in cooperation with the medical and nursing staff who are responsible for all aspects of patients' care at all times whilst they are in hospital.

Stage of illness

There is no set pattern of reflex zones which have to be treated in cancer or any other particular disease. The history of all previous unresolved illness and trauma in the patient, the treatments she has received, her personal physical and emotional capacity and temperament, and the stresses of her present social and domestic circumstances influence which painful, insensitive or disordered reflex zones are found on the feet. The outcome is influenced by her innate resilience, belief systems, purpose in living and capacity to respond to the treatments she is given.

Certain patterns of disorder in the reflex zones recur, but the individual disease history and the way in which disordered reflex zones respond to palpation dictate that each person is treated according to his individual responses.

Case study 15.1 is an example of RZT for a woman subsequently diagnosed with cancer.

Early stages

In the early stages, when investigations are still being carried out, treatments are given at regular intervals, two to three times a week, to relieve stress, relax the patient and to strengthen the GRS, with frequent

---

CASE STUDY 15.1

A physiotherapist was treating a middle-aged woman for lower lumbar pain, which was not responding well to her usual techniques. She decided to use RZT, and on assessment found the most painful reflex zones (level 5) to be those of the left kidney. The adrenal glands, lumbar vertebrae 2 and 3, the sacrum, coccyx, bladder, stomach and teeth 22 and 31 were all disordered. Soon after the first session the patient's back ache began to improve, as did all the disordered reflex zones on the feet excepting that of the left kidney. Moreover, ANS reactions became more marked each time the left kidney was palpated at each successive visit. After six sessions the physiotherapist expressed her concern over the findings to the general practitioner. A scan was arranged, which showed a tumour at the upper pole of the left kidney. This was successfully surgically removed soon afterwards.

---

harmonising strokes, holding and treatment of all disordered zones.

After surgery or therapy

During the postoperative, radiotherapy and chemotherapy periods, treatment is directed towards the same ends, as well as improving the function of respiratory, metabolic and excretory systems, and bolstering the immune system. RZT is given for some 30 minutes at regular intervals, once or twice a week, or for shorter periods (10–15 minutes) every 24–48 hours.

Aftercare

When the patient has recovered from the illness and the treatments, a longer timespan between each session is usually sufficient to maintain her progress. Treatment once a week gives way to once a fortnight, then once a month, progressing to once every 2 months until she is strong again and has no need of further regular visits. A general treatment can be arranged from time to time as suits the patient. Some patients become dependent on the therapy and are reluctant to give it up. While it is valuable for them to have regular maintenance and booster sessions, they should be encouraged to enjoy and work at their relationships, interests and occupation, and the therapist may need to broach this subject with them. However, some people have less family and social support than others, and seek a substitute elsewhere. When the time comes for treatment to be given less frequently or to end, the patient should not be made to feel that she is being rejected.

Progressive disease

When the disease is progressive and no cure is possible, e.g. multiple sclerosis, Parkinson's disease, motor neuron disease, cystic fibrosis and ankylosing spondylitis, palliative treatment is given at weekly or fortnightly intervals to foster cardiac, respiratory, urinary, bowel and muscle function. If RZT ceases to be beneficial, treatments are suspended for a few weeks before being continued again once a week or fortnight.

Terminal stage

In terminal illness, frequent, short sessions are given as often as the patient wishes for pain and symptom relief.

Treating different types of illness

Cancer

Treatment (as above) can be given over an extended period covering surgery, treatment and convalescence.

In the intensive care unit

RZT is not a priority here, but when time and opportunity allow it has been observed that patients become calmer and less restless with treatment.

Yin-Yang strokes are given at every opportunity, when washing or turning the patient and whenever there is time between essential observations, medical and nursing treatment. RZT is given circumspectly, particularly when palpating over areas corresponding to sites of trauma or surgery. Frequent short sessions have more effect than longer sessions given less frequently. The therapist should start with light treatment to whichever system is failing — usually the kidneys, adrenals, lungs and liver, and the brain structures in head injury.

After surgery

After major cardiac surgery the therapist should hold and stroke the feet rhythmically and, before giving any treatment, hold the areas corresponding to heart, sternum and thoracic spine, then lightly treat the stomach and spleen, the urinary system, the whole spine, the liver, respiratory system and then the heart zones.

After any transplant surgery the therapist should hold and stroke the spine, treat the urinary system, the liver and lungs and the areas corresponding to the transplanted organ(s). In some kidney transplants the new kidney may have been placed in a site different to that of the removed kidney. Both sites are found to be disordered and both should be treated. Such a site may remain painful for months or years afterwards, giving rise to autonomic reactions when treated.

Awaiting transplant or cardiothoracic surgery

Much holding and stroking is beneficial, with frequent Yin-Yang strokes. The therapist should give light treatment to the spine, respiratory and urinary systems, and gradually incorporate the endocrine and lymphatic systems. Short treatments can be given twice a day. For patients on dialysis RZT can help to reduce muscular twitching, drowsiness and itchiness.

Immune depletion

Immune depletion may be the result of drugs, medicines, radiation, illness, unremitting physical or emotional stress, transplant surgery, or be idiopathic. Treatment should initially consist of much stroking and holding of the feet, and light touch to each system in turn. The therapist should start with short,

frequent sessions until it becomes clear how the patient is going to respond. Many of these patients have capillary fragility, bleeding and bruising easily, and their feet are usually hypersensitive to touch. Patients coming for treatment who develop bruising with normal touch should be referred to their general practitioner for investigation. Treatment is directed at the respiratory, urinary, endocrine, alimentary and lymphatic systems. The patient is likely to need long term therapy at all levels.

Supplementary care. A positive attitude should be encouraged and the patient given small self-help exercises that are within her capacity, such as treating a small area of her hands each day.

Multiple sclerosis

Assessment can be valuable in the early stages, but is less informative once the disease has been established for some time. Treatment is non-specific to begin with until there are reactions indicating the weakest and most responsive systems. Meanwhile symptoms can be treated palliatively (e.g. the eyes if the eyelids are drooping, the respiratory system if there are many chest infections, the bladder and pelvic floor if there is poor control, and the musculoskeletal system for generalised muscle weakness). Treatment is long term.

Parkinson's disease

Assessment and treatment are directed to disordered reflex zones in the early stages, circumspectly over the head zones in early sessions, but building up depth and strength of palpation as tolerance allows. Generalised treatment is given to the spine and all systems as the disease progresses, and to relieve symptoms such as stress incontinence.

Treating different areas

The feet

In the early stages of any illness, reflex zones which reflect growing systemic disruption become painful to touch. This is usually accompanied by visual changes in the colour and texture of the skin, and by alterations of tissue tone. Since the visual changes can be slight and difficult to detect in the early stages, they should never be considered in isolation. Transient changes in skin, tissue tone and discomfort on palpation can be observed on all feet. They become significant when persistent alterations in skin colour and texture, tissue tone and pain on palpation are noticed.

Symptoms usually accompany such changes, but may not be remarked upon because of wide differences of perception in what is normal and tolerable, fear of what may be discovered, and also because people's pain threshold varies so widely. With advancing disease, widespread disorder becomes apparent in the reflex zones. Their disorder becomes more marked, but a patient who is taking many medicines or pain-relieving drugs may be unaware of increased pain in the reflex zones. Autonomic reactions are by this stage provoked by light palpation on reflex zones which mirror the tumour sites and other systems immediately affected by it.

Radiotherapy and chemotherapy as well as some medicines often effect gross changes to the tissue tone in the feet, as does advanced and widespread disease, whatever the cause, but sometimes they do not. The feet may become cold, swollen, and the patient may say that they feel leaden, the skin becoming thinned with a shiny and at times transparent or translucent appearance; the tissues feel either dense and full, soggy, unresilient or even hard over most areas of the feet, and pitting oedema develops. The reflex zones reflecting the site of the most aggravating symptoms at this time (the intestines in constipation, the bladder in retention, etc.) are usually palpably disordered and responsive to treatment, no matter how oedematous the feet. In the later stages of illness, so widespread is the disruption to the internal milieu that it is rarely possible to discover which are the most painful and disordered zones. All are disordered, and all may be painful or not painful at all when palpated. The therapist has now to rely on the autonomic responses and the pain-relieving effects of RZT to determine which zones should be treated and for how long. He is able to distinguish which are the most vulnerable by observing how quickly changes in respiratory rate,

cooling, sweating, dry mouth or pallor occur when they are being treated.

Those reflex zones which evidently provoke signs of sympathetic stimulation should be treated at each session, but only for as long as they do not provoke gross reactions. Treatment of these areas should be frequently interspersed with sedation of the solar plexus and adrenal glands and flowing stroking movements. If the patient is so sympathetically overstimulated that all palpation causes more cooling or sweating, then fewer disordered zones are treated at each session, and for a shorter time, until her condition becomes more stable. The patient should feel better at the end of each session than when it began. A treatment which provokes too many reactions exhausts and weakens her still further.

The back

If the patient has breathing difficulties, or cannot comfortably lie down, she may prefer a general, light treatment to her back.

When radiotherapy has been given, no oil or massage should be applied over the radiotherapy entry and exit points for 3 weeks from the time when she last had radiotherapy.

RZT should not be given over suspicious lumps before they have been diagnosed, nor towards a tumour site, nor over an old tumour site.

The hands

These are a comforting area to treat, particularly when the patient does not wish to be exerted or is very frail. The many accessible reflex zones on the hands provide the patient with a ready means for treatment by herself or by relatives, and can greatly help in relieving symptoms.

Treatment procedure

Assessment

The patient lies, reclines or sits in whichever is for her the most comfortable position. She should be given as many pillows as necessary to support her limbs if there is a wound, a recent operation or radiotherapy site.

Wherever feasible it is advisable to do an assessment. It is not possible to know in advance which areas will be painful on palpation or respond with autonomic reactions, whatever the site of the tumour.

Note: If a tumour has been surgically removed the tissue tone over the corresponding reflex zone feels empty or hollow. For example, a slight depression can be felt in subcutaneous tissue over the metatarsal bones on the dorsum, usually becoming palpable within 48 hours of a mastectomy.

After radiotherapy and chemotherapy the reflex zones in hand, feet and back may become less sensitive to palpation for a shorter or longer period. It is then possible to complete a full assessment with the patient barely aware that the feet are being touched. Several treatments may be necessary before touch is perceived normally again, and it is sometimes observed that normal sensation never returns. In general the patient's improvement is mirrored by returning sensation in the feet. (Yet it is possible to see patients who were treated with radiotherapy 20 years beforehand whose feet remain either barely sensitive or hypersensitive to touch. They have survived and are well, but the legacy of their illness can be traced in their feet.)

Choice of reflex zones

A clear pattern of disorder emerges when the reflex zones are painful or insensitive, when sympathetic responses are stimulated, or when the hands or feet tense up on palpation. Treatment is given to all these zones over a period of 20–30 minutes providing that this is tolerable for the patient. At the same time symptomatic treatment should be given to reflex zones which mirror pain or symptoms, and the patient should feel that those discomforts which distress her most are being treated.

If the feet are globally disordered, the therapist should treat the zones which provoke sympathetic reactions and all the symptomatic zones. If no assessment is possible or deemed necessary, the systems giving rise to the most discomfort are treated.

A note should be made of which area is being treated if the hands or feet become tense, and these should be held quietly until they begin to relax again.

The patient's feet need to be kept as warm as possible, with extra light coverings if necessary, passive movements of the feet and warm footbaths.

Apart from the disordered reflex zones, treatment of the following areas usually adds to the patient's comfort:

- the solar plexus
- the diaphragm
- the spine
- the neck
- the shoulder girdle
- all sphincters
- the adrenal glands.

Gentle traction is applied to the legs and spine as the patient breathes in, which is released as she breathes out; to be effective the traction must coincide with the patient's respiratory rhythm.

The touch is allowed to become lighter over the last few minutes, concluding with featherlight stroking movements.

Psychological factors

As the diagnosis of cancer or any disease which threatens early death or unremitting deterioration has such a devastating impact on the patient and her circle, constant and quiet encouragement are needed. Every one of the patient's inner resources has to be mobilised — hope, purpose, fortitude, determination, the imagination (using creative visualisation) and cooperation in the treatment programme, and these should be fostered by the therapist as well as the wider team.

Treatment and recovery take many months, and during this time the patient is entirely dependent on the goodwill and care of others, most of them strangers to her when she arrives in hospital. Most people feel the need to review their priorities in life at such a time — an inner process which is as urgent for them as any other treatment. As the conclusions they come to will affect the rest of their lives, they need to be given the time, space and assurance they need for evaluation.

When recovery is not expected, the value of treatment is measured by the extent to which the patient does not feel abandoned, but feels supported when she needs it, and the extent to which her pain and discomfort are eased.

Wherever possible, treatment should be conducted in cheerful surroundings. A therapist whose clothes are softly colourful is a tonic for those who are chronically sick and yearn for a little brightness in their surroundings. This might seem an insignificant detail, but the sick are responsive to such details, and much cheered by light and colour as long as they are not too bright or garish; 140 years ago Florence Nightingale (1980) described how even the very sick turn their heads gratefully towards natural light.

Symptomatic treatment

As well as the illness, the side-effects of chemotherapy, radiotherapy and many medicines may cause nausea, vomiting, diarrhoea, constipation, lassitude, coughing, hiccoughs, loss of hair and pain.

Nausea

Treatment is as follows:

- sedation of the solar plexus, diaphragm and adrenal glands, also
- the stomach and small intestine and
- the TMJ and vocal chords.

It is best to start treating these zones as soon as the patient begins to feel nauseated.

Vomiting

Treatment is as follows:

- holding of the reflex zones to the solar plexus and diaphragm on either feet or hands steadily when the patient is vomiting.

Diarrhoea

Treatment is as follows:

- sedation of the reflex zones to all sphincters, also

- the solar plexus, and diaphragm
- sedation of the stomach and small intestine against diarrhoea.

Constipation

Treatment is as follows:

- stimulation of the reflex zones to the liver, and small and large intestines, also
- the lumbar spine and abdominal wall.

Persistent, painful coughing

Treatment is as follows:

- sedation of the reflex zones to solar plexus and diaphragm for persistent coughing
- to encourage expectoration, stimulation of the reflex zones to the lungs from the bases upwards on plantar and dorsal aspects of the feet
- treatment of the diaphragm and stomach
- treatment of the thoracic spine on the feet
- massage of the thoracic spine from the 12th vertebra upwards towards the third vertebra on the back
- massage of the area over the lungs, moving diagonally from the bases towards the spine and the apices of the lungs.

Hiccoughs

Treatment is as follows:

- sedation of the reflex zones to the stomach, solar plexus and diaphragm.

Pain

To alleviate pain, specific treatment is as follows:

- sedation of the reflex zones to the solar plexus
- and those which mirror pain in the body, for example the medial arch of the foot for pain in the lumbar spine.

Supplementary care. The patient should be shown which areas can be treated or rubbed on the hands to ease any of the above.

Hair loss

Patients receiving chemotherapy are recommended to buff their fingernails firmly against each other for 5 minutes three times a day to help stimulate hair growth.

Case studies 15.2 and 15.3 detail RZT treatment after surgery for cancer.

Self-care for the therapist

Particular demands are laid on the therapist with a heavy case load of cancer patients. He must learn to eat and to breathe well, to take adequate time out for recreation and exercise, and to care for his posture when giving treatment. Finding the balance between

---

CASE STUDY 15.2

A 43-year-old woman came for RZT 2 years after having had a partial excision of oesophagus, spleen, stomach and pancreas. She had started to have a recurrence of the pains which preceded her operation. She was anorexic, nauseated, unable to sleep and distressed. Her feet were cold, pallid, oedematous and registered very little sensation on palpation. The skin was dry and flaky. Sympathetic reactions were provoked by palpation to the pituitary, kidneys, adrenals, neck and reflex zones to the surgical sites.

Treatment was given to these zones three times a week for the first 3 weeks. Only 2–3 seconds of treatment were tolerable on each zone for the first few sessions, but after four sessions her feet became slightly warmer during each treatment, and she began to feel more sensation with each succeeding treatment. She was very tired and had a slight headache after each visit. As her sleep began to improve she felt a gradual reduction in nausea and stress.

When the symptoms of pain, nausea, anorexia and distress became less severe, RZT was given twice a week. Reflex zones to the scars were treated on the feet and scar cream applied to the scars on the trunk. It

became possible to treat the disordered zones for 5–10 seconds. The first reactions appeared in the gastrointestinal tract, and lasted for six sessions. As they subsided, she began to have a diuresis, which lasted for 3 weeks, and overlapped with reactions in the respiratory system, which persisted for five sessions after the diuresis had ended. Each of these systems were treated during the reactive phase, as well as the reflex zones to the pituitary, kidneys, adrenals, stomach and spleen, which remained disordered for some 5 years.

Sessions were gradually reduced to one a week, then once fortnightly, once monthly, and then only given if she became overtired. Over the 5 years of treatment she learned to practise a relaxation technique daily, to breathe more efficiently, to do the small amount of exercise which was within her compass, and to eat more nutritious foods.

After 16 years her feet are warm, normally responsive to touch except for raised sensitivity in the adrenals (level 1 or 2), and a slight dulling of sensation over the reflex zone to the stomach. The skin is healthy, the tissue tone remains slightly full.

CASE STUDY 15.3

A 57-year-old woman had had a hysterectomy, appendicectomy, and cholecystectomy over the past 10 years. Eight months previously a lump had been removed from her right upper arm. She complained of feeling very tired, of flatulence, that the right arm was cold and painful, and of pain in the right T8 segment. She was overweight, sleeping poorly, and was intolerant of fats. The circumference of the right arm was 41 cm ($16\frac{1}{2}$ inches). She was a busy caterer.

Both feet were oedematous, the right was colder than the left, and the colour of both was mottled.

At assessment the tissue tone of all reflex zones was disordered, unresilient over the adrenals and kidneys, knotty and uneven over the small intestines, toneless over the spleen and stomach and full and bulging over the endocrines. The most painful reflex zones were those to the spleen, appendix, the lymphatics of the throat and the tonsils. The patient was comfortable until the

CASE STUDY 15.3 (*Contd*)

endocrine system was being assessed. On palpating the adrenals the feet quickly became very cold, a generalised perspiration broke out all over the body, the patient sat upright and vomited effortlessly.

She was reassured, given a warm footbath, hotwater bottles, extra blankets (as she was feeling very cold) and allowed to rest. She fell asleep for 2 hours, and woke feeling more composed. Because of this heightened response to treatment, the next appointment was deferred for 1 week.

4.10.1982. Reactions — she had felt ill for 2 days, the right arm had been less swollen for a few days, and had been tender. Treatment given to sedation to the solar plexus, adrenals, spine, arm, stimulation to gastrointestinal tract, spine and urinary and lymphatic systems.

7.10.1982. Reactions — right arm remained painful, but the swelling had subsided and it felt less heavy. She felt nauseated, tired, had a bitter taste in her mouth on waking and was not sleeping well. Treatment given to sedation of the solar plexus, adrenals and right arm. Stimulation to liver, gastrointestinal tract, spine, urinary and lymphatic systems.

11.10.1982. Reactions — still nauseated, bitter taste in mouth persists. Less pain in right arm but fourth and fifth fingers still occasionally numb. Diuresis. Pain in right hip. Earache in left ear, which then cleared spontaneously. Treatment given to sedation of adrenals, solar plexus, TMJ and right arm. Stimulation of spleen, urinary and lymphatic systems, spine, liver, shoulder girdle and left hip.

14.10.1982. Reactions — tired and breathless, persistent bad taste in mouth. Treatment given to the back. Most painful zones were those of the duodenum, gall bladder, stomach, heart, kidneys, intestines and endocrine system.

18.10.1982. Appointment cancelled as she had a headache, her bowels were active and she was sweating profusely, especially over all scar tissue. She was, however, feeling very well; there was less tingling and pain in the right arm.

22.10.1982. Felt well, calmer and relaxed. Light treatment given to all disordered reflex zones.

3.11.1982. Less abdominal discomfort and no abdominal cramp. Circumference of right arm 33 cm (14 inches) She felt tired but well. Treatment given to all disordered reflex zones, and the solar plexus and adrenals were sedated.

17.11.1982. Very busy at work and very tired, but otherwise feeling better. Sedation to adrenals, solar plexus, treatment to spleen, gastrointestinal tract, spine, urinary and lymphatic systems and right arm.

22.11.1982. Busy and tired. Treatment as at last visit.

3.12.1982. Very tired, overwrought and had a cold. Light sedative treatment given only to spleen, head zones, gastrointestinal tract, spine, lymphatic and urinary systems.

6.12.1982. Tired and resting more. Right arm throbbed for 2 days, but then felt lighter and looked almost normal. Treatment given to head zones, especially neck and lymphatics, spine, lungs, solar plexus, adrenals, urinary system.

11.1.1983. Was feeling well. Arm painful and pain down her right side due to busy period and much heavy lifting at work. Treatment to liver, gall bladder, right arm and shoulder, endocrine, urinary and lymphatic systems, spleen.

14.1.1983. Very little pain in right arm. Treatment given to the reflex zones of the right shoulder joint caused her to perspire and become very hot. Treatment also given to the reflex zones on the face.

19.1.1983. Reactions — she had felt alternately hot and cold for 24 hours after the last visit. Her bowels were active. The circumference of the right arm was 33 cm (4 inches), and it had been neither heavy nor painful. She was having fewer cramps in her legs. Treatment to all disordered zones.

21.1.1983. Was feeling well, but niggling pain in right arm and she had felt flushed. Treatment given to right arm, spleen, endocrine, gastrointestinal and lymphatic systems and spine.

26.1.1983. Feeling well. She had lost 4.5 kg (10 lb) in weight, her skin was clear and soft. The circumference of the right arm was 27.5 cm (11 inches) where the tumour had been removed, and she had had no pain. Both the feet were warm, the skin elastic, the colour less mottled, and the reflex zones less disordered, although the adrenals, solar plexus, gall bladder and spleen were still uncomfortable at level 1. Treatment was given to these zones.

28.1.1983. She was sleeping and feeling well, and had remained pain free. Treatment was given to the disordered reflex zones, and it was decided to stop treatment there.

giving the necessary care and attention to patients and self-renewal is not easy, particularly when experiencing a heavy work load. It is important for the therapist to heed warning signs of his own energy depletion and a sense of being overburdened, and not to become 'burnt out'.

Therapists are advised to have RZT or appropriate supportive care at regular intervals and whenever they are overtaxed to maintain their own good health, and to prevent stresses from building up. Treatment is a valuable experience since it reminds the therapist yet again of the effects of therapy, and serves as a teaching aid for good practice.

It is also advisable to have a working knowledge of other complementary therapies, so that an informed reply can be given when asked for information.

Most importantly, every person treating patients with cancer or other serious illness is part of an extended team, upon every one of whom the patient is dependent. Therapists should fill their place in the team without encroaching on the professional responsibilities of any other member of the team.

Summary

- The treatment should always start with light, non-specific treatment to all systems, the treatment times and depth of palpation gradually increasing.
- The therapist should slowly and circumspectly concentrate on the most disordered zones.
- Short, frequent treatments are more beneficial for the acutely and seriously ill than long, irregularly spaced sessions.
- Symptomatic treatment is given at each session to relieve pain and discomfort.
- Treatment is modulated so that reactions are kept within tolerable boundaries.
- In patients with cancer or late stage degenerative diseases, sensation may be diminished and is not a reliable indicator of which reflex zones to treat nor of the amount of treatment which is tolerable. Therapists need to be mindful of expression, gestures, respiration and the general bearing of the patient as well as the autonomic reactions.
- Pain, discomfort and distressing symptoms can be treated symptomatically as often as is necessary.
- Holding, stroking, harmonising and passive movements of the feet can be used on their own whenever necessary.
- The patient's feet must be kept warm with small, light but warm coverings and warm footbaths.
- If the time comes when treatment can offer no further help and the patient's life is ending, she should not be abandoned psychologically.
- Therapists should try to avoid becoming overtaxed, and care for themselves appropriately when their energies are depleted.

Reference

Nightingale F 1980 Notes on nursing, Commemorative edn. Churchill Livingstone, New York, p 61

Appendices

Appendix I: Symptomatic treatment for first aid

The following guidelines for symptomatic treatment can be used for first aid on the feet, hands or back by the patient, carer or therapist:

- sedation can be maintained in one zone for up to 4 minutes
- tonifying movements can be made for up to 4 minutes in one zone
- the solar plexus and diaphragm should always be sedated if there is pain or distress.

Symptoms which do not regress with a course of treatment, or which regularly recur, should be investigated.

The diagrams on the following pages illustrate the symptomatic treatment for first aid to various common complaints.

Key to diagrams

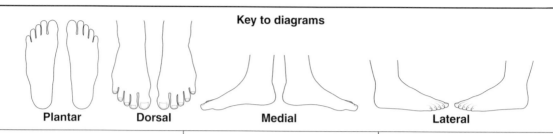

Plantar   **Dorsal**   **Medial**   **Lateral**

Sinusitis
- Tonifying of lymphatics of head/neck.
- Treatment of painful sinus areas.

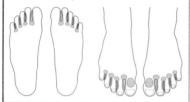

Earache
- Sedation of ear zones/eustachian tube.
- Light tonifying of lymphatics of head and neck.
- Treatment to small intestine.

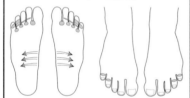

Infected/painful eyes
- Treatment to eye zones on plantar and dorsal aspects of second, third and dorsal first toes on feet.
- Treatment to hands.

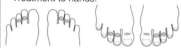

Headache
- Treatment to head, neck and shoulder girdle muscles, cervical spine, solar plexus and stomach zones.
- Sedation of painful zones.
- The patient should avoid wearing tight shoes.

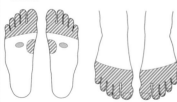

Colds/sore throats
- Light treatment to tonsils, lymphatics of head and neck, oronasopharynx and pelvis on feet and hands.

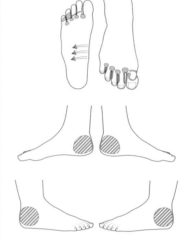

Toothache
- Sedation of painful tooth zone.
- Light tonifying of head and neck lymphatics.

Stiff neck
- Rotation of the tractioned big toes.
- Treatment to cervical spine, neck and shoulder girdle muscles.

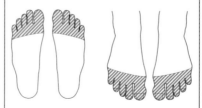

Frozen shoulder
- Treatment to all three surfaces of mtp five joint, neck and shoulder girdle muscles.
- Treatment to small intestine.

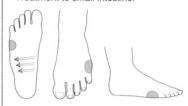

Tennis elbow
- Treatment to all three surfaces of base of fifth metatarsal, neck and small intestine.

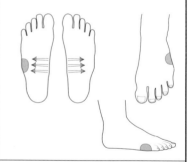

Low backache
- Sedation of lumbar, sacral spine and sacroiliac joint.
- Tonifying of abdominal wall, intestines and neck.

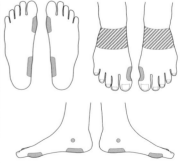

Sciatica
- Sedation of lumbar, sacral spine, sacroiliac joint, abductors and adductors.
- Treatment to the spine.
- Tonifying of intestines.

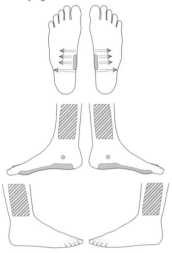

Hip pain
- Sedation of both hips, symphysis pubis, lumbar and sacral spine.
- Treatment to the gall bladder.

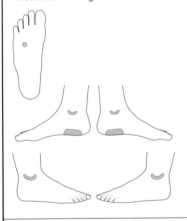

Nausea
- Sedation of stomach, solar plexus, diaphragm, cardiac and pyloric sphincters.

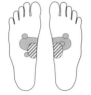

Vomiting
- Steady holding of solar plexus.

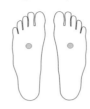

Colic
- Sedation of stomach, sphincters, duodenum, solar plexus and diaphragm.

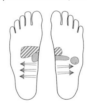

Indigestion
- Treatment to liver, stomach, small intestine, pancreas and spleen.

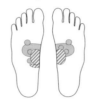

Persistent cough
- Sedation of solar plexus, diaphragm and lungs at night before sleep.
- Tonifying of lung bases, lungs and trachea during the day to help expectoration if mucus is tenacious (e.g. cystic fibrosis).

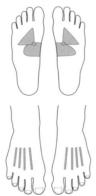

Hiccoughs
- Sedation of stomach, diaphragm and solar plexus.
- The patient should breathe into a small brown paper bag held over the nose.

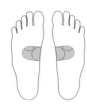

Urinary infection
- Treatment to urinary system, lumbar and sacral spine, pelvic lymphatics and oronasopharynx.

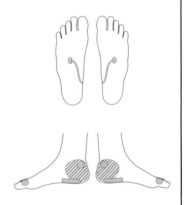

Retention of urine
- Sedation of solar plexus and diaphragm.
- Tonifying of bladder, lumbar and sacral spine for 3–4 minutes every 20 minutes.

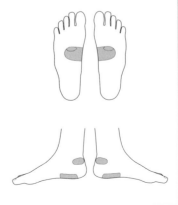

Retention with overflow
- Sedation of solar plexus and diaphragm.
- Light treatment to bladder, pelvic floor, lumbar and sacral spine and heart, every 4 hours till tone regained.

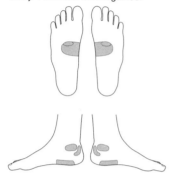

Stress incontinence
- Treatment to pelvic floor, bladder, all pelvic organs and abdominal wall 12 hourly.

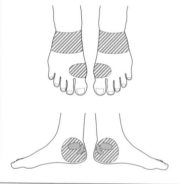

Diarrhoea
- Sedation of stomach, intestines, sphincters and solar plexus.

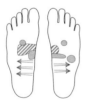

Constipation
- Tonifying of lumbar spine, small and large intestines, abdominal wall, rectum and anus.

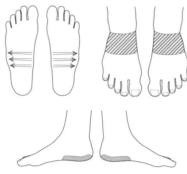

Haemorrhoids
- Sedation of anus and pelvic floor.
- Tonifying of liver and pelvic lymphatics.

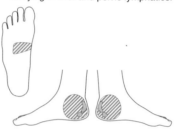

Dysmenorrhoea
- Wringing of the wrists for 3–4 minutes every 2 hours when symptoms begin.
- Treatment to pelvic organs and lymphatics on feet.

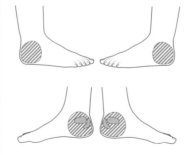

Infected wounds
- Treatment to site corresponding to wound, lymphatic and urinary system.

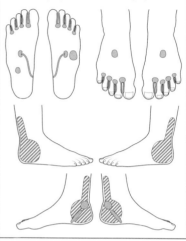

Poor milk flow
- Tonifying of breast zones on dorsum of hands and feet for 4–5 minutes every 4 hours till milk flows easily.

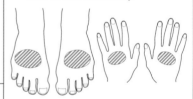

Eczema
- Treatment to small intestine, kidneys, spleen, liver and lungs.
- Sedation of adrenals, solar plexus and diaphragm.

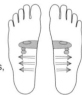

Stress
- Sedation of adrenals, solar plexus and diaphragm.
- Light tonifying of kidneys, small intestine and spine.

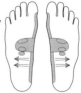

Appendix II: Nutrition

Food in combination with oxygen provides heat and energy and makes possible the growth and replacement of all human tissues such as muscle, bone, blood, hair and skin. The physical well-being of the organism depends on a balanced intake of and ability to metabolise carbohydrates, proteins, fats, minerals, vitamins and trace elements, and an equal ability to excrete their by-products.

There are strong cultural, religious, social and geographic as well as emotional overlays to eating.

People have, until comparatively recently, subsisted mainly on the foods that were locally and seasonally available. During the past century a new range of chemicals have been added to the soil. Food has been shipped over increasingly vast distances, receiving at successive stages of storage and preparation a number of bleaching, colouring, hydrolysing, emulsifying and preserving agents. In many instances the health-promoting constituents of basic foods have been removed and a host of non-nutritive substances added.

In RZT practice, the therapist quickly becomes aware of how often the gastrointestinal tract is disordered, even in those who seem to be well and believe that their diet is sound. A healthy gut lining is soon broken down when excessive antibiotics are taken orally or inadvertently in prepared foods. The liver has to detoxify all ingested material, and can become exhausted if overburdened by foods which are imbalanced, too rich or contain too many chemical additives. Proprietary medicines also pass through the liver and must be eliminated, the kidneys being the principal excretory route.

Nutrition in health is a complex subject, and diet in illness even more so, particularly as the nutritional and metabolic requirements and capacities of one person differ greatly from those of another. A sick body is often incapable of utilising foodstuffs which it needs and easily metabolises in health. In illness, normal physiological processes are impaired or break down, and a period of physical, mental and chemical (i.e. dietetic) rest is needed for them to recover. The diet in illness must be light and nutritious, while at the same time:

- making no excessive demands on metabolic or excretory functions
- providing all the substances needed to restore and renew those tissues and organs which have been damaged and
- avoiding those substances which are detrimental to recovery.

Many dietary regimes have been proposed, and all have their adherents. Peoples' health has benefited from vegetarianism, naturopathic vegetarianism, a macrobiotic diet, food combining, candida dietetics and the modest consumption of a balanced normal diet with few or no excesses.

There are none the less a few principles of healthy eating common to all regimes.

1. Freshness. All food should be as fresh and with as high an energy content as possible. Foods are living substances, and their energy content deteriorates the longer they are stored, the more they are processed and denatured and the further they are transported from the place where they are grown. Food is best prepared, cooked and eaten immediately, without being heated or reheated.

2. Additives. The addition of chemicals, artificial flavourings, enhancers, stabilisers, etc. denatures foods further. It is preferable to eat organically grown foods whenever possible, and to avoid foods to which have been added hormones and antibiotics. In practice this means seeking out free range poultry and deep sea fish.

3. Composition of the diet. The largest part of the diet should be composed of carbohydrates, with a preponderance of cereals and grains, the next largest part of vegetables, then a little protein and the smallest portion should be composed of fats. A small amount of roughage is also needed daily to keep the alimentary tract healthy. Five to six portions of fruit or vegetables (including raw) should be eaten each day. (When fruit and vegetables are being prepared they should be steamed or boiled in very little water for just as long as is necessary for them to be cooked.)

A balanced diet is healthier than an unbalanced one, so that a wide variety of ingredients are more likely to supply nutritional needs than is a monodiet. Herbs add taste, flavour, microelements and wholesome properties to food and should be a part of every diet.

4. Foods to avoid or minimise. Commercially manufactured drinks (and many fruit juices) with a high carbon dioxide and chemical content are very acid in content. Apart from having little nutritional value they overload digestive enzymes, the liver and kidneys, and use up valuable energy resources through their need to be detoxified and metabolised.

Salt should be used in moderation or not at all. It is an integral part of naturally grown food.

In nature, much hard work is required to produce sugar and honey, and then only in small quantities. Foraging for it is difficult for birds and mammals, it having been obviously designed as a delicacy, rather than a large part of the diet. Sugar is called the 'parasitic' food because it deprives healthy tissues of minerals, trace elements and energy along all metabolic pathways from mouth to bladder. In another context it was described by Professor Simon Yudkin as 'pure, white and deadly', and by Henry Hobhouse as 'wholly superfluous in the diet, a luxury when expensive and a menace when cheap'.

5. Amount of cooking. Meat and fish are more easily digested when they are undercooked and digested with more difficulty when overcooked. However, undercooked meat and especially pork may contain worms, spores or toxins, therefore a balance has to be struck between under- and overcooking.

6. Eating of food. Food should be eaten (rather than consumed) in an unhurried and congenial atmosphere. Digestion begins in the mouth, with ptyalin in saliva starting the process of breaking down starches. If this process is incomplete all subsequent starch catabolism is hindered. Food which is properly chewed is thoroughly mixed with ptyalin, warmed and processed before reaching the stomach. Thorough mastication also ensures that less air is swallowed, making digestion easier. It is surprising what a beneficial effect proper chewing has on many digestive disorders.

Food should be eaten only when sitting down, when the blood supply of the body can be evenly distributed between the smooth involuntary muscles surrounding the gastrointestinal tract and the striped voluntary muscles of activity. When standing or walking the demands of physical movement cause the SNS to direct increased blood flow towards striped muscles and to decrease the flow to involuntary muscle fibres.

It is also noticeable that hunger is not so easily appeased if one is eating and engaging in some physical activity.

Food is a part of all festivities, and most enjoyable when part of sociable and pleasurable activities. Food is recognized as an important determinant of health, and fulfils this function best when it is savoured and enjoyed. A healthy attitude towards food promotes physical and mental well-being.

7. How much to eat? In general, and cultural factors apart, it is better to eat small meals at regular intervals and at regular times, and not to overload the stomach. The body copes better with undereating than overeating, in the same way that plants are better able to withstand underwatering than overwatering.

Physiology, biochemistry and appetite in health and sickness

In health, the SNS and PNS work in tandem with and are complementary to each other. In sickness, the inflammatory response is raised and prolonged.

In the normal circadian rhythm of the body the SNS is dominant between the hours of 3 p.m. and 3 a.m. During these hours all metabolic processes, including the inflammatory response, are raised. This is obvious in sickness, when the temperature is raised at this time. The PNS is dominant between 3 a.m. and 3 p.m., when metabolic processes, including the inflammatory response, are lowered. Body temperature thus falls in the mornings.

The inflammatory response is extended when the GRS is not functioning well, as homeostatic feedback mechanisms seek to contain the infection. The SNS is stimulated, the temperature rises, muscle tone is increased, and there is an increased demand for energy (because of tissue acidosis) and for oxygen and calcium (for metabolic processes).

Unlike the healthy, who enjoy breakfast, the sick person who has not slept well, or has been restless or feverish during the night, finds it difficult or impossible to eat in the mornings.

There is a marked loss of appetite when the SNS is stimulated. Babies, children and animals all refuse food when they are sickening. It is unknown for the sick to eat fast. They have to be coaxed and cajoled and encouraged to eat tiny mouthfuls. This they will only do at intervals, and it is noticeable that they chew very slowly. Those who are sick also take only small amounts of fluid, which they sip very slowly.

Nor do they like strong flavours, salt or too many condiments. Since they have a heightened sensitivity to the smell of food, only those foods which have a light and fresh smell should be put before them. They respond to the colour and presentation of food, which they only want in small amounts. The texture of food is important to the sick. They do not like food which requires much chewing, nor do they want only bland foods.

Sick people will reject all food if there is too much of it on the plate, or if the composition of the meal does not appeal to them. They do not like talking or hearing about food, and food which has not been eaten should be removed as soon as possible.

No sick person should be left alone when eating or drinking, the effort becomes too much for them. Appetite is best encouraged when meals are brought to the bedside, the person attending the invalid sits within easy view, giving gentle encouragement. The conversation needs to be as light and easy to digest as the food, and can provide the social element of eating which is so often lacking for the sick.

Meals for the sick, who can survive on restricted or monodiets for years and for life, should be simple but tasty, without being composed of too many ingredients. There are circumstances in which foods can endanger life.

The following injunction by Hippocrates has stood the test of time:

■ *"If a man were to eat less than enough he would make as big a mistake as if he were to eat too much. Hunger is a powerful agent in the human body; it can maim, weaken and kill … A weak man is next to a sick man, while a sick man is made still weaker by indiscretions in his diet. Each one of the substances of a man's diet acts upon his body and changes it in some way and upon these changes his whole life depends, whether he be in health, in sickness, or convalescent."*

Florence Nightingale, who was no mean observer of the sick, wrote in 1859:

■ *"A great deal too much against tea is said by wise people, and a great deal too much of tea is given to the sick by foolish people. When you see the natural and almost universal craving in English sick for their 'tea', you cannot but feel that nature knows what she is about."*

Since a state of tissue acidosis exists in most illnesses, predominantly alkaline foods are needed to relieve the strain on the liver and kidneys. The body maintains the neutrality of blood tenaciously, using every available tissue and organ as a buffer when the blood becomes more acidic. (The normal pH of blood is 7.4, and in health it can move between 7.3 and 7.5.)

The enzyme systems of the body are delicately sensitive and responsive to changes in the pH of the blood and to body temperature. At temperatures higher than 37°F (98.4°F) they are inactivated, and all biochemical reactions slow down. They are similarly slowed down when the pH of blood rises above 7.4, rapidly giving rise to a sense of lethargy and dullness.

The concept of energy in the Western world is associated with light, heat, motion, electricity and chemical energy. Energy has the ability to change rapidly from one form to another, and its coherent organisation within the body fuels life.

All chemical reactions in the body either utilise or produce energy, which is expended to maintain body temperature, on movement, and the renewal and repair of all tissues. Energy needs to be constantly replenished in the form of food and oxygen. The only source of food energy available to humankind is the heat and light of the sun which has been stored in plants, which are then eaten by people or animals.

Food constituents

Carbohydrates

Carbon and hydrogen form two-thirds of plants and animals.

As carbohydrates they are needed by humans to replenish the body's stores. This inexpensive and filling food provides instant (from simple) and slow release *energy* (from the complex carbohydrates) and *fuel* for survival. In illness a carefully combined monodiet can sustain life.

Formed from carbon, hydrogen and oxygen, carbohydrates form the largest and most inexpensive nutritional source of (food) energy worldwide. They yield 70% of the fuel which is needed by the body, providing:

- energy for all cells and muscle tissue; glucose is the only form in which carbohydrate can be transported round the body and is found in

plasma and red blood corpuscles; the sole source of energy for the brain, retina and embryonic tissue is *glucose*
- heat
- essential constituents of some cells such as cerebrosides of nervous tissue and riboflavin
- protection for tissue proteins; sufficient carbohydrates in the diet spare protein (an expensive source) from being broken down to provide heat and energy
- fat if carbohydrate is superfluous.

Normal carbohydrate metabolism becomes impossible if there is a thyroid or adrenocortical deficiency, or if certain of the B complex vitamins are missing.

Proteins

Changing world patterns of eating have led to the easy availability of cheap protein. Meat, which was once considered a rich man's luxury, has become a common article of the diet.

Proteins are the only substance to contain nitrogen. They are essential in first or second class form for the renewal of certain sorts of tissues, and to manufacture enzymes in combination with fats. In order to extract the nitrogenous part, proteins have to be broken down, and excessive amounts are burdensome to the kidneys as they have to be filtered out as urea.

They are composed of carbon, hydrogen, oxygen, nitrogen, and maybe sulphur and phosphorus, and are hydrolysed by enzymes into their component parts. Apart from a few fats, only proteins can replenish the essential nitrogenous compounds in the body. Their large molecules are indispensable constituents of every cell. Neither sulphur nor certain amino acids can be synthesised by the body, and they are derived in a form which is available from the protein foods.

Proteins are essential to the body, providing for:

- the growth and repair of tissue proteins, enzymes and hormones
- energy
- maintaining the nitrogen equilibrium of the body (both a nitrogenous deficit or excess are detrimental to the body; a diet containing

enough carbohydrate and fat to supply the energy requirements of the body needs less protein to attain and maintain nitrogen equilibrium — this effect of fat and carbohydrate is called the 'protein-sparing action', and spares the function of both the liver and the kidneys)

- derivatives of protein for lubrication of the respiratory and alimentary tracts
- essential constituents found in the nuclei of all cells
- essential constituents found in the cytoplasm of all cells
- essential parts of haemoglobin, which transports oxygen.

Fats

Fats are absolutely essential to the body. They are composed of carbon, hydrogen and oxygen, and enable the body to store energy compactly. Furthermore, they provide:

- a carriage system for the fat soluble vitamins A, D, E and K, which can only be absorbed in their presence
- an insulating and packaging system, needed to conserve heat and insulate nerve fibres (it is noticeably absent in demyelinating diseases such as multiple sclerosis)
- phospholipids formed from fatty compounds are found in every plant and animal cell, and are necessary for the formation of cell membranes
- vitamin D, which is formed in the skin
- oestrogen, progesterone and testosterone sex hormones; fat packaging holds within it in solution such hormones as oestrogen, which is calcium sparing and protects against osteoporosis
- corticosteroids.

People with fat reserves survive longer in conditions of trauma and starvation.

Fat is metabolised differently when the carbohydrate stores of the body are depleted, producing acetone, which is toxic for the body. In illness, alkaline foods and fluids help to restore a healthy acid/base balance. Alkaline drinks such as water, barley water, rice water, diluted vegetable soups and diluted fruit juices and lightly steamed vegetables all help to reduce the acidotic load on all systems.

Keeping the mouth moist and clean helps to revive a failing appetite, and small and frequently renewed drinks should be offered to the sick person. Anyone who is unable to eat should have frequent sips of clear fluids.

References

Hippocrates circa 400BC Hippocratic writings. First published by Blackwell 1950. Reprinted with additional material as a Penguin Classic 1978 Penguin Books, Harmondsworth, Middlesex, pp 75, 78
Hobhouse H 1985 Seeds of change. Harper and Row, New York, pp 44–48

Nightingale F 1980 Notes on nursing. Churchill Livingstone, New York, p 61
Yudkin J 1972 Pure, white and deadly! The problem of sugar. Davis-Poyntor, London, pp 1–164

Appendix III: The lift: a gymnastic exercise or drill to relieve back ache

Many physiotherapists and therapists have an exercise or routine which they practise to keep themselves limber. These they may pass on to patients, and they will also have a repertoire of practical techniques for specific incapacities.

'The lift' is one from which I and many of the people who have come to me for RZT have benefited since our friend Dr Koni Witzig first introduced it to me many years ago. While it is recommended for back ache, it has many other advantages, and can be used by everyone to improve or maintain the suppleness of the spine, other joints and breathing.

The lift was developed by Dr Witzig during a lifetime of general practice for patients who came with neck, back and low back pain, and with infirmities of the upper and lower extremities. Its use has been proven in the treatment of patients with back ache of multiple aetiologies. Neither age, weight nor size of the patient is a barrier to its practice.

There is, however, a caution. The therapist must learn to do the lift well, under the instruction of a practitioner, and must learn it herself before giving the exercise to any patient.

It is a prerequisite that the lift has to be demonstrated to every patient, who must be instructed, supervised and corrected until adept. In general, about five sessions need to be devoted to demonstrating the lift before the exercise is properly learned and the patient can continue to exercise on her own.

The patient and the therapist should do the lift with bare feet, in light underclothing, and preferably in front of a mirror or reflecting window. It is only by seeing her reflection that the patient becomes aware of the overtaxed and distorted posture, and the muscular asymmetry causing the pain or disability.

A complex muscular and nervous system makes it possible for the spine to be bent, stretched and twisted in any direction. As the reins direct a horse, the nerves pull the muscles like a lever against the transverse and spinal processes of each individual vertebra. The physical inactivity of much modern daily life raises concerns about the function of individual muscles.

The abused spine

What happens to the spine today? If an infant is constantly laid on the same side in the cradle, the skull may become flattened, or a crooked spine, an unsymmetric thorax or an asymmetric pelvis may result.

A schoolchild who bends over a desk for 12 years or carries too heavy a satchel shows postural deterioration and feels pain. The cashier who is always at the same till in the supermarket leans on one arm while he enters the price, and with the other hand brings the goods to be priced towards him, twisting his head and neck to do so. At the end of the day he complains of pain from his neck to his fingertips.

Those who work at typewriters, word processors and computers generally sit with rounded backs, hunched shoulders and heads bent forward, turning regularly to the same side to read a manuscript.

Dentists constantly bend and turn, and suffer from loin pain because the lumbar vertebrae become overstretched and lose their natural curve.

The lifting and moving of heavy furniture, patients, mattresses or other objects without being aware of how to use the spine, joints and muscles of the body can lead to pain in the sciatic or ischial nerves.

Disturbed balance and equilibrium

All these kinds of pain may arise from faults in the frame-supporting vertebrae. The troubled musculature is not able to hold itself in a normal upright position. The balance of the flexible stretching and bending muscles becomes disturbed. The nervous system registers this disorder and admonishes us through sensations of pain. The pain-ridden person turns, stretches and bends in order to relieve the pain.

'Pain free' consumerism

The patient, wishing to be free of pain, goes to the general practitioner 'to fetch some medicine'. The doctor examines, treats, gives the desired medicines and reminds the patient of the exercises to be done. The patient feels better, has consumed the medicine to relieve the pain, is happy, and forgets the exercises.

Road to health

Soon there is a relapse. Now the patient is prescribed one of the physical therapies, which may help for a shorter or longer time, but the pain recurs if the insult to the spine and posture are not remedied. How to escape from this fiendish fix? The consumption of pain-relieving medicines does not help the strained musculature. The only help available to the patient is to be gained from conscientious training on the part of the patient.

Which brings us to 'the lift'. One single exercise removes the need to practice many exercises. One exercise can be thoroughly learned, whilst several are usually done halfheartedly. Regular exercise of the lift twice a day for 6 minutes or once a day for 15 minutes (that means doing the lift 20 times twice a day or 40 times once a day) is recommended. The unfortunate vertebrae are pressed against a firm surface such as a wall or door. Begin by circling the arms. The exercise should be performed slowly, quietly and smoothly, without excessive energy.

Keep the mouth closed and breathe through the nose to ensure that there is no overexertion.

Using a mirror

It is helpful if the exercise is done clad only in underclothes in front of a large mirror. It is soon observed that, as the flexor muscles are more used than are the extensors, the outcome is a 'gorilla posture'. Seeing this reflection in the mirror there is an instinctive tendency to straighten and extend the spine.

The benefit of the exercise

The improvement in rotation, bending and stretching of the previously rigid vertebrae when the strongly symmetrical 'lift' exercise is regularly performed is striking. The resulting physical uplift also benefits mood, digestion and disturbed sleep patterns. Anyone from the age of 6 to 90 years can do the lift.

There are no medical conditions in which it is contraindicated, and it is recommended for those suffering from asthma, rheumatism and disorders of cardiac function.

Commentary on the lift (Fig. AIII.1)

1. Starting position. The patient stands fully relaxed against a firm, flat surface. (Feet should be parallel and about 5 cm from the wall.) Children and youngsters should adopt an upright posture. Round shoulders make it difficult for the head to touch the wall. In this case the head is held lightly in a neutral position which does not cause pain. The patient should try to hold the head with the chin drawn towards the neck, and not jutting out, against the wall.

2. High frontal armlift. The arms hang loosely by the sides. First the arms and fingers are stretched out; the person begins to breathe through the nose. The doctor or therapist observes whether the posture of the patient is perpendicular. The strongly overdeveloped musculature in a right-handed person can pull the spinous process of a vertebra out of true in such a symmetrical exercise. The doctor or therapist therefore controls the spinous processes of the vertebrae on the back. The arms are then lifted upwards in front of the body in a half circle until the upper arms touch the ears. The fingers are spread widely.

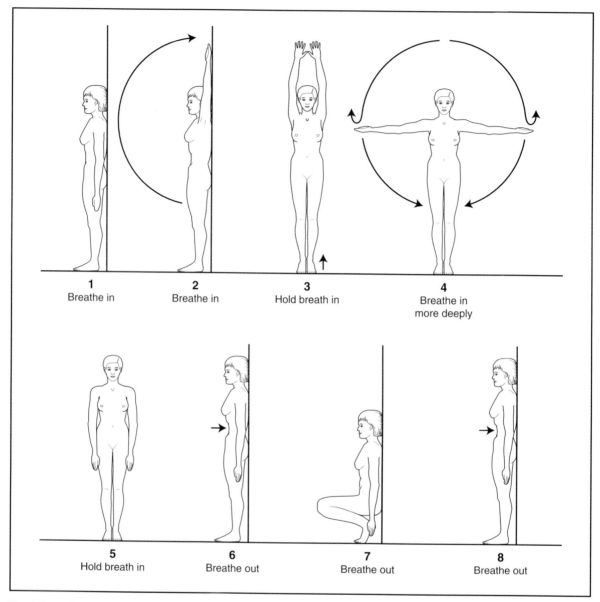

Fig. AIII.1 *The left exercise: 1 starting position; 2 high frontal armlift; 3 standing on the toes; 4 sideways arm circling; 5 resting; 6 correcting the pelvic position; 7 knee bending; 8 rising*

3. Standing on the toes. Keeping the thumbs touching, the patient stretches upward and stands on the tips of the toes. Raising oneself for a short time on tiptoes is a controlled, symmetrical and thorough stretching of the body right through to the fingertips. For this reason the head should not be tilted backwards.

4. Sideways arm circling. Standing flat on the floor again, the arms are brought down sideways in a half circle. (The palms are turned up when horizontal.) The doctor or therapist encourages the patient to stretch the circling arms fully, and to separate the fingers as widely as possible. Existing pain or discomfort, such as may be found in the left shoulder blade, can be alleviated by a light, conscious stretch to the right. This 'pulling away of the pain' towards the healthy side encourages symmetry.

5. Resting. The lungs are full of air, stretching the intercostal spaces, the sternoclavicular joints and the sternocostal joints. At this moment of maximal inspiration, the patient should endeavour to let the arms and shoulders hang loosely down by each side of the body and allow them to relax completely. It is usually necessary to practise the exercise a few times before this can be accomplished.

6. Correcting the pelvic position. Keeping the mouth closed, expiration now begins. The patient must be encouraged to draw in the muscles of the stomach wall and to press the hollow in the posterior pelvis lightly against the wall. She should become aware of how the symphysis pubis is lifted forward, and how the pelvis is tipped backwards. This forward tilting of the pelvis often relieves pain in the sacroiliac joint.

It is important to follow the breathing technique faithfully, and many patients and therapists have to learn how to do this.

7. Knee bending. Keeping the spine against the wall and the knees touching each other, the patient slowly bends her knees. With the arms hanging loosely by the sides, the patient holds the breath in and keeps the stomach muscles drawn in. She bends the knees only to the extent that she can raise herself up again without falling forwards.

8. Rising. The patient now rises slowly from the squatting position, keeping the back lightly pressed against the wall and stomach muscles fully contracted. The expiration is completed. (Breathing in and out should be done through the nose only.)

For patients who are confined to bed, convalescent, arthritic, or who have disease of the hip, this exercise can be done on the floor, otherwise on a firm bed.

Once it has been mastered, 'the lift' can be done without the supervision which is necessary in the early stages until it has been properly learned. If the pain recurs, the exercise has probably been neglected. When practised conscientiously and regularly, the lift is neither time consuming nor costly. Often patients have to learn that neither the consumption of medicines, physical or other therapies are as effective as intelligent, self-motivated care.

Appendix IV: The Sitz bath

When the skin is warmed, arterioles near the surface of the skin dilate and fill with blood. When the skin is cooled, the arterioles constrict and blood returns to the deeper circulation. Since unstriated muscle fibres form the walls of the arterioles, this dilating (as they fill) and constricting (as they empty) restores and maintains muscle tone. The stimulus given to the circulation improves the oxygen supply to the surrounding tissues, and the local lymphatic drainage is also improved.

Regular Sitz baths will assist the circulation when the patient has varicose veins or haemorrhoids, or suffers from dysmenorrhoea or menorrhagia.

A bath should be filled with about 8 cm (3 inches) of cold water, and also a large bowl with water which is as hot as the hand can bear. The buttocks are immersed in the bowl of hot water, and the feet in the cold water in the bath, for 60 seconds, then the position is reversed so that the feet are in the hot water and the buttocks in the cold, again for a further 60 seconds.

This is repeated twice more, and the buttocks should have their final immersion in the cold water.

When menstruation begins the Sitz baths are stopped until 24 hours after the period has stopped, when they should be resumed.

For menorrhagia, 8–10 cm (3–4 inches) of cold water is run in the bath, and the patient sits with the heels and buttocks in the water for 30 seconds every night. This is stopped for 72 hours when menstruation begins. After 72 hours this procedure is resumed four times a day for 30 seconds each time.

When the period ends, the heels and buttock should be plunged once more into cold water every night for 30 seconds before going to bed.

This regime is continued until the periods last for only 4 days.

Appendix V: Anatomical terms

I have throughout this book employed the anatomical terms in common medical usage. These will be familiar to all readers and thus lend ease to description.

Plantar — pertaining to the sole (in RZT the sole of the foot)

Dorsal — pertaining to the upper surface (in RZT the upper surface of the foot)

Medial — in or towards the midline

Lateral — on or towards the outer border

Longitudinal — running lengthwise, in a direction parallel to the long axis of the body (i.e. from head to foot)

Transverse — in the horizontal plane (i.e. parallel to the ground when standing)

Border — the edge or boundary of a mass of tissue

Margin — the edge or border of a structure

Proximal — nearest to the centre of the body

Distal — furthest from the centre of the body

Anterior — that aspect of the body which faces the viewer and is visible

Posterior — that aspect of the body which is hidden from view, such as the back when you are facing a person

Superior — the upper end of the body is the superior part

Inferior — the lower part is the inferior part

Aspect — the part of a surface which fronts a particular direction, e.g. *dorsal* aspect, facing towards the dorsum or back, or *medial* aspect, facing towards the medial sagittal plane of the body

Superficial — that which is closer to the skin surface

Deep — that which is beneath the superficial

Flexion — bending the body or the limbs or any joints so that an angle is formed (in plantar flexion the toes are angled towards the sole or plantar aspect of the foot; in dorsiflexion the toes are angled toward the dorsum of the foot)

Extension — bending the body or a limb so that the the dorsal surfaces of the body are brought closer toward each other (e.g. allowing your head and neck to stretch backwards extends the neck)

Rotation — the act of turning round an axis

Pronation — the hand rotated so that the palm faces downward

Supination — the act of rotating the forearm and hand so that the palm faces anteriorly

Eversion — (of the foot) the act of turning the whole foot so that the plantar surface faces laterally

Inversion — turning the foot so that the plantar surface faces medially.

Warning note: No joint should ever be flexed or extended beyond the limit of comfortable movement. Disease or injury may have caused joints to become rigid, and they may be damaged further if they are overextended.

Appendix VI: Useful addresses

Further information can be obtained from:

South Africa
Trudi Kaiser
15 Sunning Dale
Old Mutual Drive
Stellenberg 7530

UK
British School of Reflex Zone Therapy
Enquiries to Ann Lett
23 Marsh Hall
Talisman Way
Wembley Park HA9 8JJ

USA
Angela Haviland Yorath
4026 West Patterson Street
Chicago
Illinois 60641

Further reading

Bieler H 1966 Food is your best medicine. Ballantyne Books, New York

Froneberg A, Fabian M 1982 Manuelle Neurotherapie/Nervenreflextherapie am Fuss. Haug Verlag, Heidelberg

Lorimer D L 1993 Neale's common foot disorders, diagnosis and management: a general clinical guide. Churchill Livingstone, Edinburgh

McKenzie R 1980 Treat your own back. Spinal Publications, Waikanae, New Zealand

McKenzie R 1983 Treat your own neck. Spinal Publications, Waikanae, New Zealand

Madders J 1997 The stress and relaxation handbook. Martin Dunitz, London

Marquardt H 1984 Reflex zone therapy of the feet. Healing Arts Press, Rochester

Marquardt H 1993 Reflexzonentherapie am Fuss. Hippokrates Verlag GmbH, Stuttgart

Mennel J B 1940 Physical treatment by movement, manipulation and massage. J and A Churchill, London

Miller B, Goode R 1961 Man and his body. Gollancz, London

Murray M 1998 The encyclopaedia of natural medicine, 2nd edn. Michael Little Brown, London

Selye H 1956 The stress of life. McGraw-Hill, New York

Simonton C, Matthews-Simonton S, Creighton J L 1980 Getting well again. Bantam Books, New York

Trattler R 1987 Better health through natural healing. Thorsons, London

Index

Page numbers in bold refer to illustrations and tables